THE SECOND PART

OF THE POPULAR ERRORS

T0136471

THE SECOND PART

OF THE POPULAR ERRORS

LAURENT JOUBERT

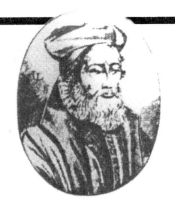

TRANSLATED AND ANNOTATED BY

GREGORY DAVID de ROCHER

THE UNIVERSITY OF ALABAMA PRESS

•

TUSCALOOSA AND LONDON

Copyright © 1995
The University of Alabama Press
Tuscaloosa, Alabama 35487-0380
All rights reserved
Manufactured in the United States of America

∞

The paper on which this book is printed meets the minimum requirements of American National Standard for Information Science-Permanence of Paper for Printed Library Materials, ANSI Z39.48-1984.

Library of Congress Cataloging-in-Publication Data

Joubert, Laurent, 1529–1583.
    [Seconde partie des erreurs populaires. English]
    The second part of the Popular errors / Laurent Joubert: translated and annotated by Gregory David de Rocher.
    p. cm.
    Includes bibliographical references and index.
    ISBN 0-8173-0758-3   978-0-8173-5415-2 (pbk: alk. paper)
    1. Medical misconceptions—Early works to 1800. 2. Medicine, Medieval.   3. Medicine, Popular—France—Early works to 1800.
I. Rocher, Gregory de. II. Title. III. Title: Popular errors. Part 2.
R729.9.J68213 1995
610—dc20   94—4708

    British Library Cataloguing-in-Publication Data available

Leur santé mesme est alterée par la contrainte des regimes.

— Montaigne, *Essais*, II, 37

CONTENTS

ACKNOWLEDGMENTS ix

ABBREVIATIONS x

INTRODUCTION xi
The Second Part of the Popular Errors.
Editions of *The Second Part of the Popular Errors.*
Inventory of the 1587 Micard Edition.
Brief Description of the Contents of the Micard Edition.
Index and Notes of the Present Translation.
Selected Bibliography.

PRELIMINARY MATTER 3
Extract from the King's Authorization to Print.
Letter by Barthélemy Cabrol to Nicolas de Neufville.
Letter by Barthélemy Cabrol to Antoine de Clermont.
Index of Chapters and Subject Matter Contained
in *The Second Part of the Popular Errors.*
Liminal Poems.

THE SECOND PART OF THE POPULAR ERRORS
CONCERNING MEDICINE
AND THE REGIMEN OF HEALTH 25

APPENDICES 231
A. A Common Question: What Language Would a Child Speak
If It Had Never Heard Speech?
B. On the Beverage of Monseigneur the Maréchal D'Anville.
C. The Health of the Prince, Containing Two Parts.
D. On Nightfall, What It Is, and Whether It Falls on Us.

INDEX 283
Micard Index 305

ACKNOWLEDGMENTS

I wish to express my gratitude to the Research Grants Committee of The University of Alabama for grants-in-aid that have made it possible for me to gather materials for this translation. I am also indebted to James D. Yarbrough, dean of the College of Arts and Sciences, and to James G. Taaffe, provost and vice president for Academic Affairs, for a sabbatical leave allowing the preparation of the manuscript. I express once again my indebtedness to those colleagues whom I thank throughout the notes for their invaluable assistance in their areas of expertise, and to my research assistant Geraldine Bailey for her painstaking editing and countless trips to the Gorgas Library. For their careful reading of the manuscript and their numerous valuable suggestions I thank especially Professor Natalie Zemon Davis of Princeton University and Professor Joseph Allaire of Florida State University. Happily, this second volume has benefited, as did the *Popular Errors*, from the vigilant copyediting of Trinket Shaw. In the final analysis, it was the diagnostic skills of Dr. Robert Pieroni of The University of Alabama Capstone Medical Center that made the completion of this fifteen-year project possible. The errors that remain are, finally, not Joubert's but my own.

ABBREVIATIONS

PE   Laurent Joubert. *Popular Errors*. Translated and annotated by Gregory David de Rocher. Tuscaloosa: University of Alabama Press, 1989.

TL   Laurent Joubert. *Treatise on Laughter*. Translated and annotated by Gregory David de Rocher. University: University of Alabama Press, 1980.

INTRODUCTION

THE SECOND PART
OF THE POPULAR ERRORS

The Second Part of the Popular Errors differs considerably from the preceding volume and differs also from what Laurent Joubert himself had projected in terms of its content. The second part of *Les Erreurs populaires* was to have been devoted exclusively to the discussion of a proper health regimen in the areas of personal conduct, the maintenance of one's surroundings, dress habits, and diet.[1] Fortunately for us, Joubert did not adhere to his plan; rather, in what was to be his last work, the celebrated Montpellier physician furnishes us with a rich variety of subjects drawn from nearly each of the thirty books that were to constitute the ambitious enterprise of *Les Erreurs populaires*. Thus, although perhaps only a ghost of what the treatment would have been had Joubert been able to bring his conception of the remaining parts to

---

[1]See Joubert's "Division of the Entire Work into Six Parts Containing Thirty Books" in appendix A of *PE* (245-54).

completion, *The Second Part of the Popular Errors* now reveals his main ideas concerning complexion, air and clothes, appetite and thirst, along with meals and digestion, topics that were to have appeared in the second part as first promised by the author.

Also present in various parts of several chapters are those subjects found in the projected Third Part, namely, the preparation and order of food, the importance of beverages and, surprisingly, the problematic nature of wine in the diet (chapters 1, 4, 9, 10, 12, 21, and the tract "On the Beverage of Monseigneur the Maréchal d'Anville"). From the Fourth Part come the proper use of food during illness, various diseases, prognosis, and the importance of sleep (chapters 6, 7, 8, and 18). The Fifth Part finds all of its projected chapters actualized in his sections on "Metaphorical and Extravagant Remedies," "Fabulous Stories," and "Superstitious, Vain, and Ceremonious Remedies." Finally, the Sixth Part of the "Entire Work" as envisaged by Joubert before the publication of *The Second Part of the Popular Errors* is also almost completely represented in miniature in the chapters on purgation and evacuation (chapters 3, 16, and 20), and in those on bloodletting (chapters 13, 14, and 15). Ironically, the subject that is not present, the subject that was to constitute the ultimate chapter of Joubert's *magnum opus*, was the one that came to interrupt the author in his progress in 1582: death.

EDITIONS OF *THE SECOND PART OF THE POPULAR ERRORS*

The first edition of *La Seconde partie des erreurs populaires* is that of L'Angelier, published in Paris in 1579. A second edition appeared the following year, published by L. Breyer.[2] Of the eight editions that followed, the most carefully reproduced is that prepared by Claude Micard and published in Paris in 1587; it is the edition that serves as the base text for the present translation. The Micard edition was seen as the definitive version of Joubert's *Erreurs populaires*; all later editions offering The First and Second Parts of the work were wholly or in large part reproductions of the Micard.[3]

---

[2]For the location of collections holding these editions, see the introduction to *PE* (xx).

[3]For a discussion of the Micard edition, see the introduction to *PE* (xxi).

INVENTORY OF THE 1587 MICARD EDITION

The Micard edition contains all the elements of the previous printings of the work, although the order is slightly changed; all items are translated herein unless otherwise indicated.

1. Joubert's letter to the reader ("Au lecteur d'esprit libre et studieux"), which also appeared in The First Part. A translation of it is given in *PE* (24-25).
2. A reproduction of Joubert's "Division de toute l'oeuvre en six parties, contenant trente liures"; this table is translated in appendix A of *PE* (245-47).
3. The title page, bearing the "BONA FIDE" colophon of Claude Micard, the date of publication, 1587, and the location, *"rue S. Iean de Latran, á la bonne Foy"* (herein reproduced).
4. A copy of an extract from Joubert's permission from the king, dated 30 August 1577, to have printed any of his works.
5. Barthélemy Cabrol's letter to Nicolas de Neufville, bearing the heading of dedicatory preface, dated 3 February 1579.
6. Barthélemy Cabrol's apologetic letter to Antoine de Clermont.
7. Table of contents of the twenty-five chapters contained in *The Second Part of the Popular Errors*.
8. Three dedicatory poems.
9. Chapters 1 through 21.
10. Christophle de Beauchastel's letter to François Joubert.
11. Chapters 22 through 25.
12. "Medley of Common Expressions and Popular Errors" (seventy items previously published in 1578 and translated in *PE* 16-19).
13. "Gathering of Common Expressions and Errors with a Few Problems Sent by Various Individuals to Monsieur Joubert" (333 items).
14. "Catalog of Several Different Popular Errors and Sayings Gathered from Several Individuals and Given to Monsieur Joubert by Monsieur Barthélemy Cabrol" (123 items in French, 9 in Catalan, 1 in Spanish, 30 in Italian, and 6 in Latin).
15. Jean Imbert's letter to Étienne de Rate, dated 20 February 1579.
16. "Summary of What Is Treated in the Following Sections."

17. "Explanation of Some Popular Terms and Phrases Mainly Concerning Illnesses" (twenty-three items).
18. "Metaphorical and Extravagant Remedies" (four items).
19. "Superstitious, Vain, and Ceremonious Remedies" (thirteen items).
20. "Fabulous Stories" (four items).
21. Isaac Joubert's letter to his father, Laurent Joubert, dated 1 January 1579.
22. Isaac Joubert's French translation from the Latin of Laurent Joubert's last *Paradoxe* of the Second Decade, on the subject of poisons.
23. Isaac Joubert's French translation from the Latin of Laurent Joubert's second *Paradoxe* of the First Decade, on the subject of how long one can live without taking nourishment.
24. Laurent Joubert's treatise on the nature of language, "A Common Question: What Language Would a Child Speak If It Had Never Heard Speech?"
25. Index of the Contents of the First Part and the Second Part of the *Popular Errors* (of the Micard edition).

BRIEF DESCRIPTION OF THE CONTENTS
OF THE MICARD EDITION

Any understanding of the complex printing history of *Les Erreurs populaires* entails a critical reading of the two letters by Barthélemy Cabrol serving as dedicatory epistles of the Micard edition.[4] Their status as precious documents of history or as the most crass of hawking strategies could be argued. Both letters attest to what has been called the scandal of *Les Erreurs populaires*: the persona of a saddened and depressed Laurent Joubert is presented in the first, and the second contains a laborious reprise of the gynecological vocabulary of which much was made in the Fifth Book of *Popular Errors* (PE 208-22).

---

[4]*LA/ PREMIERE ET/ SECONDE PARTIE/ DES ERREVRS POPULAI-/ res, touchant la Medecine & le/ regime de santé./ Par M. LAURENT IOVBERT, Conseiller/ & Medecin ordinaire du Roy, & du Roy de Na-/ uarre, premier Docteur regent, chancelier & iuge de/ l'uniuersité en Medecine de Montpellier./ AVEC plusieurs autres petits traictez, lesquels/ sont specifiez en la page suyuante./ SE VENDENT/ A Paris, Chez CLAUDE MICARD,/ rue S. Iean de Latran à/ la bonne Foy. 1587./ Auec Priuilege.*

The conventional liminal poems grace this edition before the presentation of what might be called the first half of *The Second Part of the Popular Errors*: twenty-five chapters on subjects as varied as the nutritional and therapeutic value of wine, fevers, practical care for the ill (changing of linen), the nefarious role of women attendants, proper times and quantities of administering broths, excessive bedcovers, the rapid deterioration of sausages, bloodletting, purgation, proper diet and conduct when taking medication, excessive care, loose bowels and a healthy digestive system, the aphrodisiac nature of oysters and truffles, and alternate versions of four chapters, which had appeared in the 1579 edition of *Les Erreurs populaires*, on the abilities and failings of physicians.

There follows a considerable section devoted to common sayings and expressions: the first list is merely reproduced from the 1578 edition of *Les Erreurs populaires*; the second contains 333 items gathered from various sources; the third was supplied by Barthélemy Cabrol and contains 123 items, plus 9 in Catalan, 1 in Spanish, 30 in Italian, and 6 in Latin. After this a rather interesting section tenders an "Explanation of Some Common Expressions and Phrases Mainly Concerning Illnesses" in which are listed various expressions for menstruation, abortion, circumcision, suffocation of the womb, and a score of common pathological conditions. "Fabulous Stories" heads Joubert's refutation of popular misconceptions concerning the viper, the beaver, the salamander, and the bear.

The final pages of the edition contain two invaluable windows on the scientific discourse practiced during the Renaissance in France. The first is in the form of translations of two of Joubert's *Paradoxes* (written and published in Latin) furnished by his son, Isaac: the first is on the subject of poisons, a subject of great concern to monarchs, princes, and other powerful individuals during the troubled times of the Reformation; the second discusses the possibility of living without taking nourishment, walking the thin line between medical and theological authority. The last item of the Micard edition is a tract that appears in all of the works Joubert published in the French language: "What Language Would a Child Speak If It Had Never Heard Speech?" Since this piece cannot be said to be specific to any particular work or edition, it appears in this volume[5] in appendix A.

---

[5]As indicated in the introduction to *PE* (xxiii).

Also appearing in the appendices are three items that had appeared in the 1579 Millanges edition of *Les Erreurs populaires*, but which, because their subject matter is more related to that of *The Second Part of the Popular Errors*, were kept for publication in the present volume.[6] In appendix B appears my translation of Joubert's thinly veiled criticism of Henri de Montmorency's concoction of what today might be called a health drink ("Du breuuage de Monseigneur le Marechal d'Anville"). Appendix C contains an enchiridion for the ruling prince in which are spelled out the extent of the monarch's responsibilities, as well as those of the court physician. The last text of the present volume is appendix D, a brief discussion of the possible dangers of nightfall and an excellent example of the discourse characterizing error books.

INDEX AND NOTES OF THE PRESENT TRANSLATION

The index I have compiled resembles that of *Popular Errors* (names, places, works, and subjects, including all anatomical, medicinal, and pathological terms). It also includes a translation of the index of the contents of *La premiere et la seconde partie des erreurs populaires* as it appeared in the Micard edition. This allows today's reader not only to ascertain which topics were deemed to be of interest to sixteenth-century readers but also to have quick access to them.

The notes follow the same format as that delineated in the translator's preface to *Popular Errors* (*PE* xi), namely, all notes appear together. Joubert's marginal notes are easily distinguished from my own in that they always are preceded by the phrase "Joubert's note: . . ." In some cases my own commentary follows, set off in brackets (e.g., "Joubert's note: Chapter 11 [Joubert is referring to Lactantius's *De opeficio dei*]). All the notes in the present translation are at the bottom of the page, not at the end of the volume, as was the case in *Popular Errors*.

SELECTED BIBLIOGRAPHY

The following works are a supplement to the selected bibliography at the end of the introduction to *Popular Errors* (xxv-xxvi).

---

[6]See the introduction to *PE* (xxiii).

Anonymous. *The Mirror of Coitus: A Translation and Edition of the Fifteenth-Century* Speculum al foderi. Translated by Michael Solomon. Madison: The Hispanic Seminary of Medieval Studies, 1990.

Ferrand, Jacques. *A Treatise on Lovesickness*. Translated and edited with a critical introduction and notes by Donald A. Beecher and Massimo Ciavolella. Syracuse: Syracuse University Press, 1990. An exemplary model of the annotated translation.

Rocher, Gregory de and Geraldine Bailey. "L'Épitaphe de François de Montmorency par Laurent Joubert." *Bibliothèque d'Humanisme et Renaissance* 55.1 (1993): 77-80.

Siraisi, Nancy G. *Medieval and Early Renaissance Medicine: An Introduction to Knowledge and Practice*. Chicago: University of Chicago Press, 1990.

THE SECOND PART

OF THE POPULAR ERRORS

LAURENT JOUBERT

PRELIMINARY MATTER

EXTRACT FROM THE KING'S AUTHORIZATION TO PRINT

Through the grace and privilege of the King, granted in Poitiers on the thirtieth day of August fifteen hundred and seventy-seven to Monsieur Laurent Joubert, physician and chancelor in the University of Montpellier, for having all his works printed during a period of ten years as is more completely provided for by the license of said privilege. Signed Henry [and further down], certified and registered at the presiding seat of Agenois, on the seventh of November fifteen hundred and seventy-seven.[1]

---

[1]This extract is from the same privilege used by Simon Millanges in Bordeaux, who claimed to have a signed document from Joubert granting him and him alone permission to print Joubert's works for a period of five years, starting from the last day of the printing (1578). See *PE* (280) for translations of these documents.

LETTER BY BARTHÉLEMY CABROL
TO NICOLAS DE NEUFVILLE

To my most honored Liege, Monsieur de Neufville, Seigneur de Villeroy,[2] the King's Councelor and Secretary of State, Grand Treasurer of his Majesty's Accounts, from Barthélemy Cabrol,[3] his most humble servant, Greetings

My Liege, I have taken refuge in you in order to save me from the displeasure Monsieur Joubert has suffered because of me over a second part of his *Popular Errors*, which I was having printed a bit on the sly, in view of his decision not to bring any more of them to light. He caught me at the print shop and was most angry about what I was doing.[4] Yet when he learned that I intended to offer it as a present to you, he was so satisfied that he granted on the spot Lucas Breyer, a book merchant (and whose services I had sought), permission to continue and gave him in addition two handsome texts translated by his eldest son, Isaac, from his Latin *Paradoxes*.[5] Through this gesture I came to understand the great respect he bears you and the venerable authority you have won over him through your kind deeds and intercession in his behalf, which he continually proclaims privately and publicly, counting you among the best peers of France and one of his

---

[2]Nicolas de Neufville (1543–1617), who with his wife held one of the literary salons of the period but later fell from grace because of his Protestant leanings. Clément Marot had served for a time as page to Neufville's father around 1515 when composing his *Temple de Cupido*.

[3]Barthélemy Cabrol, from Gaillac in the diocese of Albi, authored the *Alphabet anatomique* (Tournon, 1594; Geneva, 1602; Montpellier, 1603; Lyon, 1614), later translated into Latin (Geneva, 1604; Montpellier, 1606). He accompanied Joubert to Paris when the physician was called by Henry III for consulting on the question of the monarch's sterility. Cabrol was the first royal surgeon of Henry IV and the first royal anatomist, a post created by Henry IV in the University of Montpellier in 1595.

[4]What was suspected by historians concerning this so-called piracy seems to be borne out upon reading this letter. Joubert and Cabrol were too closely allied in friendship for such "disloyalty" not to have been prearranged. See Pierre-Joseph Amoreux, *Notice historique et bibliographique sur la vie et les ouvrages de Laurent Joubert* (Montpellier: J.-G. Tournel, 1814), 121.

[5]On Joubert's *Paradoxes*, see the introduction and the index to *PE* (xiv–xv, 342).

best friends. This he does, says he, because without his ever having rendered the slightest service either to you or to yours, you have in his affairs always been so gracious, kind, and favorable that never could he expect another thing from a person he would have served willingly the rest of his life. Such, Monsieur, is your greatness, to have thus acquired a large number of sympathetic servants, among whom I know Monsieur Joubert counts himself, and who will never spare himself any pains should any obligation call him to show you his indebtedness.

One of the ways (and one not to be scorned) of showing it is to honor his benefactors through his writings. And I am certain that if he himself had put forth this work he would have sooner dedicated it to you than to any other I know of. It is therefore lawfully yours, especially in view of the author's permission, which is his complete consent: it is as if he were giving it to you, and as if I were presenting it to you on his behalf. May my actions show you the strong desire I have to be known by you, putting me before your good graces and presenting me for your service when it will please you to honor me with your commands. My Liege, you will find that in this I will be more devoted than you could ever wish from the most devoted and trustworthy servant you have ever had. I am so moved to serve you, both because of the praise from Monsieur Joubert and because of the general reputation of your rare and excellent virtues, which have made you pleasing in the sight of our Lord the King and of the other princes of this kingdom, you who manage the greatest and most important affairs of the Crown with dexterity and prudence, accompanied by a singular confidence, discretion, loyalty, soundness, integrity, sincerity, wisdom, diligence, patience, vigilance, promptness, honesty, gentleness, grace, goodness, gentleness, humanity, kindness, courtesy, modesty, generosity, constancy, magnanimity, frankness, excellent memory, subtle invention, profound and sound judgment, cogent and deft reasoning, good advice and council, along with every other virtue required for your station, position, and responsibility. Oh happy is the king who has such a counselor next to him! Oh how infinitely fortunate the monarch who could have as many as there are seeds in a beautiful pomegranate, as King Darius wished for as many Zopyres! Happy the nation, happy the people, [when they have] one with such an ability to obtain from the king what can be justly requested or hopefully expected, an ability so consummate, so sure and true as has ever been seen in France, in a personage who is so affable, so approachable, so faultless, so worthy of his charge, more so than anyone in the world ever was.

My Liege, I would be too prolix (I see it only too well) if I wished to recount only a tenth of the praiseworthy actions the public knows about, not to mention those which I myself could not worthily cover. I think, therefore, it would be much more pleasant for you to cast your eyes immediately on the beautiful and delightful works of Monsieur Joubert, knowing as I do that you have already taken great pleasure in reading the first part, which he himself had published one year ago. I trust that you will not take smaller pleasure in reading these, but whatever the case, may you interpret in a positive manner my boldness and accept the present I offer you in all reverence and humility, kissing your hands and praying God that you be granted the best of your fondest wishes in good health, along with a very long and very happy life.

From Paris, this third of February, 1579.

LETTER BY BARTHÉLEMY CABROL
TO ANTOINE DE CLERMONT

Letter by Barthélemy Cabrol, Master Jury Member of the School of Surgery in the University, Municipality, and City of Montpellier, and Royal Surgeon

Repelling the envious and venomous remarks made against the author of the *Popular Errors*

Addressed to the most virtuous, magnificent, and generous Lord, M[onsieur] Antoine de Clermont,[6] Baron de Montoison and Gentleman of the King's Chamber

---

[6]Antoine II, Compte de Clermont-Tonnerre (1525–78), served in 1551 as grand-master of France's water and forest resources, then as governor of Dauphiné, and finally as lieutenant general of the king's armies in Savoy. In 1569, during the battle of Moncontour, he was wounded, and his son, Antoine III, sometimes confused in biographies with his father, Antoine II, was killed.

It is commonly held, and very true, that "Envy will never die." For Envy was engendered by Lucifer at the very beginning of the world and will know no end, not any more than the devils of Hell, fathers of calumny and detraction, after which they have been named. I have felt the hard and painful sting of it on occasion on my own account, but I have always taken consolation and no small courage upon seeing myself in such an affliction in the company of the most worthy, virtuous, studious, and erudite people in the world, and upon hearing constantly that no one but the miserable is exempt from Envy and that it is better to be subject to Envy than to pity.

But what I felt deep within myself because of these stings and bites is nothing compared to the assaults and attacks visited upon Monsieur Joubert as soon as he began to become prominent, enjoy a reputation, and be considered among the most erudite and rare personages of his profession. It began when someone published the first decade of his *Paradoxes* without his even knowing anything about it, and then again when he recognized the work as his own and published it along with the second decade. Good heavens, what detractions and calumny did envy not incite in his regard for that work! I knew it well for having seen it, and how sad it made his friends and all those who knew his virtue, worth, and discretion. In spite of such slander the work was a huge success and earned him a lot of notoriety, just as the palm branch bears up and straightens under the load pressing down on it and trying to crush it, so much so that today his *Paradoxes* enjoy such fame and demand that they are debated and defended on the other side of Germany, as are the works of the most erudite of our time. Yet Monsieur Joubert, having promised a great number of other *Paradoxes* (according to the listing found at the end of the first decade in the second and third edition), has not tried to continue in this endeavor because he was disgusted and justly angered by the mean things envy had incited against him.

It is true that in diverse works, as the subject comes up, he treats these other *Paradoxes*, but it is only in passing and not in any depth, which causes considerable sadness among the more studious. Such was the case (unfortunately) in one of his more recent works, the *Popular Errors*, with common sayings that were criticized and corrected by him, containing sixty chapters and promising another three hundred, as is clear from the catalog that he published therewith.[7] But having heard through true reports that he was the subject of much envy, detraction, and calumny, and even that his reputation was suffering in several quarters, he became sad and resolved to abandon this endeavor also, even though, in the opinion of the most sensible and trustworthy who speak about the matter without any excess of emotion, the work is most worthy of praise, and its continuation is desirable in view of the great good the public will draw from it. They excuse very wisely and interpret very positively what the reproachful find faulty in it and deflect the violence of their stings so that no harm can come to the author's reputation or diminish it in the slightest. On the contrary, it is strengthened by the attacks, as virtue is made vigorous by attempts made upon it, or as plants that exude sweet-smelling tears (that is, resins or gums) only produce them when they are strong and have been wounded.

The principal reasons for the reprehensions (to no longer say biting attacks) launched by those who tax Monsieur Joubert for having been vulgar in his book, *Popular Errors*, were two. The first was because he dedicated it to the Queen of Navarre, most virtuous and generous princess, true mirror and model of honor, when he had to treat disgusting material (as it was called) and the shameful parts in the opening pages, writing about conception, reproduction, pregnancy, and birth. The second was because it all would have been better in Latin than in French for two reasons: the one is that these words do not sound as bad in a foreign language as they do in one's own, and women and girls, who are more ashamed about such things, would not have understood them; the other is that it is not good to divulge our art to common people and to let them understand what physicians wish and ought to retain for themselves, namely, the understanding of several things common people do and say without knowing the why and wherefore. As for the first reason, it is adequately explained in the second edition, both by Louys Bertrauen and by the author himself, who was willing to change the person addressed and present the entire affair to Monsieur de Pibrac, chancelor of the Lady in question so that he could pick and choose the terms Her Majesty might be familiar with and

---

[7]See the division of the entire work in appendix A of *PE* (245–68).

decide without the slightest doubt, the chancelor in question deciding for himself as to the rest since it was proper to his own condition.[8]

It has been said that Monsieur Joubert thus made honorable amends in the matter. Indeed, it is honorable and most praiseworthy to show such self-restraint and to refrain entirely from using the freedom common among writers lest the most delicate of readers be offended. And after all, when we speak familiarly, we are constantly having to say (since we do not wish to offend anybody, even if it be an inferior), "Please excuse me!" Must one back away from saying it to a princess, or to others of any estate, when one learns they were in any way offended? If there ever were an occasion to say "Please excuse me," it is when one thinks one has done something kind or thoughtful and finds that it was not at all viewed as such. And so for remarks that we said in jest but that were taken quite otherwise, we say we are sorry: "Please excuse me, I didn't wish to be offensive"; or "I wasn't thinking anything bad"; or "I didn't mean it the way you understood it." Well, such expressions are reparation and honorable amends, about which one should not be ashamed, as if they were ones used for absolution or expiation of a felony, which is a matter of criminal punishment and is binding. But the deed in question is of an altogether different order. Indeed, someone with the intention to please, honor, and serve people of the highest rank, right up to the princess (to whom his work is dedicated, presented, and offered in all humility, reverence, and devotion), receives in return for it a sound detraction and public calumny.

As for the subject matter, I have heard people of all kinds, from every class, station, rank, and estate speak about it, who did not refrain from telling me their frank opinions of it; most of them did not even know the affection I have for Monsieur Joubert. I met very few who do not have an infinite admiration for his work, and who do not wish to see the continuation of it. People say it is the most interesting subject they have seen treated in a long time, both useful and delectable, which are the two principal requirements for a perfect and fulfilling work. And as for the type of language, they say there was no harm in it and that it was even honest and proper. Still, Monsieur Joubert (as he is most wise,

---

[8]Cabrol seems to be saying that Pibrac would discuss with the princess (Marguerite de Valois) the appropriateness of sexual terms pertaining specifically to women and would decide for himself on the appropriateness of such terms referring to men. See the translation of the two letters in question in *PE* (3–10).

prudent, discreet, and circumspect) did well to change the dedication so as to please everyone, as he explains in his letter to his friends and to those who speak well of him.[9]

I now come to the matter of the second question,[10] that it would have been better to write these things in Latin, for the two reasons I mentioned above. Concerning the first, it was adequately taken care of by Monsieur Joubert in the letter I just cited, in which he argues pertinently that the most chaste women in the world may read it and learn nothing in it but proper things, as well as of their duties in marriage; the same is true of their husbands. As for young women, they can know nothing of the matters of the flesh if they are virginal in mind and in body, so to speak. But in addition, in order to please everyone in all matters, he has since removed everything that could offend in the slightest the most delicate consciences, knowing full well that one must not only abstain from evil but even from the appearance of it, that it is necessary to abandon and reject anything that might scandalize another, even if it means dismembering oneself, cutting off one's arms and legs, plucking out one's own eye, as Jesus Christ says, if any of them are a cause of scandal.[11]

The other reason is that matters of medicine must not be divulged, made familiar and clear, because people could make improper use of such information, knowing more than they should, to the point that they will want to contest the opinions of physicians on all points of medicine. Those who say this are modest, discreet, and trustworthy friends of Monsieur Joubert and they have told him this directly, as friendly advice. But it seems they have not read carefully his letter "To the Broad-minded and Studious Reader,"[12] in which he claims that he undertook this work to keep people in the places assigned them by their vocation, and to stop them from trying their hands in the area of medicine, so that they would no longer be as overconfident and as presumptuous as usual. He claims that he understands better what he learned from the ancient physicians and can use it more wisely for their

---

[9]See *PE* (6–10).

[10]The second of the two reasons for which Joubert was attacked by his critics.

[11]Joubert's note: Matt[thew] 18: [8–9].

[12]See the translation of this letter in *PE* (24–25).

own benefit, that it is within his grasp, and that they should not make trouble for physicians by trying to explain to them their duties when they treat and serve their patients. He wrote so that patients might know what he knows, or believes he knows, and abandon the errors that have had such a hold on them.

The work is full of such remonstrances and exhortations, without going into the extremes required by imbeciles. Monsieur Joubert knows full well that the mysteries and secrets of medicine, along with the principal points of the art (obscure matters, and of considerable importance), must not be communicated or revealed to the profane. That is just what he calls, somewhere in his work, all those who have not sworn and taken the oath in the school of medicine, subscribing to the sacred oath of Hippocrates, which he follows every day of his life. He makes scores of medical students who wish to take courses or earn degrees at the University of Montpellier swear to it each year. He who is the chancellor and regent of the University of Montpellier, who is solely responsible for the strict observance of its laws and statutes, will certainly not fail in discharging his duty. It is not, then, divulging or revealing medicine to the profane when one teaches them how to do well what they already are doing and explains to them what they know without really understanding it, so to speak.

And furthermore, who can find any evil in each person's knowing how to maintain his or her own health so as not to have as frequent a need of a physician? Will people say that Monsieur Charles Estienne, and after him Monsieur Jean Liébault, his son-in-law, both most erudite and humane individuals, did evil in writing their *Maison rustique* in French, in which there are a lot of family recipes, called common remedies, not only useful in preserving one's health but in warding off several illnesses?[13] Likewise the book entitled *Thresor des pauvres* has

---

[13]Charles Estienne (1504–62) was the third son of the famous printer Henri Estienne. He was the author of numerous medical works, among them *La Dissection des parties du corps humain* (Paris, 1549), *Dictionarium historicum ac poeticum* (Paris, 1544), and, in collaboration with his son-in-law, Jean Liébault, *Praedium rusticum* (Paris, 1554), translated as *L'Agriculture et maison rustique* (Paris, 1572; Lunéville, 1577; Lyon, 1583).

Jean Liébault (1535?–96) was a physician from Dijon who also wrote, among other works, *Quatre livres des secrets de medecine et de la philosophie chymique* (Paris, 1573, 1579, and 1582) followed by *Trois livres de la santé et fecondité et maladies des femmes* (Paris, 1582; Rouen, 1649).

been highly regarded and well received by all,[14] likewise the beautiful work by Monsieur Simon de Vallembert, on the food and the illnesses of children, and several other similar works that were written only in French.[15] On the contrary, there would be a need for everything concerning ordinary people's health and the ability to care for it themselves to be written in French so that they can profit from it, without begrudging them it, which would be an envy completely hostile to humankind. Would it be good if one had never revealed to people how to use wheat and grapes in order to make bread and wine, how to cook meat and prepare other foods, but that only a few had kept all that secret among themselves, so that all the others would have to pass through their hands and be at their mercy in order to have bread, wine, and food? Likewise (moving up from earthly goods for the body to the heavenly ones for the soul), there are complaints about some theologians who do not wish to allow the translation of Holy Scriptures into French, so that ordinary people might only have access to it through the mouths of the theologians, denying the ignorant this spiritual food, which they themselves nonetheless dole out from the pulpit and explain as profoundly, as subtly, and as clearly as they are able. And what difference is there in reading the same texts alone at home or in hearing them read publicly and in French? I do not see a great deal of difference between such distinctions and that of hindering people from learning for their own benefit as much as they can about the art that teaches them how to live in health and care for themselves when they are sick, under the guidance and care of a physician.

---

[14]The *Thresor des poures qui parle des maladies qui peuvent uenir au corps humain et des remedes ordonnez contre icelles. Auec la cirurgie et plusieurs autres praticques nouvelles* (Paris, 1512; 1517) was the first French translation of the vast work of Arnau de Vilanova (1235-1311). Much incertitude surrounds this Catalan physician and alchemist. He studied in Spain and in Paris, taught in Montpellier, and practiced in Barcelona, before being excommunicated by the archbishop of Tarragon and later declared a heretic by the Inquisition. Fortunately, he was protected by the pope (Boniface VIII), but his philosophical works were burned. The most important work of his to be published during the Renaissance was the *Breuiarium practicae* (Milano, 1483), and the first edition of his complete works was published in Lyon in 1504.

[15]Simon de Vallambert (dates unknown) was a French physician who published, among other works in Latin, the two following works in French to which Cabrol is referring: *De la conduite du fait de chirurgie* (Paris, 1558); and especially *Cinq liures de la maniere de nourrir and gouuerner les enfans des leur naissance* (Poitiers, 1564).

Now I ask you, what does Monsieur Joubert write other than what physicians instill and inculcate in their patients, friends, relatives, acquaintances, servants, guards, and other domestics almost every day? Is it worse to write it down than to say it? Do we not want people to keep it straight? Here is the way, by putting it in print, for voice fades away, but what is written endures. I do not see, then, that this reprehension has any foundation or is applicable in any way, or else I have misunderstood it. These are the principal areas, it seems to me, of the censures I have heard here and there.

There is yet another point over which Monsieur Joubert has been calumniated in a most absurd manner. It is over the depositions of the midwives, which some have dared to say were fabricated by himself.[16] He totally refutes this in his "Letter to His Friends and to Those Who Speak Well of Him,"[17] naming the person who furnished those from Paris and Béarn. As for the one from Carcassonne, I know for myself that he obtained it from a man who was the principal secretary of Monsieur the Marshall Damville, who quoted it often in jest.[18] And Monsieur Joubert is greatly hindered in understanding even the terms used by these midwives and knowing how to apply them to the diverse parts constituting the female genitalia. For he is not at a loss to distinguish as many parts as the midwives. We isolate sixteen or seventeen of them in public dissections. I shall present them in the order of appearance: (1) the *os Bertrand* or *Barré*, also known as the *os pubis* or *os du penil*;[19] (2) the pubic hair covering the aforementioned part; (3) the mound, called by some the *mons Veneris*; (4) the two labia or lips, which form the mouth or opening; (5) the two pterigomes or great

---

[16]These depositions appear in the fourth chapter of the fifth book of the *Erreurs populaires* (translations of them are in *PE* 211–13).

[17]The translation of this letter is in *PE* (6–10).

[18]Henri I, Comte de Damville (1534–1614), one of the sons of Anne de Montmorency, was an opponent of the Guises and the leader of the *politiques*, the Huguenots who had had considerable power and prestige toward the end of Charles IX's reign.

[19]The *os pubis* was also called the *os sans nom* during the Renaissance (see *PE* 318, n. 18).

wings, commonly called dewlaps;[20] (6) the two smaller wings under
the great ones, called nymphs, from a Greek word;[21] (7) the tentigo,
thus named by Fallopio, which is like a wart near the top of (8) the
mons Veneris and covered by the great wings—it is the head and acorn
or glans of the clitoris, which corresponds to the virile member, and it
is composed of two cavernous bands of tissue; (9) two muscles, which
support it and make it stand erect; (10) the orifice of the bladder, which
is a fleshy opening; (11) five or six little pieces of flesh or carneous
nodes, similar to warts; (12) the great canal corresponding to the length
of the virile member, with several circular ridges; (13) the hymen,
called the *dame du milieu*;[22] (14) the mouth or opening of the womb,
or *amarry*,[23] rough and as though with small teeth, resembling the
mouth of a lamprey; (15) the neck of the *ammary*; (16) the internal
orifice, which is the opening in the *ammary*; (17) the center and body
of the *ammary*, without any division into sections or pockets. I do not
mention the testicles and the wings supporting them, along with the
spermatic vessels, since these parts are farther back, hidden from view
unless one opens the belly. All the rest is visible and can be observed
in any woman who has had a child without making any incisions. The
matrix speculum reveals all of them. And whoever has the time and
wishes to verify what I claim will be shown most willingly by myself
every one of them (I have only to be furnished a subject), inasmuch as
I have pointed them out publicly in the medical schools in the University
of Paris. It must not be believed that these are imaginary or contrived
things, but I confess along with Monsieur Joubert that I simply do not

---

[20]Cotgrave gives translations of Cabrol's *aislerons grands*: "Ailerons grands. *as*
Landies." Under "Landie" Cotgrave gives: "*The deaw-lap in a womans Privities (as in
Landies;).*"

[21]Cotgrave also gives the gynecological sense of the term, "Nymphe: f. *A Nimphe;
also, a little excrescence, or peece of flesh, in the middle of a womans priuities.*"

[22]Literally, the "lady of the middle."

[23]Cotgrave translates this term of Cabrol's very generally as "the wombe, or matrix
of a woman." During the Renaissance the cervix was known as the *arrierefosse* or
reffiron (both terms appear in Joubert's *Popular Errors*). Cotgrave translates *reffiron* as
"the third gate of the wombe; or the mouth of the matrix, which is cleft acrosse, and
not lengthwise, as the Hymen, &c."

understand the terms midwives use and consequently cannot apply their terms to these parts.

And so all has been calumny, untruth, imposture, and detraction, which pale and gaunt Envy has launched against this good doctor and master because of the great popularity and currency of the *Popular Errors*, which has been printed in six months in four different places, namely Bordeaux, Paris, Lyon, and Avignon, and in each place no fewer than sixteen hundred were printed. This book has enjoyed such a great reputation that it started out selling for ten or twelve sous and has since sold for an *écu* and even four francs, in much the same way (as in a sort of famine) that the price of wheat goes up every day. Moreover, everyone is asking in bookshops and at printers' for the sequel to this work; even the author is importuned on a daily basis to make the rest of it available, at least in groups of five books at a time (if he does not wish to bring them all out at once) according to the divisions he has already promised, not to mention what more he will yet promise the public.[24]

But he is so angry and stung by the aforementioned attacks, and is so sensitive and jealous of his honor, that he has often—I know it for a fact—thought about burning everything he has done. Oh what a loss! So much is he upset that nobody has been able to make him give in and agree to the publication of the other parts, which he keeps so secret and locked away that there is no way even to see them or read them in manuscript form. For I know, and he is only too aware of it also, that several people would very willingly undertake publishing them on the sly without asking his permission. Now, in view of this firm resolution (not to say obstinacy), I have decided to have a few chapters of his printed that I have had for some time now, promising myself I would try to get from him explanations about a few matters on which I wished to have his opinion and a better understanding. There are not very many chapters, but most of them are quite long and have so many subheadings that if one wanted to divide them up there would scarcely be less than thirty. Monsieur Joubert traced them out long ago, before publishing Part One of the *Popular Errors*, and they deal with certain topics that have since been put elsewhere by the author in the "Division of the Entire Work," both generally and particularly, some finding themselves

---

[24]The first part of the *Popular Errors* contained five books. For the "Division of the Entire Work into Six Parts Containing Thirty Books," see *PE* (245–68).

now in the seventh book, others in the eleventh, the seventeenth, the twentieth, the twenty-third, the twenty-fifth, the twenty-sixth, and those which follow even in the thirtieth. I am not further concerned with their order, since we cannot have anything else from the author that had been promised, at least for the moment. We have to deal with him as one would with a debtor whose payments are not forthcoming, taking what can be had. I did the best I could in following and observing his orthography, just as if it had come from his own hand. In this his nephew Christophe de Beauchastel has faithfully and most willingly assisted me, and to whom I have given for his efforts as many *écus* as he gave me copies of chapters.

I know full well that Monsieur Joubert will not be pleased with what I have done with his work, but I was forced to do it by my great affection and my good intentions, which might be able to put me back into his good graces, especially when all is done through the care of a great friend of his and the result is a work well printed in his own style. For very often circumstances remove the evil from something that is inherently reproachable, as is said of honest deceit. And this is why I decided to communicate all this to you, my Liege, you (as I say) who have the power and the means to appease Monsieur Joubert in the event he complains about this enterprise of mine, since I clearly see how much he respects, reveres, honors, and cherishes you, you who are so friendly and helpful that he will never be displeased by it if he knows you think highly of it. On the contrary, he will be grateful for my having done it when he sees that it was only after having revealed my reasons to you, as well as to Messieurs de La Roche and de Beaufort, your very dear brothers, Messieurs de La Baume, de Mon[t]perroux la Verune, de Vontais, de Pardillan, du Moutet, de La Coste, de Brete, de La Bastie, Messieurs de Sagnes, Fevol, the two Girard brothers, du Vaure, Alian, Renier, and other friends of theirs who see more clearly in this affair than Monsieur Joubert, as people do who are not involved. And besides the burden I lift from him by acting in this way, and the worrying he might do about it, I even bring him the relief of freeing him from the responsibility and of challenging the bites and stings of accursed Envy (which by itself halts the completion of the entire work, promised in such an orderly fashion). I take upon my own shoulders all the indignation of the despiteful envious.

I have added to this Second Part of the *Popular Errors* a catalog of several diverse common expressions, which I have gathered from several contributors. The person who furnished me with the most to be sent to Monsieur Joubert was Monsieur Guillaume Capel, doctor of medicine from Paris, a most erudite and humane man who is keenly interested in quaint things. I do not doubt that Monsieur Joubert will be most happy to accept this catalog, since he himself requested readers to send him from all parts of the world popular sayings that are not included in his list. And so I will at least gratify him in this, which I offer to him as a sign of my sympathy.

My Liege, I beg you most humbly to be ready to take my defense if perchance I encounter reproach in this endeavor and to protect me with your shield, the good graces of Monsieur Joubert, who loves and admires you. Let him know that I did not do it without justification, and that I was bound by the public good, which I chose over my own personal pleasure. For it weighed upon me to see myself possessing and enjoying alone such fruit. I preferred to share it with those who were desirous of it because of the taste they acquired for it from what the author himself had published. I was also brought to it because I wished to have something to offer my Liege Monsieur de Villeroy, to whom I had nothing of my own to offer that was worthy of his grandeur, and so I borrowed the fruits of someone who is a very highly regarded servant of his and who will not be displeased (I trust) when he looks into it.

My Liege, I kiss your hands, praying God grant that you obtain your most noble desires, in perfect health and with a long and happy life.

From Paris this twentieth of January, fifteen hundred and seventy-nine.

INDEX OF CHAPTERS AND SUBJECT MATTER
CONTAINED IN
THE SECOND PART OF THE POPULAR ERRORS[25]

That one often can and should do without wine, since it is not as necessary as people think.   Chapter 1

Against those who think all fevers are cold except for those called *hot*. Where the shivering comes from, and the return of limited fevers.   Chapter 2

Concerning colds and the voiding of grease or fat in one's excrement, and how people err in thinking that all or most of the illnesses of workers come from colds.   Chapter 3

Why undiluted wine is prescribed for people who are very hot, and why pissing is prescribed before going to bed when people have strenuously exerted themselves.   Chapter 4

That it is necessary to change the linen often for the feverous.   Chapter 5

That women kill the feverous by giving them too little to drink, too much to eat, and too many covers. And what diet is appropriate for the feverous.   Chapter 6

Against those who do not allow the feverous to drink during an access, and those who want them to drink hot liquids to make them sweat more profusely and more often.   Chapter 7

Concerning broths and barley soup administered at midnight or in the morning, most unadvisedly.   Chapter 8

Whether it is bad to drink before going to bed.   Chapter 9

---

[25]Joubert, drawing from the longer title, adds in this heading the words *"and Popular Expressions"*; I have supressed this addition to make the title agree with the English translation I have given it. For the full title of the Micard edition, see the introduction (xiv, n. 4).

Whether liquids should be drunk at as warm a temperature as the blood, even in summer, and whether it is bad to cool wine.

Chapter 10

Against those who complain of hot nights in summer and yet sleep on a feather mattress with the windows closed.   Chapter 11

That blood sausages do not keep well, whence the custom of giving them as presents.   Chapter 12

Against those who have an inordinate fear of bloodletting, and think that the first use of it saves one's life.   Chapter 13

That bloodletting can be used on pregnant women, children, and the elderly.   Chapter 14

Against those who use bloodletting rashly and too often.

Chapter 15

That purgation can be appropriate in any season, even during the dog days.   Chapter 16

How one should conduct oneself on days when medicine is being taken. Whether one may sleep afterward. Concerning the time of day for administering a laxative broth. Concerning the meals that should be taken on such days. And why one should not go out of one's room.

Chapter 17

Why it happens frequently that patients who receive the most care most often die.   Chapter 18

Against those who maintain that death never comes without regret.

Chapter 19

Against those who in order to have loose bowels walk barefoot on cold surfaces or drink lots of oil, and what constitutes having a healthy stomach.   Chapter 20

Whether or not oysters and truffles make a man more lusty in the venereal act.   Chapter 21

Against those who measure the ability of a physician by the success he enjoys, which is often due to luck more than to knowledge.[26]
                                                            Chapter 22

That laymen have little respect for a physician who does not treat according to their diagnosis; that the last-used remedies gather all the glory; and happy the physician who arrives as the illness is weakening.[27]   Chapter 23

Concerning the importunate and the distrustful, who calumniate the procedures of the physician. Concerning the overconfident and the presumptuous, who are dangerous around a sick person.
                                                            Chapter 24

That it does not usually profit patients to have several physicians.[28]
                                                            Chapter 25

LIMINAL POEMS[29]

Maius Io captas nostris Ioberte camoenis
    Io triumphe, fas Io.
Aut (clari suboles patris) e stige Maeona solve,
    Aut monstra clava figere
Desine: vel fuerit tantis ingrata tropaeis
    Nostri camoenae seculi.

---

[26]A longer and more elegant form of this chapter appeared in *PE* (12, 63-65).

[27]This chapter also appeared in a more elaborate version in *PE* (11, 53-56).

[28]A longer version of this chapter appeared in *PE* as follows: "That it does not usually profit patients to have several physicians, but that one physician must be most assiduous in treating them" (12, 70-72).

[29]I wish to express my gratitude to Geraldine Bailey, my Research Assistant, and to Arthur Robinson, Assistant Professor of Classics, both of the Department of Romance Languages and Classics at the University of Alabama, for their gracious assistance in translating these liminal poems.

Monstra quidem Alcides stupido metuenda popello
   Partu deorum discidit.
Monstra sed errorum tu Coa cuspide scindis,
   Turbae timenda Delphicae.
Ergo tuis ut Io par sit Ioberte triumphis.
   Emitte Plutus e favis
Maeonidem: patris solium vel Apollinis, aulam
   Stellis coruscam scandite.
                        —*Io. Edoardus du Monin, Burg.*

A greater shout of praise do you receive from our Muses, Joubert.
   Hurrah! Rejoice! It is fitting! Hurrah!
Illustrious offspring of the father, free Homer from the Styx
   Or cease to bludgeon monsters with a club!
Else it will be but a hollow victory
   For the Muses of our age.
Hercules, offspring of the gods, did indeed tear asunder
   These monsters for the foolish, fearful commoners.
You, however, cut apart Errors' monsters with your Chaonian spear
   For the fearful Delphian throng.
Therefore, that the hurrahs be equal to your triumph, Joubert,
   Release Homer from the Plutonian labyrinth
Or ascend the throne of our father Apollo
   In the glittering palace of the stars.
                  —Jean Edouard du Monin, Burgundian[30]

Illudit [m]iseris varius mortalibus error:
   Et nullum errores non genus artis habet.
Sed non quam medica, damnosior error in arte:
   Unde salus doctis, mors rudibusque venit.
Non ducis indocti duplex datur error in armis:
   Cui semel erranti tota caterva perit.

---

[30]Jean Edouard du Monin (1557?–86) passed for a prodigy of erudition. A student of Latin, Greek, Hebrew, Italian, and Spanish, Monin also studied theology and philosophy, letters and mathematics. He came to Paris in his youth and studied at the Collège de Bourgogne, where he wrote Latin and French poetry as well as a tragedy. He was assassinated at only twenty-nine years of age.

Non sibi commisso medicus bis aberrat in aegro.
  Errorem cuius mora aliena luit.
Ergo magna tuis, decus o Ioberte medentum,
  Gratia debetur tempus in omne libris.
Qui non contentus praecepta docere medendi,
  Qua schola doctorum, Regis et Aula probes:
Errores etiam, quos ignorantia vanis
  Invexit populis in sua damna, doces.
Quod pietas est si qua viam monstrare vaganti,
  Quam pius arte tua est vita [med]enda labor.
                              —*Io. Auratus Poëta Regius.*

Ubiquitous error is a bane for our unfortunate race:
  And no profession is free of error's offspring.
But there is no more damaging error than in medicine:
  Health follows the skilled, death the unskilled.
The same error twice committed by a leader is forbidden:
  In erring once he condemns his entire army to death.
So too with a physician to whom the sick is entrusted:
  The death of another atones for the error.
Therefore, Oh Joubert, you the glory of healers, thanks
  Are owed to your books until the end of time!
You are not content merely to teach the arts of healing,
  Teaching in schools of the learned, of kings, of courts,
But also dispelling the errors ignorance has provoked
  Among the common people to their great loss.
What greater piety, as in showing the way to one who is lost,
  Than the pious labor in your life-healing arts.
                              —Jean Dorat, King's Poet[31]

Chacun monstre sa faute, un monstre à faire mieux.
Infinis sont de mal, un chemin de bien faire.
De IOUBERT & l'auis & l'exemple à mieux faire,
Tance, de faire mal, aprend de faire mieux.

---

[31]Jean Dorat, sometimes spelled d'Aurat (1508–88), was a philologist who was most famous for serving as teacher of the young members of the Pléiade at a school in Paris called Coqueret. He wrote several volumes of Latin poetry and some Greek verse as well.

C'est bien fait, auertir l'egaré d'aller mieux.
Le remettre au chemin, est encore mieux faire.
Auiser l'homme cheu de sa chute, est bien faire:
Et luy tendre la main, est faire encore mieux.
Tant de lampes estaindre, Apollon n'a que faire,
Menteuses és couleurs, aprises de les faire,
Pallir aux yeux trompez, sinon qui luyse mieux.
En vain l'homme deffend, & reprend de mal-faire,
Sinon qu'en faisant mieux, il enseigne à mieux faire.
Bien fait qui bien reprend & mieux fait qui fait mieux.
                                                —DV PERRON

Each man shows his error, one shows how to do better.
  Countless are the ways to do badly, one way to do well.
  Joubert's thoughtfulness and example for doing better
  Chide for doing badly and teach to do better.
It is a good deed to show those who stray the way,
  But putting them back on the path is still better.
  Pointing out his fall to a fallen man is a good thing:
  But holding out your hand to him is better yet.
So many lamps going out, Apollo could care less about
  Those deceptive in their color, those clever in going
  Pale to the untrained eye, save the one that shines out.
In vain do men forbid and reprehend doing things badly,
  Unless by doing better they teach how to do better.
  It is good to reprehend but much better to do better.
                                    —Jacques Davy du Perron[32]

---

[32]Jacques Davy du Perron (1556-1618) was born in Berne of a Normandy family
whose members had taken refuge in Switzerland to avoid religious persecution. He
learned Greek, Hebrew, and philosophy on his own and Latin and mathematics from his
father. He was a physician, and Henri III called him to his service as a reader. He
became a member of the clergy and was made cardinal.

THE SECOND PART OF THE POPULAR ERRORS CONCERNING MEDICINE AND THE REGIMEN OF HEALTH

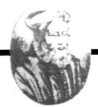

CHAPTER ONE
THAT ONE OFTEN CAN AND SHOULD DO WITHOUT WINE, SINCE IT IS NOT AS NECESSARY AS PEOPLE THINK

Wine is without question a very nourishing food that not only engenders of itself lots of blood but also causes proper digestion of other foods, revives the spirits quickly, kindles and invigorates natural heat, maintains natural moisture, purges liquid waste through sweat and urine, while dissipating into vapor those most subtle poisons called the black ones.[1] In short, it is infinitely profitable to the person who uses it properly and in moderation. But if its good qualities are abused by drinking it more for pleasure than through necessity, then wine can do just the opposite, engendering in the body and in the mind a thousand evils, which have as their related cause indigestion, phlegm, chills,

---

[1]The French term used by Joubert for "black" is *fuligineux*; Cotgrave translates the term as "sootie, blacke; smoakie." On Joubert's use of the term *vapor*, see *PE*, bk. 2, chap. 8, n. 2 (298).

obstructions, and other indispositions wholly the opposite of wine's characteristics. Experience sufficiently demonstrates this fact when we see that drunkards are frequently victim to colds, the falling sickness, apoplexy, numbness, paralysis, the shakes, cold sweats, dropsy, and other similar conditions.

We must therefore use wine with discretion, accommodating the nature of its properties to the needs we have of them. First of all, children who are well born ought to abstain from it because they enjoy naturally such a great amount of heat and moisture that these qualities cannot be augmented in them without serious consequences to their health. Besides, wine fills the head with an abundance of vapors, and overheating their boiling brains, it damages their minds. Once over eighteen years of age, one may have wine in very small quantities, and girls more than boys, contrary to popular opinion. The amount must be increased little by little until one is forty years old. I say "little by little" because otherwise it troubles the understanding and either deadens it or makes it wild, driving youth to anger, lust, and all manner of license. But for the elderly it is most appropriate; for them it is what milk is for children. Even Plato (the divine philosopher) said that God gave it to man as a remedy for the bitterness of old age, a most health-preserving medicine. For it makes the old young, makes them forget their worries and problems, suspicions, and concerns, rendering them more tolerable by softening their harsh and dire condition, just as fire softens iron and makes it malleable.

From this reasoning it can be seen that wine is not so necessary that many would be unable to do without it, whether ill or in good health. For those with hot complexions especially, and for the elderly as well, it is dangerous because it increases their natural heat beyond due proportions, threatening to set fire to the whole house, so to speak, and burn it to the ground. But leaving aside all such reasons, I wish to show by an inquiry that one can live a comfortable, healthy, and long life, whatever one's age is, wherever one lives, in whatever time of year, all the while abstaining from wine. From time immemorial the world has been divided into three parts (today a fifth and sixth part have been added), of which Europe, which we inhabit, is, according to the cosmographers, so small in comparison to the others that if the entire world were a city, such as Paris, Europe would only be one or two houses. Asia, Africa, and America would among themselves account for the rest. Now, this small bit of land is the place where the most wine is consumed, for in the other countries either there are no vineyards or the people abstain from this drink (unless it is taken on the sly) because of the order of Muhammad, whose sect has grown to such proportions that Christians are but a small handful compared to such a huge multitude. Are they any more sickly, weak, or fragile? No, on the contrary, we admire their strength. Do people not say, "He's as strong as a Turk"? As for agility, dexterity, vigor, and other physical virtues, they are in no way behind Christians, if they do not surpass them altogether, besides which they lead healthy lives and live to a ripe old age.

If it is maintained that Africa and America are countries that are too warm for wine to be drunk there, but that in cold or temperate climates one cannot live without such drink, I will answer that a portion of Asia is also in a temperate clime and indeed in the best of climates in the opinion of the most renowned geographers. Those regions near the north are freezing cold, yet wine is completely unknown there, and everywhere people live very well. What will we say if in our Christian Europe as well there is to be found an infinite number of people who have never drunk wine, and still others who have hardly ever drunk any, such as in the cold northern regions, where it is not produced but, imported from elsewhere, costs so much that poor people never taste it except on grand occasions, for their ordinary drink is plain water, beer, ale, cider, pear water, apple water, and other beverages made from grain or fruit? They live no more poorly because of it than do the rich; they are as healthy and spry, if not more so. In our mountainous regions (I am speaking of those which are a little farther away from the hillsides and plains that produce wine), poor people drink nothing but water and yet live longer and are ill less often than those of the lower regions, in which there are still several individuals who from birth despise wine and reject it outright or others who have stopped drinking it of their own will out of concern for their health, as if they were avoiding chills, colds, and gout. This is so much the case that if we put together all the wine drinkers we will find their number so small that if the world were divided into a thousand parts there would scarcely be ten of them.

Yet one does not hear that for all our wine we live longer or stronger than others from hotter, colder, or more temperate climes. In spite of this, ordinary people, and especially peasants, have such an affection for wine that they do not think they can live without it. Whether healthy or ill, they still want it, even when suffering from a burning fever. If it is forbidden them because it obviously increases their already excessive

warmth and doubles their thirst, their headache, their backache, putting
them in danger of frenzy, they think we wish to weaken them and push
them down so as to make the illness last longer. These poor people
absolutely believe that wine alone sustains their strength. And so in
order to drive out illness they seek to drink the best. I remember
treating twenty-five years ago a gentleman near Aubenas in the Vivarez
region who sought to prove to me that when he suffered from a high
and persistent fever resulting from a severe pleurisy he should not
abstain from wine, claiming that it took its very name from life, as if it
were its essence.[2] And when I had refuted his idea, this is what he
answered: "How is it possible that wine, so good and gracious to
everyone, even the most uncouth, could possibly hurt me, who during
my whole life have loved and cherished it so much? Would it not then
be most evil and not at all good, as everyone considers it to be?" There
are the sound arguments given by the most clever of imbeciles who
follow only the sensual and animal appetite. The others simply think it
is good for them and are not moved by any pleasure in it, not even
finding that wine has a pleasant taste, no more than does medicine; these
people, because of their innocent simplicity, deserve to be rescued from
their error.

Let it be known by such as these, then, that physicians forbid wine
in two cases, mainly. In the first, when the patient is warm in all or in
part of the body. Do you not suspect that wine obviously increases heat?
If you complain of feeling as if you are on fire, do not take anything
that can cause heat. Someone will reply that the wine has been so mixed
or (as people say) drowned that it no longer tastes like wine. And what
good is it if water completely wipes out its strength? You will say that
it corrects water by means of its quality, and the little bit of substance
that it contains confirms and maintains the strength of the patient. It is
therefore necessary that this small amount of wine retain its quality in
proportion to its quantity, and that it will always be a little bit harmful.
This is speaking most strictly and not as a gentle physician who is
humane and of a considerate nature. Such a physician, the above
considerations put aside, must be understanding with respect to the
habits and desires of the patient and must remember the maxim
delivered so wisely by the good old man: "Food and drink, although

---

[2]The argument is linguistic, based on the similarity of the French words for "wine"
and "life": *vin, vie.*

somewhat worse for you but so much more pleasant, are to be preferred to their opposites!" And this same physician prescribes for acute illnesses that are accompanied by a persistent fever weak wine, called *oligophore*, which we can reproduce with large doses of water and small ones of wine. I will further add that wine with a lot of water quenches thirst better, is more refreshing, and moistens more thoroughly than water alone, as Galen has proved to be the case with *oxycrat* for those who are very thirsty.[3] For wine and vinegar make water penetrate more deeply, and this refreshes and moistens, and so it follows that one's thirst is better quenched. In fact, if I did not fear the abuse and the importunateness (for if one ounce is allowed today, two will be wanted tomorrow) and the reproaches one can encounter because of it or at least the suspicion that one has not followed proper procedure, when afterward there arrives some break in the ordinary course of the illness (which will be attributed to a drop of wine), I would allow a small amount to be taken by people with a fever who desire it strongly and who assure me they will feel the better for it. But we fear so many things that we prefer to have the patient endure some discomfort than to have the physician's honor put into question. For one easily abuses what is enjoyable, and if ordinary people are allowed something that is a little suspect, everything is calumniated. Besides, there are several other means of sustaining a very weak patient that are free of all danger and suspicion, such as soups, bullions, consommés, broths, strained meats, extracts, meat juice, fresh eggs, and purées, all of which are far more nourishing than a little wine.

It is true that wine brings about digestion and facilitates the absorption of the other things eaten; it relaxes us, picks us up, makes us sleep better, and, when well diluted with water, also quenches thirst better than water alone or water mixed with syrup does. I simply warn against becoming so attached to it that one only wishes to drink it full strength and still longs for it even when the physician forbids it, or (what is worse) to drink it on the sly, as if to fool ourselves. One tries every means to withdraw the wood and remove the coals in order to stop a fire; these people, on the other hand, pour oil on it. They are concerned about feebleness, but how can strength be returned to the body if it is the heat, intensified by the wine, that is weakening it? We all see that

---

[3] *Oxycrat* is Galen's term for what Cotgrave calls "a potion, or drinke, made of vineger mingled with water."

the heat of summer, of the baths, or of hothouses makes us feel weak, aimless, and tired. Fever causes similar effects, more because of its very nature than because of the bad humors. If in scorning our reasons they would at least heed the warnings nature gives them, they would behave much more wisely than they do. For just as we lose our appetite when the stomach is full of liquid (which denotes that nothing more should be put in it until it is empty), so too when wine seems bitter to us or to have some other bad taste, as happens during almost every fever, it must be supposed that for the time being wine is not helpful and that the body has no need of it. Indeed, nature has given a coarse sense of recognition to the stomach and to its mouth (which is commonly called the heart, in imitation of the ancient Greeks)[4] in order for us to know what is fitting to eat, along with the appetite, which also warns us about what we eat, so that, governed by them through an instinct they control (if we are wise and heed it), we might be able to take proper care of ourselves whether sick or healthy.

But the intemperance of man is such that in spite of these warnings he will follow other desires. I take it for granted that people who are ill (especially with a fever) and find that wine has an unpleasant taste scorn and offend nature if they try to drink any. But I do not on the other hand maintain that it cannot be drunk if it is not found to be distasteful. For the second case, which forces us to take its defense, does not always make it lose its delightful flavor. When one has a cold or chills not centered in the head, these conditions cannot transmit their awful characteristics to wine that is drunk. Yet wine is not allowed, and rightly so, when one is in such a condition, because the humors, warmed, broken up, and freely flowing because of the heat of the wine, exit more easily; this same heat, moreover, enlarges the passages by making the pores and tubes dilate. Besides all this, wine penetrates so deeply that we sometimes feel it in our very fingernails almost as soon as we have swallowed it. And so when wine meets up with thick, heavy, slow-moving humors in its path, it pushes against them, stirs them, and makes them thinner. For these reasons we advise people with colds, chills, and gout to abstain from wine. It is not that we take any pleasure in torturing people and treating them roughly. It is the illness that shows

---

[4]French still retains the expression *avoir mal au coeur* (literally, "to be sick in the heart") in the sense of being sick to one's stomach.

us what it thrives upon, and we in turn point it out to our patients. Is it not a grave error to give the illness the arms it needs to conquer you?

It is therefore necessary to accept the conclusion that wine is not as good for man as it is often made out to be, whether in good health or ill, especially since there are a great number of people who have never drunk a drop of it and live no more unhealthily because of it. It is a gross mistake to consider wine so important in sustaining our strength that we do not wish to abstain from it when it clearly hurts us. For those with delicate health, milder beverages are made in the place of wine, such as metheglin (called *bouchet*)[5] and coriander water. Barley water and hydromel are to be used ordinarily. I mean hydromel made with water and not with wine, as it usually is when it resembles malmsey in taste and strength, for in that case it would not be any less harmful to fluxion than wine. Hyppocras made with water is properly called *melicrat*,[6] and that made from wine *hydromel*, according to Dioscorides.[7]

---

[5]Joubert uses the term *hippocras d'eau*, which Cotgrave translates as "metheglin; wine, or drinke made of honey and water." Cotgrave also translates the common term *bouchet*: "a kind of broth for a sicke bodie; also, the sweet drinke, Hydromel; or, a drinke made of water sweetened with sugar and cinnamon; or, as; *eau de bouchet*. A certaine compound water, which with that of Corianders, makes a kind of Hipocras."

[6]Cotgrave translates *melicrat* as "metheglin, or Mede; drinke made of water, and honie sodden together."

[7]Joubert's note: Book 1, chapter 17.

Dioscorides was a Greek botanist of the first century A.D. He wrote a famous *Materia medica* in which five hundred plants are named and described. This work remained the principal source for medical students and botanists until the seventeenth century. Pietro Andreo Mattioli (1500–70) wrote *Commentarii in sex libros Pedacii Dioscoridis adjectis quam plurimus plantarum et animalium imaginibus* (Venice, 1544), while Benoît Textor (date of birth and death uncertain) published a work based on Dioscorides, *Stirpium differentiae ex Dioscorida secundum locos communes* (Paris, 1534).

CHAPTER TWO
AGAINST THOSE WHO THINK ALL FEVERS ARE COLD
EXCEPT FOR THOSE CALLED *HOT.*
WHERE THE SHIVERING COMES FROM,
AND THE RETURN OF LIMITED FEVERS[1]

The abuse one commits in giving wine to those with a fever, as we have just shown, is based not only upon the maintaining of strength, but on another common mistake: the belief that a fever is an illness of the cold type. The reasoning (I think) is that this illness is caused by cold and is accompanied by cold, unless (perchance) the fever is continuous, in which case it is called hot fever. For clearly after a long labor or exertion that has caused the body to become hot, if one is surprised by cold there is a danger of fever. And, in fact, ordinary people will not believe in any other cause for this illness, which they call "catching cold."[2]

If the fever is limited, such as the quartan, the tertian, or daily (be it simple, double, or compound), because the access begins with a shiver, stiffness, trembling, or quaking, people conveniently think that the illness is caused by the coldness enclosed within the body and that it must be ousted by heat, since nature teaches them that one contrary drives out another. And so these good people are of the opinion that the fever is this great cold caused by coldness, to the extent that, if they are asked after it passes if it lasted very long, they will answer, "An hour or two at most," not realizing that the heat that comes after the cold is part of it. This is why all their attention is directed to keeping warm, and so they cover themselves all up, heat up stones and tiles for their feet, drink good undiluted wine, sip spiced broths seasoned with saffron or with very old cheese that stings like pepper. In short, they only try to overpower the cold and in one way or another to bring on sweating, as if the illness were caused by a frozen humor that had to be melted and turned back into liquid. Thus when they begin to feel warmth, they think the fever is over and they have only to wait for the sweating to

---

[1]Limited fevers, also called cold fevers, as is seen in this chapter, are opposed to continuous (or hot) fevers. Cotgrave translates *fievre continuë* as "a continuall feuer, whose fit neuer ceaseth till the disease, or diseased, end."

[2]Joubert's term is *morfondement*, which Cotgrave translates as "a cold; or a taking of cold."

begin. This explains why the better informed among them endure patiently the awful suffering of being almost stifled with covers during hot weather to squeeze out the humors, just as one wrings out a sponge with two hands. They think that the excessive heat that bothers them so severely and so long after their short-lived shivers is but the result of their own procedures with their covers, from trying by every means to subjugate the cold, which they hold to be the very essence of the illness. This is why they nourish the burning heat as much as they possibly are able until sweating occurs. It is not surprising, then, that they use spices, since this is what they believe. But these poor people are gravely mistaken as to the nature of their illness, and this is why all these errors spread so wildly. For they do not know that a fever is burning heat, and that coldness is its precursor, or herald, which proclaims its arrival, which I shall make them understand very easily with the following argument, by demonstrating the cause of such diverse effects.

Our skin is everywhere pierced by small holes whose existence cannot be suspected except for the sweat that comes out of them and the hairs that take up most of the opening. Wise nature has done this in order to allow free passage to the vapors our heat generates, and this heat would be stifled by them if they were hindered, just as fire is if it is not given air. These vapors are like soot, thick, heavy, made up of burned matter, undetectable because of its fineness if it were not for its nature, which is foulness, blackness, and greasiness, transferred to our shirts and other clothes. Moreover, in winter, because the cold tightens and contracts, the skin of our hands (which are less covered, so we can use them, than other parts of the body) is rough and black because of this retained excrement. For it does not exit with ease when the epidermis is constipated. This therefore is their function, and the reason we have openings in the skin, namely, to provide an exit for the continual fumes, vapors, and exhalations of the heat, which is always at work on humors in the body, making them into food. If these pores become plugged, or so restricted that the fumes stay inside because they are unable to pass through, our heat becomes excessively sour, stinging, strong, and burning, like a fire smothered with ashes, and if this condition lasts a long time, these poisons stifle and overcome the body.

When we have exerted ourselves, the increased heat warms up the humors, exciting and driving out a great amount of exhalation, of which the moist ones often become water and make up the sweat while the dry ones dissipate in fumes. At such a time it is necessary that the pores (thus do we call the openings in the skin) be open imperatively. For if the cold surprises them and constricts them, the ordinary and ongoing warming will make of our natural heat (which is gentle, benign, and muted) a fire disrupting all the humors. This is the source of continuous fever (which lay people call hot), when the disorder, imprinted deep within the humors, continues several days without intermission and no longer is dispelled when the cause is removed. For the exhalations, which have built up in great quantities, need to be voided, and the blood, which has become overheated, must be cooled. Sometimes the matter made vile because of the heat stoked by the constriction of the skin is dissipated in an access of fever, which results in sweating; but a certain amount of external heat (which can be called *empireume*, in the sense of a trace or vestige of fire)[3] left over from the first disorder, after a time, provokes a similar inflammation and adulteration of humors. This is what causes intermittent fevers every twelve hours, every day or every two days, unfailingly returning regularly until the corrupt quality left in the heart by the first blast of heat is entirely extinguished and dissipated.

This is how external coldness causes high-intensity fevers, which, burning within the humors, persist for a long time. Thus from one contrary its opposite is engendered, because of the circumstances. For the cold, which causes the skin to contract, hinders perspiration, whose task it is to maintain natural warmth in its proper normal state. One must not therefore think that fever is a cold condition because it can be caused by coldness, especially since there are many other causes ordinary people rightly suspect and attribute to cases of fever, such as food poisoning, anger, sadness, worms, sunstroke, and similar things that cannot be likened to common chills. Among them are indigestion, obstruction, infection, internal aposteme,[4] thirst-breeding, heated air, excessive activity, late hours, and other causes no less responsible for fever and unknown by ordinary people. All of them share this common point of engendering a great quantity of exhalations, of upsetting the humors by

---

[3]Cotgrave defines both *empireume* and *empyreume*: the former as "a marke of fire, scorching, or burning; a remainder of warmth, or heat; a sparkle, or small fire"; and the latter as "a drie, and accidentall heat, or fierie qualitie; or, as *Empireume*."

[4]An aposteme was an abcess. Cotgrave defines it as "an inward swelling full of corrupt matter." See *PE*, bk. 4, chap. 11, n. 4 (314).

overheating the blood, the spirits,[5] or solid particles, with a pernicious heat, which is the very essence of fever. It is therefore not cold, as is thought, because external cold is sometimes the cause of it, since we see that it most often springs from other causes.

But how would it be possible (you will ask) that a condition springing from heat should manifest shivering, stiffness, chills, and shaking, even the chattering of teeth? This is the other cause of error among those idiots who, when they fail to see the cause of such strange symptoms and thinking it to be more serious than all the rest, look absolutely no further and call it a fever. This is why it is essential to teach them what it is that causes such symptoms, and what it indicates, so as to correct the errors that ordinary people commit with such imprudence. The average physician (with whom I wish to part company momentarily, having concern only for lay people) holds that the feverish, hot quality of intermittent fevers (commonly called limited) corrupts the humors found in the blood vessels; and when the heat becomes so excessive and vile that nature is disgusted by it, the veins force these humors out by means of a violent expulsion, which spreads them throughout the body, the vessels, the tissues and membranes, and other sensitive organs. This matter moves with such violence and heat that the places it rushes through have so much pain that patients feel as though they are being stabbed, torn, sliced, or burned. It must not be thought strange that a humor hot with waste matter or some other element will cause chills and stiffness, for boiling water thrown suddenly on naked skin makes it shake just as will cold water. Sparks of fire have the same effect, and if one is jabbed hard with a needle, the entire body reacts. So too do the sentitive parts of the body when irritated by hot and caustic humors, making the person shake while trying to twist about and resist what is being done to them. This is what causes yawning, stretching or pendiculation,[6] and coughing, symptoms that prefigure the access and persist until this matter is consumed and dissipated in sweat or in exhalations.

---

[5] I have translated as "spirits" instead of "humors" because Joubert uses the word *esprits*; the distinction between the terms is minor. See *PE*, bk. 2, chap. 7, n. 2 (298).

[6] Cotgrave translates *pendiculation* as "a pendiculation; or, a stretching in th'approach of an Ague [fever]."

For coldness is virtually nonexistent,[7] but humors are pushed violently about from one place to another and will start to turn foul in confined places, for inasmuch as the limbs have already become used to them just a short while after having first opposed their arrival, they are no longer so very much upset by them. And when the substances are hotter yet, after penetrating the heart, their heat spreads throughout the body. This disorder always goes from bad to worse until the humors are completely vitiated; then, weakened by the heat, they finally are dissipated, discernibly in part, but in part indiscernibly, when their influence fades. And so the condition of a fever that has subsided is nothing other than humors, fouled and made corrupt by excessive heat, which causes them to become burning hot, and burn they do as long as it takes for them to be consumed. The shivering that precedes is the indication, or arrival, of the substances that will cause the access. And so it is a gross error to maintain that shivering is the essence of fever and not the burning that results from it, especially since its name clearly indicates to which of the two fever must be attributed. For fever is not so named because of the cold, but because of the fervor, after the Latin, which has it derive from *ebullition,* just as Greek has it derive from *fire.*

I think I have sufficiently shown that fever, whatever its source, and whatever its type, is entirely founded in heat, so much so that the poor idiots go too far in keeping people warm, torture their bodies in vain, make their condition worse, and often kill themselves by abusing spices, undiluted wine, and heavy covers. They think everything comes from cold and that it is only a matter of causing profuse sweating. They call a continuous, burning fever that is not accompanied by chills a hot fever, as if there were any cold ones, unaware of what the word *fever* means. And if I were asked why it is that continuous fevers are not accompanied by shivering, I would give the answer that our school maintains, that the corrupt substances are all kept in the veins and do not move out to the more visible parts of the body, unless it be at the very end, at which time there is also stiffness.

---

[7]There is a lapsus in the 1587 (Micard) edition at this point. The text reads as follows: *Car le froid n'est, sinon tandis que l'humeur est poussée d'vn lieu à autre violemment, & qu'il commeance mieux à pourrir en lieu estrois: car depuis que les membres l'ont ja accoustumé, vn peu apres sa venue qu'ils refusoyent, ils n'on sont plus tant offencez.*

There remains to be explained (since several people are curious to
know) why it is that intermittent fevers return with such regularity, one
every day, another every two days, and still another once every three
days. I am happy to give them the common opinion of physicians. It is
because the body, needing four different humors in order to sustain so
many of its parts, which are all different, produces more of one than
another, according to need. Thus it makes a large quantity of blood and
less phlegm, yet still more choler, and more choler than melancholy.[8]
Now, if the phlegm happens to go bad, adulterated by the feverish heat,
the disorder will return on a daily basis. For phlegm is produced easily
in a short amount of time and is therefore very copious. We do not have
as much choler and still less melancholy humor so as to make the fits of
fever return as quickly; it takes a longer time to build up a sufficient
quantity of them. Let us suppose (for example) that all fits require one
ounce of matter. The first fit provoked by that ounce of matter consumes everything; the second fit cannot begin until enough humor to
upset nature is generated, namely, when (as we suppose) there is
another ounce of it, for neither a half nor three-fourths can provoke an
access. In six hours the phlegm becomes so abundant that scarcely the
rest of the day taken up in a fit of fever is able to consume the excess
humor. It takes more than thirty hours to make an ounce of choler, the
amount required for an access of tertian fever, and two days to renew
the small amount of melancholy humor, which causes the quartan fever.
For it is thought that the humors correspond with each other and
become fever breeding little by little, not all at once, and that during the
intermissions of the total amount that has been in the body for some
time, as much as is needed for an access goes bad (unless still more
completely corrupt matter has recently been produced) during the fever's
remission. Thus if the ounce always happens to be built up at the same
time, the fever will return punctually and will be difficult to cure, as
Hippocrates has said.[9] Now very often the fever is delayed or advanced

---

[8]Joubert reiterates the doctrine of the four humors, using the terms *sang* ("blood"),
flegme ("phlegm," or "mucus"), *cholere* ("choler," or "yellow bile"), and *melancholie*
("melancholy," or "black bile"). For the relation between the four elements (earth,
water, air, and fire) and the four humors, see *PE*, bk. 5, chap. 6, n. 2 (322).

[9]Joubert could be referring to any of several places in the works attributed to
Hippocrates: *Prognostic*, xx; *On the Nature of Man*, xv; *Aphorisms*, IV, xxxvi–lxx;
Epidemics, I, xxiv–xxvi; *Diseases* I, xxiii and II, xl–xliii.

because our body undergoes thousands of changes in what we do, what we excrete, ingest, or apply topically, such that a simple quartan fever can, because of a severe disorder, become double or triple, depending on whether an amount of melancholy humor equal to the ounce is completely generated every two days, just as it is in a tertian fever, or every day, as in a daily fever. For the essence of fevers (at least the simple ones) does not always correspond to their names, and we do not consider tertian every fever that returns on the third day, nor daily one that is common. But I am getting too far into things, more than is necessary for ordinary people, who will be satisfied knowing that fits of a limited fever are in proportion to the amount of humor causing them, as we have argued. I could furnish several other proofs if my discussion were for physicians. I skip over them lightly and do not go into the great subtleties the matter deserves. If I wished to argue these points more soundly, it would require questioning all that we said about the cause of shivering, which is a sign of heat. For this is commonly believed (something we refute in our *Paradoxes*[10]), just as is everything we said concerning the adulteration of the fever-begetting humors. In all of this I am firmly upheld by Professor Simon Simoni,[11] a most learned and intelligent philosopher-physician who has beautifully elaborated upon the subject I have barely touched.

It is time to conclude. One must no longer distinguish between hot and cold fevers, since the word *fever* implies ebullition. It is a burning and a blistering heat that cannot properly be called cold. Also, the word *hot* is superfluous, for there is no other kind. Heat, and not cold, is the true disorder that must be treated.

---

[10]On Joubert's *Paradoxes,* see *PE,* bk 1, chap. 2, n. 12 (286).

[11]Simon Simoni (1532?–1602) was a physician, philosopher, and theologian who began his career in Geneva, holding chairs in philosophy and later in medicine, but, after an argument with Thédore de Bèze, went to Paris to teach at the Collège Royal. His writings touched on Aristotle's *Nicomachean Ethics,* fevers, rabid dogs, sneezing, infertility, and the plague. Simoni was expelled, however, for his Protestant leanings and afterward taught philosophy and medicine in Prague and finally in Krakow.

CHAPTER THREE
CONCERNING COLDS
AND THE VOIDING OF GREASE OR FAT
IN ONE'S EXCREMENT, AND HOW PEOPLE ERR IN THINKING
THAT ALL OR MOST OF THE ILLNESSES OF WORKERS
COME FROM COLDS

Because we mentioned above a cause of a disorder called colds, on which lay people blame almost all their illnesses and especially fevers, it would be most appropriate to point out what they are, and that they must not be thought to be so common. From what I am able to understand from the remedies the peasants take for them and from what they say about them, colds come about when, after excessive exertion, working the entire body into a sweat, people are suddenly exposed to cold. A fever develops rapidly in those who are replete with large quantities of excrement if the skin is quick to contract for the above reasons. In others the muscles ache, and even the bones, as if they had been severely beaten; there is fatigue, a bloated feeling, and difficulty in breathing. These are the most common ailments related to the condition of a cold, and they are caused by the vapors stirred up by the heat that is unable to pass through the skin, contracted by the cold, and that remains in the sinews, muscles, and tendons allowing for movement; because these parts are gorged and hindered, they fail in their function. The pain resulting from this condition is either like having needles stuck everywhere in the body, like being skinned, or covered with apostemes, or like having one's body inflated or stretched, according to the nature of the exhalations, fumes, and vapors. Difficulty in breathing results from the lungs' being shocked by the cold air after having overheated, for the bronchial tubes stiffen and cannot easily dilate as usual, and so people with a cold become pursy.[1] In other cases the pores of the skin are so open that cold penetrates to the very muscles, seizes and beleaguers the veins, which it is able to obstruct and plug no less than a slight chill can do to the openings in the skin. And this is what sets off a fever, caused by internal obstruction brought about by nothing more than constriction.

---

[1]Joubert's term is *poussifs*; Cotgrave translates the term as "pursie, short-winded; also, broken-winded."

Sometimes the cold stiffens the veins such that during a violent effort they are unable to respond and either split open at the end or burst somewhere else. Then blood spurts out or bleeds into an internal cavity, where it clots and turns black; this happens most often in the lung and in the stomach. The result is that the ill spit up or vomit blood in the type of cold ordinary people fear the most, for they think that the blood, thus blackened and clotted, is coming out of the veins, in which the penetrating cold has frozen it. But this is an error quite easy to expose, first of all because blood could not get through the narrow parts at the end of the veins if it were already clotted, and there would have to be a large rupture for the huge clots that are expelled. Moreover, it is impossible for blood to freeze in the veins because of the cold, otherwise, when our extremities, our hands and our feet, are as cold as ice, we would think that the blood in them is frozen. Still more easily would it be able to freeze in the bodies of dead people, in which it nevertheless remains liquid, as we see through dissection in bodies after ten or twelve days. It is not the warmth of the veins (whatever Aristotle says)[2] that keeps the blood from freezing. For the entire body is considerably warm, and yet it is only in the veins that blood can be kept from hardening. It is a property and natural characteristic that makes veins in this way fitting to preserve the blood. As soon as it escapes, wherever it may fall, it will inevitably clot, and if it is inside our bodies, it will bring about a thousand complications similar to those caused by poison. It is therefore imperative to stop such an unfortunate thing from happening, and when such a condition is suspected, all measures must be taken to keep the blood from clotting, or to make it thaw, as ordinary people say.

Whatever the case, as soon as they feel a little sick after strenuous exertion and then cooling off too quickly, and suspecting that their blood may be beginning to clot or that it has already done so, ordinary

---

[2]The section from the *Meteorologica* (IV) to which Joubert is doubtless referring is the following humoral argument: "Blood, on the other hand, and semen are made up of earth and water and air. If the blood contains fibres, earth preponderates in it. Consequently it solidifies by refrigeration and is melted by liquids; if not, it is of water and therefore does not solidify." This translation is from the E. W. Webster edition of *The Works of Aristotle* (Oxford: Clarendon Press, 1931), 3: 389.

people take doses of mummy,[3] pitch, parsley, walnut brandy, alcohol, whole mustard with undiluted wine, sulfur or saffron, powdered savory, parsnip juice, and other similar things that can thin the blood. Or yeast water with some mithridate, or blessed charcoal and broom flowers in order to provoke sweating. Others drink salt water, as though it were holy water, or watered ashes as lye. There are several other big secrets kept among these poor people, of which the aim is none other than to thaw the blood, which they always suspect of being clotted by their colds, whether accompanied by fever or not, for colds can cause both conditions, separate or in combination.

From these remarks I wish to conclude that the main property of colds is to chill the blood in the veins. I maintain that it is a property given to this cause, and that few if any other disorders cause the same congealing. For it is necessary for the skin and for the entire body to be completely unobstructed, such that the cold will not encounter any hindrance, which is precisely what happens in the above case. This is what I consider a true cold to be, for which the remedies commonly taken can be of considerable worth. For as far as fevers are concerned, they have so many means of being produced (as we have said in the preceding chapter) that it would be abusing people to argue always for this or that particular one. Fever is most often caused by something other than a cold and, with the exception of a fall and in a different way, only a cold can cause the blood to clot. It is for such a reason that this word must be used in the most strict sense and not loosely applied to all sorts of fevers. For colds can cause two sorts of disorders, one of which springs from no other source, and the other from several different ones. Thus people are very mistaken in the way they name them and are in grave error when they attribute to them all kinds of fevers and several other illnesses that in no way spring from cold, internal or external.

---

[3]Joubert uses the word *"mumie,"* which Cotgrave translates as "mummie; mans flesh imbalmed; or rather the stuffe wherewith it hath beene long imbalmed (whether it be Pissasphalte, or Mirrhe, Saffron, Aloes, and Balme incorporated together.)"

There is another disorder or condition named *larfondement*[4] in several places where I have been, and people are called *larfondu*[5] when they pass melted grease in their excrement (such as urine and stool), as well as lard, whence the term. This occurs in burning fevers, which physicians call colicky because the extreme heat weakens the healthy organs and brings them to a hectic state.[6] When ordinary people know a person is *larfondu,* they have no hope for a cure, and they think that the cause for this disorder, called *larfondement,* is an excess of things that are too hot or poisonous substances. Thus there is a notable difference between colds and *larfondu,* even among ordinary people, who are the ones who invented these terms.[7]

Enough arguments have been presented to show the error of those who preach at length about their colds without knowing what is revealed by them; yet they attribute to them the source of all illnesses, or very nearly. I said that it is the cold that shocks the heat resulting from exertion, as ordinary people understand it. But if the cold were to come right after a bath, a fit of anger, or some other strenuous activity, its name would not change, for we are talking about nothing but heat, where it comes from and where it goes.

---

[4]Cotgrave translates this term as "the disease wherein one voids his fat, or grease in his excrements."

[5]For the adjectival form of this pathological term, Cotgrave insists on the same definition: "that voids his fat, or grease in his excrements."

[6]Joubert uses the term *hectique,* translated by Cotgrave as "sicke of an Hectick, or continuall feuer; (hence) also, meager, leane, dried up, in a Consumption."

[7]The French terms for the two conditions are very similar (*morfondement* and *larfondement*), thus explaining Joubert's remarks about their differences in spite of similarities in appearances, either symptomatically or terminologically speaking.

CHAPTER FOUR
WHY UNDILUTED WINE IS PRESCRIBED FOR PEOPLE WHO ARE VERY HOT, AND WHY PISSING IS PRESCRIBED BEFORE GOING TO BED WHEN PEOPLE HAVE STRENUOUSLY EXERTED THEMSELVES

To those who do very hard work, undiluted wine is given to drink in the hope (as I see it) of hindering and diverting the cause of colds, which result from a sudden chill coming upon heat, with the consequent thickening of the blood. Their intention is good and their actions are more apropos than their words, for they say that drinking wine cools them off and keeps them from catching cold. In the first place, wine most obviously heats; how, therefore, could it cool them off? If it is the case, it is a coincidence, just as if one were to say that fire cools our bodies because we become colder after we have been warmed by it and then go out into the cold air. The reason is that the pores, dilated because of the heat, allow entry to its contrary to a much greater degree than before. Thus wine can cool us off by extinguishing with its great heat the lesser heat produced by the exertion, and maintaining the natural heat in its first condition. [Second,] we can also say that the coolness is caused by the undiluted wine if the wine hinders the cold, which shocks the heat from bringing about a fever that would engulf the entire body in flames. Third, it also cools the body when it causes an emotion and its inherent heat to be calmed down little by little, not all of a sudden, which would cause considerable danger, as does every sudden and unexpected change, something nature cannot endure without injury and displeasure.

We can also say that if water is drunk after strenuous exertion there is a danger of hydropsy, as Galen maintains,[1] which the wine counters because of its potential heat, sustaining the natural heat of the liver and stomach, yet also refreshing them with its actual coolness when it is drunk. Refreshment, moreover, sometimes means a fresh supply of food and some reconstitution, for one properly says "to refresh" meaning "to supply with victuals" or "to renew munitions." It also means "to dress up and adapt the old," such as when one says "to redo the hem of a garment." Now just such a meaning fits our discussion, for strong

---

[1] Joubert's note: Book 5, *Of the Affected Parts,* chapter 6 [*De locis affectis;* on Galen, see *PE,* bk. 1, chap. 1, n. 10 (284–85)].

exertion causes a massive dissipation of humors and vapors in the blood, from which the remaining humors are dried and depleted. Wine corrects all these disorders, reconstituting the humors, repairing the damage done to them, and engendering fresh ones inasmuch as it is active and vaporous. This is how it refreshes the body, replenishing it with humors, which are the source of our strength.

And so, for all these reasons, ordinary people speak much more cogently than they realize and act even more wisely when they prescribe wine after strong exertion. In the second part of their reply they claim wine stops them from catching cold. There are two kinds of colds, as I have argued above: the one is when we are caught by a chill and our skin contracts and increases the intensely burning heat such that a fever follows; the other clots the blood, not that which is in the veins (as lay people think), but that which bleeds into the stomach, the bowels, or elsewhere. For it is impossible (except perhaps in the most rare and unknown case of this condition) that blood clots within its natural vessels. But outside of them it immediately or shortly thereafter congeals. For both of these types of colds wine is a fitting remedy, because it is active, penetrating, and fiery, just what the disorder requires. For penetration, conducting the heat inside, keeps the pores open for the cold, until such time as the vapors generated have been removed through exhalation and the fumes of hot blood have been released. By these means the fever is avoided when there is no constriction, either without or within.

As for the congealing of the blood, wine likewise limits it with its active heat, which keeps this humor in its red and liquid state. For once cold comes upon the blood, it becomes black, since its vermilion nimbleness is as though deadened, and it gathers into clots, which are very difficult to dissolve and so very dangerous, causing such effects as to have them classified among poisons. For the body in this condition becomes cold and almost dead, the pulse weak and nearly stopped; weakness seizes the heart, making it faint, and is accompanied by a cold sweat, and so on. This is why it is a good thing, when one can foresee that the blood can escape from the veins (either through dilatation and scarcity, which accompany exertion, or through splitting or rupturing, when coldness has stiffened the veins), to prevent the blood from congealing. To counter these dangers lay people use the remedies we mentioned in the chapter on colds, but they do not know how to use them properly. They are used as soon as they feel a cold coming on, and wine is prescribed before feeling the slightest symptom.

It is all well and good to give [wine] to people who are overheated because of long and strenuous work before they take their rest. Lay people are not the inventors of this good remedy. It comes from the advice of physicians given in the past, and as it was very easy, people retained it, practiced it, and kept applying it right up to our own time. Several of them are unaware of what it helps, the others do not understand how it can accomplish what they say. They speak of cooling off and of colds without knowing what either is about. Now they will see more clearly in their affairs and will be so assured, knowing through explanation the fruit that comes from it, that they will be able to use this antidote much more effectively. But concerning this condition, to which all the disorders of workers and laborers are attributed, I remember one man who used to say, "All disorders are a result of cold"; he was speaking of all illnesses in general. Then a good fellow answered him in his particular dialect, "They sure aren't from scorching," meaning burns, as from fire or boiling water, and other such things. For it is most certain that this ailment is not from a cold.

Let us now see why people prescribe pissing before resting. When a person has worked, or walked for a long time, or been running about and worrying, ordinary people recommend pissing before taking a rest. This is very good advice, and I think they picked up this rule from their grandparents, who found it in the ancient physicians, as is the case in everything that is well done still today in the maintenance of health. It has been handed down from father to son for so long that its origin is no longer known; yet it is highly likely that the old physicians taught this. But ordinary people do not understand the reason behind what they do and always follow custom, whether it be good or bad. This particular one is among the most praiseworthy, and I wish to point out why it is so beneficial.

When our bodies make a strenuous exertion, the humors become stinging and concentrated because of the heat that makes them more active. This is what causes the feeling of needles pricking throughout the whole body after a strenuous effort if one is the least bit of a hot complexion. The urine is consequently more burning, which is quickly noticed upon pissing, for it stings more sharply coming out and causes a certain disgust expressed in a shivering in the body, especially with the last few drops. Being in this way so biting, it could do harm to the bladder if it were retained a long time and could eventually burn through it (since it is soft and tender tissue, like that in children), causing an ulcer. It is therefore a good idea to empty the bladder right away without waiting to feel the need for it. For one does not feel clearly what can do harm to the body in its overheated state.

I have another explanation that is nearly as weighty: it is that one must be watchful, after strong exertion, that the urine already sent down to the bladder does not become absorbed by the neighboring parts and harm the body with its toxic nature. For the exhausted members, strained by the exertion, attract humors from wherever they can find them. The organs next to the bladder can draw out some of its contents, which, converted into vapors, exit from the highly dilated pores. Now sweat and urine are of the same nature; when one has lost a lot of sweat, it is therefore to be feared that, in order to fill the lack, urine will begin to follow. And if it spreads throughout the body, it does a poor job of cleansing, since it is a wholly superfluous and useless humor that can only have the title of excrement. It must therefore be voided immediately. By so doing, two complications will be avoided: one the danger issuing from its stinging concentration, and the other from its possible recirculation in the body.

Lay people knew very well they must watch over themselves in this way; now that they know the reason for it, they will know how to make their kind do it even better. Aside from the above reasons we can mention another which is of great importance, for this is the procedure used to keep from getting kidney stones. When the body has made a strong exertion, all the vessels are so wide open that these gross substances pass through; for heat dilates to an incredible extent. Now, since the passages and tubes conducting the urine are greatly enlarged, a lot of thick matter comes down with it into the bladder. This is viscous phlegm and the filth or dregs from yellow bile, from which kidney stones are formed by means of a drying heat, just as manure is dried by the sun when its moisture evaporates. During the agitation and movement of the body these thick humors are carried along and arrive in the bladder with the urine; there they separate and harden from the stinging portion while one rests, and the urine also becomes still. For the weight of such matter causes the thicker portion slowly to fall to the bottom, and thus when the urine itself is later voided, leaving in the bladder the deposits that had been carried down to it, they are retained because of their viscosity and their weight, which make them stay behind.

If it happens often that a person works under improper conditions (especially immediately after eating) and leaves such a mixture of urine in the bladder while resting, before long there will be enough residue to form a kidney stone. For today one as large as a lentil will form, tomorrow another, such that soon there will be enough to make for a large blockage. It is therefore essential to urinate after strong exertion before inactivity gives the thick humors time to be isolated and deposited on the bottom of the bladder. If one pisses right away, one sees that the urine is opaque because of the mixture of these substances. And if one looks at it in a glass, after separation takes place, left on the bottom will be a deposit that resembles those we said remain in the bladder if one puts off urinating.

These remarks make it easy to understand how important it is for children not to hold their urine (as when they are in a hurry, especially after a meal), so as to keep them from developing kidney stones, to which they are more subject than older people (I mean those which form in the bladder) because of their insatiable appetite and frenetic activity at all hours. Of the three pieces of advice I gave, that of the common practice of having people piss after exerting themselves, especially children when they have exerted themselves, is the most urgent. The second is of some importance, and the third even more so. Whatever the case, the custom is very beneficial and must be observed by all who are careful and concerned about their health. I can add still another reason that will be no less important, in my opinion. It is that urine retained in the bladder, once it later becomes warm, transmits heat to the body. Thus to cool off in a healthy and proper way it is good to urinate. Stop and think! We bleed off and spill a portion of the blood overheated by a fever in order to cool off the body, just as nature on her own will often relieve the head's boiling with excess blood by letting it flow out of the nose, causing considerable relief and refreshment. Urine, voided and discarded without regret, must not be thought of differently.

CHAPTER FIVE
THAT IT IS NECESSARY TO CHANGE THE LINEN OFTEN
FOR THE FEVEROUS

Our natural heat (principal instrument of all activities required to sustain life) is founded in moisture and never ceases to be operative as it prepares food for the body, refining the humors and separating the good from the bad. The good is sent to the parts that need nourishment, the bad is shunted into the places set aside for excrement, of which there are several kinds and diverse receptacles for each. The most rarefied and active excrements (which are the subject of my discussion) have no vessel other than the skin itself and turn into nothing but fumes and vapors drawn from the substances that our natural heat works upon. Their lightness carries them from the innermost parts of the skin covering the body, since all exhalations move upward.

Now among the functions of the skin is the most natural and most necessary one of allowing to pass through without obstruction these airy superfluities that are sent to it from all parts of the body; upon receiving them, this thin membrane, which is open, spongy, and without obstacle, furnishes them passage to the outside (by means of its invisible pores and caverns), so that they may be dispersed into the air. The thicker and stickier portion of these superfluities congeals in these narrow passages and after a time becomes hairs. Such excrements are sweat and the fumes that soil our shirts and other clothes with a black, greasy, and clammy filth. They are quite abundant in people who have an active body heat because of the dryness of the complexion brought on by the dry warmth that burns off much more than just moisture, for the arid heat converts a lot of matter into sweat and fuming vapors. Moist heat, such as that found in children, dissolves a lot more of this matter; but in this case it is such a mild, gentle, and subtle exhalation that it is invisibly dispersed, like the steam coming off hot water. Wood produces a fire that burns hotter than the heat of water and produces such a thick smoke that it leaves soot deposits, and from its burned substance the coals finally become ashes.

Such superfluities abound in the time of a man's virility; women and children, being softer, have far fewer and do not smell like a goat or a shoulder of mutton after strong exertion. For such odors come from these dry excrements, which for the above reasons are very copious in summertime and in men who have been through adolescence. If, then, dry heat produces a large amount of soot (black, greasy, smelly vapor), fevers are very likely to generate much more of it. And in fact we see that the shirts and sheets of feverous people become soiled immediately, because their disorder is one of natural warmth converted into a dry and burning heat. Now these fumes are much better outside than inside our bodies. Yet nature, most concerned about our welfare and wishing to purify the blood, causes this infection to be voided as soon as it is born. And to this end she has formed arteries with two types of movement: one for rejecting and driving out, as when she disperses the superfluities of a burn; the other for receiving coolness by widening. For nothing conserves natural warmth better than voiding these vapors, which could otherwise stifle it, and moving the blood about, which is its very hearth.

Since such is the case, and since these excrements must be voided for the purity of the humors and spirits, which would otherwise be clouded by them, the passages of the skin must be kept open and clean by making sure there are no obstacles in them. This is the purpose served by rubdowns and baths, of which the ancient Greeks and Romans made common use. Moreover, one must ensure that what comes in contact with the body, such as linens and all clothing, be very clean, so that the waste matter already transmitted through voiding will not be reabsorbed by the opening of the pores, which indiscriminately suck in everything presented to them. The pores have expelled these vile fumes through their contraction. If you allow the skin to keep this filth next to it, the pores will certainly reabsorb it, for they draw in air on all surfaces, whether it be good or bad, sweet or foul, pure or infected.

It is therefore good to change linens after sweating, for fear that the superfluous humor be reimbibed by the body, which finally ridded itself of it, since black and dirty linen returns to us what it took from us. Since, then, it is so essential that this matter be voided in order to dissipate our heat, it is most damaging if it is reabsorbed. Is it not great stupidity, knowing that it is important for such impurities to be driven out, to leave them where they can easily reenter? It must not be doubted that they contaminate with their foul quality the air that is between our bodies and our linen. The pores upon opening draw it in just as they find it and infuse it, mixed up together with all the fine substances in it. The proof of this is that when you step naked out of the tub and stand in a place where the dust is all stirred up, you will immediately feel something stinging you (like thorns and needles) all over your body. It is the fine particles of the dust that the openings suck in, drawn by the widely opened pores. One must therefore be most careful about the condition of the air that comes in contact with us, as with everything that has to do with our natural heat and that which maintains our spirits. Now, the air that is in close proximity to dirty sheets cannot be very clean; and if the pores return it to the body, it is a more serious error than the previous one. It is therefore essential to use fresh linen very frequently when it comes in close contact with the body, in order to rid ourselves of what was deposited on it, not only putting on some that is white and clean but that smells sweet also. For that makes the ambient air pleasant for our humors, which are delighted and restored by sweet odors, such that if you pay close attention, you will see that we are revitalized, rejuvenated, and strengthened after changing the linen and putting on clean clothes; it is as if it reconstituted our spirits and our natural heat, which the ongoing infection had been befouling, upsetting, confusing, mingling, troubling, and injuring. For our spirits require a high degree of purity, cleanliness, and integrity (since they are celestial and divine) to fulfill their function and show their power.

From whence then comes the notion of ordinary people, who dare not change patients' linen but rather make them endure for a long time a smelly odor, like swine wallowing in the mire? Perhaps it is because they were once forbidden to move them too much during fevers for fear they might catch cold, and ever since these good people think that white linen is bad for them. Oh the great error, from which come the cruelty and barbaric tyranny with which the poor patients are treated! There is nothing that makes them get better more quickly or that renews better their strength than keeping them clean by all the means at one's disposal and in refreshing sheets smelling of roses and other such things when they are feverous. Each time the bed of a person with a fever is made, it would be fitting to change the sheets, the linen, and the nightshirt. For the fever would then be of shorter duration and the pain less severe. We wish to purge the humors by means of drugs, so as to extinguish the heat that is burning them up. One must therefore be no less careful to remove the fumes and subtle impurities that sustain such a fire. Stop to think! Without being at all sick it is possible to catch a fever by sleeping in a sick person's sheets if one is the least bit predisposed. It is because our pores, by drawing in air, let into our bodies the vile quality of the filth encrusted in the sheets and cause our natural heat to become feverous. Will they do any less harm to the person who has soiled them? At the very least they will maintain the disorder in its present state. Let us waste no time then in changing our minds about this! We must not go on allowing the ill to be mistreated because of this awful practice of keeping them confined and wound up in their filth and corruption since this is doing them no good whatsoever but, on the contrary, causing them considerable harm. The linen of the feverous and other ill people must be changed frequently when it is dirty, and it is essential to realize that these poor patients must be kept as clean, if not more so, than the healthy, for they must be treated kindly, so that they may better be able to bear the discomfort of their illness.

CHAPTER SIX
THAT WOMEN KILL THE FEVEROUS BY GIVING THEM
TOO LITTLE TO DRINK, TOO MUCH TO EAT,
AND TOO MANY COVERS. AND WHAT DIET IS APPROPRIATE
TO GIVE THE FEVEROUS

Having discovered and corrected the error of those who get too warm during a fever as a result of the use of wine, spices, and a lot of covers, because all their ills are thought to come from cold, and the error of those who do not wish to allow them a change of linen, it would also be good, in order to conclude these remarks, to show those importunate women the three notorious mistakes they make in torturing the ill by refusing them drink, forcing them to eat, and heaping too many covers on them.

Common folk in general are of this opinion and follow this practice; but women especially take it to an excess that is unbearable and upsets the patient more than the others do. This is due to a natural condition that drives them to overstep the limits of common sense and always to be excessive, more so than men, in their affections and actions. For if they love, it is to perfection, just as they hate to the very death. If they fall victim to avarice, it is extreme; if to mad spending, it is prodigality itself. In gentleness, sweetness, and graciousness, if they are willing they are unsurpassed; likewise, in anger and spite they can display a great rage. I am not saying this to blame them (as most men relish speaking ill of the feminine sex, the refreshment and true consolation of this earth) but to declare the cause of their abuse. In the same manner I will rebuke those who disparage women and I will give to those who praise them unfoundedly arguments that show their imperfection. For these extreme affections flow but from one subtle, penetrating, nimble spirit, concealed in a soft, delicate, and highly purified body. The proof of this is that we see other materials sustain with ease diverse qualities and changes because of their purity. White is the only color that will receive all the others in its perfection, just as woman receives all sorts of fashions. And just as water is highly prized for its lightness, which is ascertained by its quickness to boil or be cooled, so too do I maintain that the complexion of those who are quick tempered and change quickly from one extreme to another is simple, clear, and pure. For the opposite comes from a thick and dull heaviness, which makes for contumaciousness and immobility.

Women are of such an unfettered, clear, and pure substance (as witnessed by their softness, tenderness, beauty, and delicateness) that they have a great promptness and surpass men both in quick apprehension and in superlative affection. Thus they have less hesitancy in their words and thoughts because of this mobility, which results from a lightness that comes from pure simplicity, with which the sky, above all other bodies, is also endowed. Likewise, their quickness of mind in understanding and in resolving every difficulty is such that men cannot manage to approach it. And yet one scorns her answer if it is premeditated, and people say that the first reaction of a woman is to be heeded, before she is able to think about it. For they have this perfection of being quick and very subtle, which allows them to resolve a matter very quickly. If a woman thinks about it at length, she comes up with a thousand diverse and unstable arguments because her sharp and penetrating mind is never happy with itself and always wants to arrange the parts in a better way, such that it mixes everything up and ruins everything. Just as a good painter who has a lively mind will make a beautiful portrait in a first draft that will meet with everyone's approval; if it is not immediately taken from him he will find a few lines that need to be redrawn and will not stop until he has made the whole thing much worse.

It is therefore a most praiseworthy quality in women to be so quick and witty, since it comes from their most subtle matter, which causes them to be called flighty. But one must not belittle their having such an unsurpassed nimbleness. They rarely ever stop before going to extremes, which men, hindered by their heaviness, are unable to attain as easily. This is why we find women so excessive by nature, not only in their ways of doing things and in their affections, but in their care of the ill, where I will now stop for the time being. For if we order a hot bath, they will make it burning hot. We mean for the heat to be tepid, and it is enough if it does not feel cold. They think that because heat is required, the more the better; and indeed you would think it was for skinning a pig. If you forbid patients to drink excessively and if they are taken care of by women, they will die of thirst. If you say, "Give them plenty of nourishment," enough said; they will be completely gorged with food. Are you recommending that they be kept covered? You will see them henceforth stifled. Thus nearly in all things women go beyond our orders, rushing toward excessiveness, unable to hold to the medium. These errors must be pointed out to them so that they will keep from repeating them. The theologian and the moral philosopher will preach against certain practices and will claim that extremes are evil and that virtue lies in the middle. The physician will make known the evils that come from their excesses as I have sought to do here. I am speaking only to the ignorant ones and to those who make use of such practices; the more wise, then, will not be offended by it. It is enough if I have allowed for the nature of all women; I only rebuke the errors, and so those who do not think themselves guilty of them have no reason to be concerned by these remarks. But let us return to the path I have abandoned somewhat in order to make clear to women that I am not blaming their sex (which I find most pleasant), but in an attempt to make it more perfect, I wish to try making it rid itself of what can be calumniated in it.

Being attentive to the manner of caring for the ill, I put together some important points indicating where dolts err frequently, and especially concerning the feverous, such as when to change linen and prescribe wine, about which I have written two separate chapters. As for eating, drinking, and the use of covers, women, among others, are terribly mistaken, and all the while thinking they are providing relief, sustenance, and a cure for their patients, they are torturing, overwhelming, and stifling them, often making their ills incurable. To hear women talk, their patients drink too much, eat nothing, and are never sufficiently covered. I hope they will, upon reading my arguments, correct this error that blinds them. But because I wish, aside from the reasons I will be providing, to give common folk a little guide on how to care for fevers, it will be best to put everything together so as not to be too lengthy, which might become boring. Along with teaching what must be done for the feverous, we will be able to become fully acquainted with the ignorance of lay people, for the straight reveals the crooked. Thus in handing over my notes on how to take care of oneself when one has a fever, I will in the same stroke be fulfilling my promise and modestly admonishing those who proceed differently.

I presuppose that a physician always prescribes, according to the needs of the case, the purgations, the bloodletting, and other remedies that must be used because of particular illnesses, because of the condition of the patients, their complexions, their ages, the climate, the season, etc. My intention is to discuss only the treatment of the patient inasmuch as we turn it over in most cases to women who see to implementing it. This instruction will be most useful; if they will learn it well, they will relieve physicians of the task of having to repeat it daily and will supplement what physicians might sometimes forget, since they have several patients to think about. Fever is an illness of heat, as its name signifies, which I show above as having been derived from the word *fire*, or *fervor*. It afflicts the entire body after seizing the heart, source of our natural heat, and afterward becoming so burning hot because of its augmented character that one is horribly consumed by it. The heart, because of its very nature, is incomparably more heated than any other part of the body, to the point that the arteries are unable to cool it through their operation alone. Nature had to surround it with the lungs, in the guise of fans or bellows to bring it cool air and to empty it of its fumes when it is overheated. Now when this heat is greater than normal, one must take breaths more often and even pant to satisfy the requirements of cooling and to draw in more fresh air, for otherwise the excess heat cannot be dispersed. If, then, in fevers the whole body is burning, and fire proceeds from the heart, one has great need of coolness in the air in our rooms, just as when one is forced to take short breaths.

Ignorant people, who think that all their ills come from cold and that fever is brought about because of cold, heat the room as much as they can, closing every opening and starting a huge fire, next to which they place their sick ones, as if to roast them. So much so that the air from their lungs heats the heart even more, increases the illness and often turns a limited fever into a continuous one. We are presupposing here that the season is summer, in which fevers are more frequent, and even that the weather is very hot, such as during the dog days; otherwise, some of what we say about cooling the air sufficiently must be taken back. In view of the above reasons, then, we suggest that the feverous be kept in a spacious and well-ventilated room so that the air will be free to circulate. In small chambers and dressing rooms the enclosed air is quickly heated, and if one stays there a long while, one is forced to breathe in again the fumes that our lungs expelled. The room should be most clean for our purposes, on a lower floor and with vaulted ceiling (provided the story is not a damp one) to be more suitable.

Once the room is well chosen, it is a matter of stopping anything that might cause it to get hot. Lots of people and dogs must not be allowed in, for their breath gives off a great deal of heat. No fire should be lit, and not even a candle should be burning if one can do without it. The sun's rays should not be allowed to come in, nor even touch the panes on the outside. The best thing for the room of the sick person would be to have windows on two or three sides, so that when the sun strikes one of them, the two remaining ones may be kept open to bring in fresh air constantly, which is important to have right from early morning. Evening also brings fresh air, and it must not be scorned. If there is a door through which a nice wind comes in, it must be kept open at all times, but only halfway so as to make the wind stronger. And if that is not enough, fans must be used and the air in the room kept moving, as one does with a wet sack, constantly shaking it and making the air circulate and remain cool. Movement of the air is essential so that there is always new air in contact with the patient. Besides such agitation (which obviously cools, as is the case with moving air), other means can be used to the same end. Take some cool well water and pour it back and forth continuously from one bucket into another, changing it from time to time. This moves, cools, and humidifies the air, and the noise coming to the ears of patients unable to sleep sometimes induces them to sleep. It is also important to moisten the floor with cold water constantly, afterward pouring good vinegar on it. The more wealthy will use rose vinegar, rosewater, or March violet water, for fresh odors mitigate the heat and revive the spirits.

The floor should be strewn with roses, violets, vine shoots, lettuce, water lily leaves, and other flowers that have been soaked in very cold water, rose water, and rose vinegar. The walls should be garnished with boughs, especially willow branches that are always fresh, for when they dry they are harmful. The bed set aside for the patient (placed in the coolest and most unlit part of the room) should be high and spacious, so that he may stir unhindered as he moves about, as is often perforce the case. Alongside, a small couch is needed for cooling off when the bed has become hot from a long rest or when the linen is being changed as required, for the sick must be kept in very clean conditions, as everything upsets them because of the illness that makes them fussy. This is also why they must be kept in absolute cleanliness, why they must not smell anything unpleasant, why the covers must be soft and light, in no way soiled or coarse, the sheets fine, sweet smelling, and very white and changed every day if the patient has a high fever or sweats profusely. Sleeping on a featherbed is pure folly for those who complain about the heat since they are obviously warm. I grant that it is necessary for the feverous to have a soft bed because they are wholly broken and undone by their illness, but they must sleep on something that holds less heat, such as cotton, wool, or hair, from which mattresses are made that are very soft. Cooler material is found in chaff and oat, barley, millet, or other brans. I would gladly sleep on straw to be more at ease. Some put their mattresses on cots to sleep cooler and more comfortably, but I would not recommend any kind of featherbed whatsoever, because any heat that gets into it stays there for a long time.

Under the sheet it is good to put at the small of the back a piece of water camlet or goatskin or to make a very flat pouch half full of chaff to sleep on. Plutarch says that in Babylon the most wealthy would sleep, as a great luxury, on leather skins full of water during the hottest times of the summer. We find such coolness a little dangerous for the feverous; it would perhaps be better to fill these skins with air, in the manner of a balloon, as I hear a few rich sovereigns do with their beds in Italy. But these are dainty practices that we can easily do without. I am very much in favor of a bed suspended by ropes for two advantages gained in being rocked: one is that air is free to circulate and it is cooler, for the reasons mentioned above; the other is that the movement makes patients sleep, as if in a cradle. The canopy of the bed should be rather high, so that there is plenty of air. Portable beds with their low tents are so oppressive for the sick that they cannot breathe.

If the windows or doors blow wind directly on the bed when the room is to be aired, the curtains must be drawn (which otherwise serve no purpose) for fear that the sharp cold might shock the skin and cause the pores to close, through which the waves of the burning heat need to exit. For we do not want to cool externally; that would only increase the internal fire. We want cool air for the lungs, which cool the heart burning with fever. This is why the entire body, except for the face, must be covered in accordance with the quality of the air, so that the skin will always remain open. Patients must not be engulfed in a pile of covers, for this torture serves no purpose and makes them more thirsty. It is sufficient if they are covered just enough to counter the closing of the pores and to allow free passage for the fumes and vapors and for the sweat that seeks an exit. They have enough covers, then, with a sheet when they have a high fever; as it subsides, when they feel the moisture (which means the sweating is about to begin), they must be given more covers to assist the heat in expelling this humor, in spite of the unpleasantness of enduring this pain.

But it must be realized that it is the remains of the foul matter that caused the paroxysm and that if some of it stays behind the patient will take a lot longer to be completely rid of the fever, for as long as a drop of this matter remains, the body is upset by it. Convinced, then, that it is finally coming to an end, one must bear the suffering patiently and not remove the covers. For if the pores become constricted and the sweat is retained, the fit will last longer; and there is sometimes the danger that a limited fever will turn into a continuous one because of the retention of excrement and the constriction of the skin. This is when covers are needed, when the patient is about to sweat, not during the access and the burning heat, as these importunate women insist. For as long as the body is not feeling the coolness of the room and is somewhat covered everywhere except the face, one should be satisfied and not torment the patient any further. At the beginning of the access, when they feel the chill, the stiffness, and the quaking, they can be covered as much as one likes, and in this their wishes should be observed: warm their feet with covers, tiles, and stones; use whatever methods and applications are necessary (but not hot beverages, as common folk do, for all that does is cause them to be extremely thirsty, because they are too warm internally) to make this fearful quaking stop as soon as possible. When the heat begins to manifest itself externally and the covers begin to be a burden, they must be removed little by little, and the patient made as comfortable as possible until a single sheet remains.

This is how limited fevers should be dealt with. As for continuous ones, which always have the same heat, or nearly so, at least until they are completely cured, they must be treated according to their nature, and patients should be only slightly covered so as not to make them thirstier, only enough to stop the skin from tightening. Thus if the heat is severe, they must only be covered halfway through the access of limited fevers; and the advice of these women must not be followed, for the sick never want too many covers. But it is essential to note the following rules in order to understand when, how, and how often we must air out the room and change the amount of covers, especially since the season, the time of day, and the nature of the illness (the variety is considerable) call for much prudence at every moment, for the number of remedies cannot be fully listed in writing, and they must be closely followed, as we shall now argue.

In this matter our sole objective is to maintain the opening of the pores and to allow the lungs to get fresh air. Thus if it is in winter we must keep more covers for fear the skin will contract, and we are at no loss to keep the air fresh but rather attempting to keep it warm, so that when the restless patient turns over in bed the air that gets in will not shock the skin with its freezing coldness. Also, the patient must not be kept close to the fire as peasants do; it is enough if the air of the room is not as cold as the season's. In summer it is rather difficult to cool it so much that it will close the pores (especially if one is covered with a sheet). Now in this matter the extent of the heat that the patient endures and that is in the surrounding air must be considered; for if the heat of the fever is extreme, we will make the air as cool as possible; if it is less, we will work at it less, observing the proper proportion in the opposition of contraries. When the heat of the air is moderate, very little is needed to keep it in check; if it is excessive, it must be countered in several ways. Thus if the heat of the fever and of the air are both just as burning hot, nothing that can cool them must be neglected; if they are less so, proportionately fewer means are to be used. For the elements present must be taken into account and equal remedies used, without regard for a fixed rule. We will therefore not be concerned about fresh air unless it is summer, and then it will be a case of going about it more or less, according to the extent it is needed. In winter it is necessary to heat it somewhat. In spring and in autumn it is quite temperate and we should be satisfied with it. For this, in our opinion, is the kind we call cool, and it is very suitable for fevers.

The same is true for covers, which must be accommodated to the temperature of the air; in summer fewer are needed, in winter more. The temperate season is between the two. Also, at night it is cooler than during the day, and so more covers are needed, proportionately, at night than during the day. And when one sleeps, because the external members get cold, more covers are needed whatever the hour might be, but far fewer if one is very hot because of illness. The best thing to do is to wait until the patient is asleep and then add covers, for if they are added before he dozes off, it annoys him so much that he becomes completely unable to rest.

Used with some discretion and common sense, these rules allow us to remove or add covers and to bring in fresh air in the treatment of all sorts of fevers, at any time of day and in any season. Also to be considered is a person's complexion, age, and sex, which flow from his temperament. For by the same fever, some persons will be made very hot, others less so, according to whether their natural heat was great or small before the fever. Those who have a sweet and gentle natural heat, such as women and children, do not feel it as much as young men thirty years old, whose bodies are by nature hotter. And of these the sanguine or choleric surpass the others in heat. Old people are cold and are unable to have such hot fevers, as Hippocrates says.[1] Moreover, because of their very tight skin, in women and children the excessive softness hinders the pores from opening. Young people strike the medium, and it is unlikely that their skin will constrict. For these two reasons one must not fear bringing in fresh air when a young man with a very hot complexion (and who in his very health seems to be all ablaze) has a fever, as would be the case if he were of a different temperament, nor when a strong old man does, or a woman. In all this there are still several distinctions, for all women, all old men, and all children are not in the same condition: some are hotter than others.

Thus it is (to be brief) with all rules, according to which one must try to approach as closely as possible the condition of each individual, for it is not possible to set limits on these particularities. It is enough for one to know in general the rules for treating the feverous. As concerns the air and use of covers, I have gone over it so thoroughly

---

[1] Joubert's note: Hippocrates, Book I, chapter 14 [for references to fever in the works attributed to Hippocrates, see n. 9 of chap. 2 above; the specific reference is *On the Nature of Man*, chap. 15 in modern editions].

that the discussion has become prolix. But I shall be more brief in pursuing the rest, in which the above arguments can be used if one has the least bit of imagination in knowing how to accommodate them.[2]

CHAPTER SEVEN
AGAINST THOSE WHO DO NOT ALLOW THE FEVEROUS
TO DRINK DURING AN ACCESS, AND THOSE
WHO WANT THEM TO DRINK HOT LIQUIDS TO MAKE THEM
SWEAT MORE PROFUSELY AND MORE OFTEN

I have shown elsewhere how fevers must be treated to get the better of them as soon as possible. Here I shall treat succinctly the error of those who do not allow the feverous to drink during the access, either forcibly or through scolding. Our Hippocrates says clearly in his *Aphorisms* that during the access it is necessary to abstain.[3] But there it is a question of broths and other food, for he adds that it is dangerous to have them take food at that time. But as for drinking, it is essential in order to quell the fever when it is at its highest point, and even Galen prescribes drinking large quantities of cool water at the peak of burning fevers and of synochal fevers.[4] Now, the state of the access corresponds to the state of the entire continuous fever. And what is the danger in drinking a considerable amount when the access is in its full strength? None. On the contrary, it is of great benefit and quells the fever, as when much water is thrown on a fire. Still, it is important to point out that the drink given the feverous be very cool (and not hot as several would wish) so that the patient will sweat sooner because of it. For those who prescribe hot drink are mistaken on two accounts: drinking hot liquids does not quench thirst; and drinking cold liquids provokes sweating as much or more than hot liquids. This fact can be

---

[2]A note at the end of this chapter reads as follows: "This chapter was left unfinished, but the two or three that follow can serve the purpose and be adjusted."

[3]Joubert's note: *Aph[orisms]* 2, Book 1.

[4]Joubert's note: *On the Method*, Book 9, chapter 5 [*De methodo medendi libri XIV;* a synochal (or synochous) fever is a continued, or unintermitting fever (*Oxford English Dictionary*)].

proved by anyone who doubts it; it will be seen that if one drinks cool liquids when very hot and thirsty, beads of sweat will form on the forehead, even in winter.

Thus, since there is both pleasure and profit, we allow, indeed we order, patients to drink liquids as cool as can be obtained, and one or two long swallows, according to the duration of the access. Common folk, since everything is suspicious to them because of their ignorance and because they are fearful even in things that allow every assurance, have an unfortunate trait of not allowing anything pleasurable for the sick. They are afraid to comply with the wishes of patients, as if they were always unreasonable.

CHAPTER EIGHT
CONCERNING BROTHS AND BARLEY SOUP ADMINISTERED AT MIDNIGHT OR IN THE MORNING, MOST UNADVISEDLY

With broths and barley soup the sick are most often annoyed. They take no pleasure in them, and at times their sleep is interrupted most indiscreetly for the purpose of administering such nourishment, either at midnight or in the morning, which can never have as much worth for the patient as a good rest. That is how common folk are wrong in two ways: one, when they do not allow the feverous to take liquids in a reasonable way, and the other, when they force food upon them inappropriately.

Certainly not a single thing can be prescribed with enough care to avoid being easily abused, especially when it is something that is the slightest bit pleasurable, and even more so when it is a matter of nourishment. For the question of food is so fair and pleasant that common folk take it up most readily. The term *drugs* is extremely odious and horrible to them, even anything that comes from the apothecary shop, except for sugar, hippocras, biscuit bread, teasel,[1] tartar, preserves, and other sweetmeats. This does not astonish me, nor do I condemn it,

---

[1]Cotgrave translates the term Joubert uses (*le pignolat*) as "the preserued kernell of a Pine-apple; or conserue of Pine-kernells"; and *Pignolat. Chardon pignolat*: "The Teazill, card Teazill; Fullers Thistle."

for that is very natural. I am a man and I share our common weaknesses; I am not a stranger or foreign to anything human.[2] I know that medicine is contrary and an adversary to the natural good, and that if medicine were familiar or friendly to nature it would not have such effects but, rather, subdued by the body, would be converted into the body's substance. Thus the dread it causes us is a most natural reaction and not reprehensible. What I have said is said lightly, so I will not be seen as an unpleasant and disgruntled druggist, inasmuch as I myself have recourse to them often, aware of the need I have of them. I merely wished to touch upon this point as much to excuse common folk with respect to physicians, who do not have much pity on those who cannot stand physicians, as to blame those excessively dainty people who will have nothing other than broths and barley soup as a cure or to prevent illness. Even then they fail to use them as they should, for in adopting such a remedy, they do not cut back on other meals. This is what I wish to criticize, showing them not only what physicians intend in this practice (at least those who first instituted it) but also the way I prescribe it.

These broths and barley soups at midnight or in the morning are given for three reasons. One, to help those who lack appetite and are unable to eat at the noon or evening meal, but especially at supper, and to whom, in order to make up for it, something is given at midnight or the next morning. The second reason is nearly the same, it is for those who are ravenously hungry and almost insatiable, such as when they are just recovering from a serious illness. For inasmuch as they have a weakened stomach and are unable to digest as much as they would like to eat in one sitting, they are advised to divide up their meal. And because at night (because of sleep, which retards the action of the stomach) one does not digest as well as during the day, we prescribe that they sup lightly and that in recompense we give them a broth the next morning, as if one had held back the soup normally taken at supper and returned it to them the following morning after they had slept. What I say about sleep's slowing down the action of the stomach is amply proved in my *Paradoxes* with cogent arguments, of which I

---

[2]The phrase is altogether too reminiscent of Terence in his play *The Self-Tormentor* (I, i, 77): *"homo sum: humani nil a me alienum puto."*

shall only cite one, in that it concerns this subject.[3] It is that from the noon meal to the evening meal there are normally but eight hours, and from supper to the next meal there are sixteen, without our being any more hungry afterward than one is after the eight hours. Let us suppose now that both these meals are identical in quantity and quality, in food and drink, in short, that the only difference between them is that one of these meals is followed by night and sleep, and the other is not.[4] The third reason is that such a diet is used to modify or prepare the body through gentle means, namely, to cool, moisten, purify, and thin the humors, to break up and void kidney sand and stones, to provoke sweating or the menses, and [to relieve] other minor complications of an importance not great enough for the use of stronger and more unpleasant remedies.

A lot of people use these in the spring, especially in April and May, but with such indiscretion that they do them more harm than good. And so I was constrained to point out this error, according to the conditions of my charge. The mistake lies principally in that they cut nothing back from the ordinary dinners and suppers for these broths and barley soups. For if they dine and sup as much as usual, it is certain that by the next morning the stomach will not be empty, and that consequently the broth will encounter undigested matter, which it will render even more indigestible while it sees to its own digestion, right up until dinner arrives, which, mixing up with all the preceding, takes on the foulness and contagion of what is underdone. This then meets up with supper, to the point that there is no end to such disorder, which more than anything else spawns a quantity of phlegm. If the bouillon happens to be made up of clarifying, purifying, and thinning agents provoking any excretion, then it does far more harm, for it drives and forces the rest of the undigested supper to precipitate in the veins and arteries, where they cause obstruction and bring about colds, fevers, and a thousand other conditions, which is far worse than if the raw liquids languish or decompose in the stomach and bowels, where

---

[3]Joubert's note: Decade I, Paradox 8 [on Joubert's *Paradoxorum decas prima atque altera* (1566), see *PE*, bk. 1, chap. 2, n. 12 (286)].

[4]Joubert leaves his conclusion unstated here. It is of course that since the two equal meals leave us equally hungry after different spans (eight versus sixteen hours), the action of the stomach must therefore be slower during sleep.

they cause colic, sharp cramps and stomach noises, queasiness, nausea, vomiting, and so forth.

And so, whoever wishes to proceed correctly in using these thirst-breeding broths (which is also the nature of our barley soup) must sup lightly, so that the stomach can digest more thoroughly than usual and can be completely empty. One must act as if one were holding a portion of one's supper for the next morning. And if afterward one were to eat a little less at dinner this would be the best thing one could do. This is how to go about caring for oneself in this matter so as to come out of it ahead and not behind, as is the case with most who abuse these remedies. Some feel good using them because, for lack of appetite, they hardly eat anything at dinner or at supper, which is the first circumstance mentioned above. And I have no doubt whatsoever that this is how the first authors of this regimen understood and practiced it. From this very fact we can understand that if one has to take, on the following day, some julep, apozem,[5] or syrup (preparative agents, for the most part), it is necessary to have eaten lightly, so that they will come upon an empty stomach. Otherwise, if they are aperients, they will force the undigested food into the veins and into the arteries, strengthening the root of the illness we are seeking to destroy. And if this unfortunate condition were not to persist (since all such drugs are not penetrative), they still should not meet up with anything in the stomach. For that would weaken the potency of the remedy, diluting it unduly.

I will show elsewhere how important it is to keep the stomach empty when one takes medicine, and that many people do not do well to eat and drink as much as they please the evening before, hoping that the medicine will take care of any excess; such a discussion cannot be easily joined to this one.[6] For whatever it might be, broths, barley soup, milk from a she-ass or some other animal, juleps, or any other

---

[5]I have used "apozem" to translate Joubert's *Apozeme*, which Cotgrave defines thus: "*Apozeme* or, *Apozime*. A decoction, or water with diuers sorts of hearbes and spices, used instead of a syrop."

[6]It is obvious from this sentence that Joubert was not wholly responsible for the organization of *The Second Part of the Popular Errors*, as might indeed be inferred from the two letters written by Barthélemy Cabrol and published in the Micard edition (herein translated, pp. 4–17). Chapter 17 below treats the question of the proper diet when taking medication.

drug, if it comes upon a stomach that is not empty and free of the food of the previous day, either it does little good or causes a lot of harm. Thus one might ask me what use there is in taking thirst-breeding broths and barley soup alone in the morning, as opposed to having them at dinner or supper with other foods, since both are foods that can mix with the rest. I answer as I have above, that if such things are mixed with other food, either their strength is attenuated, or (if they are aperients) they conduct the food out of the stomach before its complete digestion and do more harm than good. It is therefore better for each thing to be taken separately, and not to mix food with what is medicinal.

CHAPTER NINE
WHETHER IT IS BAD TO DRINK BEFORE GOING TO BED

The custom is, in France (at least in the best families), always to have wine with the evening meal and never to be without wine in one's bedroom. Although some abstain from this drinking, the others drink on occasion or regularly just before getting into bed, more out of habit than driven by thirst. The common folk of Languedoc have a popular proverb speaking against this practice: one who goes to bed thirsty wakes up healthy. Hippocrates seems to be in agreement with this, saying in his *Aphorisms*: "Those who have great thirst at night, if they go to sleep thirsty, they do well."[1] But one could interpret his words as meaning those who wake up thirsty, and not those who are thirsty before going to sleep. For it makes more sense not to drink throughout the night and upon first waking up than before going to bed. And as for me, I do not find it bad at all that those who are in the habit of drinking upon getting into bed continue to do so, as I have seen my late father do for more than twenty years. And I have heard that in one of the most noble and illustrious families in France it is a common practice, since they believe it contributes to their health, to the point that their children also are nourished by the practice.

It is true that habit is a powerful tyrant, often having more influence over us than nature itself, although nature rules legitimately and habit

---

[1] *Aphorisms*, I, ii.

by usurpation. Still, custom must not be scorned because of the hold and sway it has gained over us. Moreover (as Galen says), those who acquire some habit choose for the most part a practice that befits their nature, especially since when they are constantly annoyed by something that upsets them they reject it.[2] Yet some, either won over by pleasure and voluptuousness or (out of wild folly) not being bothered by them, maintain their bad habits. But there are only a few of these; there are far more who do not persevere in them. And in another passage he says that no one is so stupid as to turn drinking cold water into a habit if the practice is distasteful.[3] For if upset and sickened by it, one will abstain from it completely.

One might well reply that there are very few people who are willing to control their appetites or, indeed, to refrain from anything at all, unless their physicians expressly forbid it and do so in writing. Otherwise it seems to them that they are not bound by it. That is the grand folly: not wanting to abstain from something one knows and admits to be harmful to one's nature unless the physician has expressly forbidden it, and even then there is still a lot of convincing to do. A wise and reasonable person can easily make up a regimen all by himself, based on his own experiences and observations concerning the quantity and quality of all its elements, with more assurance than the most knowledgeable physician in the world, if he is willing to look into the matter without deceiving himself. But let us set aside custom, and even childhood food habits; let us see whether there is some semblance of reason in entreating or allowing one to drink when going to bed.

It seems to me that the practice can be defended in the case of those who take great pleasure in it and do it willingly. For as Hippocrates says, concerning eating and drinking, that practice that is a little worse but brings more pleasure is better than its opposite. Furthermore, supposing there is a fair time span between supper and going to bed (such as a minimum of three hours), digestion is half over. Taking a little wine, then, is not harmful. For wine mixes well with what is half digested, since wine needs very little time to be broken down because it is a liquid that is easy to convert and that facilitates digestion. Thus

---

[2]Joubert's note: Book 5, *On the Conservation of Health* [De sanitate tuenda].

[3]Joubert's note: *On the Method,* Book 9, chapter 10 [*De methodo medendi libri XIV*].

it does not slow down what is already in an advanced state but will be ready to exit the stomach as soon as the rest, to which it will moreover do the favor of helping along more quickly so that its chyle will penetrate the liver more easily. And so the most informed among those who make use of such a regimen do so (as I have understood it) for the purpose of hastening distribution and moistening of the liver. From this it follows (according to them) that one rests better and has a more pleasant sleep. To this end the sweet vapor of the wine contributes, moistening the brain, which causes deeper sleep and hence a more successful secondary digestion along with the production of a lot of good blood. One cannot argue here for indigestion, something to be feared, because of an interruption of the digestion the stomach had begun. Indigestion is not from drinking liquid (and especially not from drinking wine) as would be the case for something else that takes a long time to digest or that would thicken the chyle more, which, because of such thickening, might linger too long and be difficult to disperse. The wine one drinks is like the water one adds to a thick soup, which would otherwise burn in the pot. And in order not to interrupt its cooking, good cooks dilute it with hot broth or boiling water. Wine, the natural heat of which maintains and speeds along digestion, acts in the same way, without such an interruption lasting or being detrimental. For immediately the digestion starts up again, going stronger and finishing more quickly. The stomach empties better when its chyle is more liquid, and the liver has a larger portion of it.

From this we can gather and conclude that such a combination can be good only for those who drink little with their meals, especially at supper, and who, eating well, do not become thirsty. Such people do no harm to themselves drinking a few hours later; I think it is healthy for them. However, I am not writing this to persuade anyone to take up this habit; still less would I like to acquire through my arguments the reputation of introducing drinking after supper as a regimen of health, becoming a sort of advocate of nocturnal banquets (for it is much better by far to drink reasonably with one's meals and in proportion to what is eaten). But I do point out with these remarks that those who have the custom of doing so are supported in part by good reasons, and if they have been so raised from childhood they can certainly continue to do so in good health.[4] And so one must not be astonished over his not becoming ill from it. I had an aunt, my father's sister, married to the Villars family in Condrieu, and who died very old. She never failed to drink, just before going to bed, a large glass of water in which she had soaked a big crust of bread for about an hour. She did this for forty years and was always in good health. They say, however, that she finally died from hydropsy, which could have been for some other reason. But I do not approve of this drinking of water at bedtime, and still less this practice many women and girls have of giving in to their appetites and cravings and drinking without any hesitation two or three large glasses of plain, pure, cold water before going to bed. They sometimes brag about it, but there is not always cause for laughter, especially when from this excess they end up with a bad stomach and the liver and spleen plagued with obstructions, causing them to have pale and vile coloring, shortness of breath, palpitations, suffocation of the uterus, and, for some, the misfortune of sterility.[5]

CHAPTER TEN
WHETHER LIQUIDS SHOULD BE DRUNK AT AS WARM A TEMPERATURE AS THE BLOOD, EVEN IN SUMMER, AND WHETHER IT IS BAD TO COOL WINE

Most common-folk opinions are taught by older people who, having lived a long time and seen many things, want to control everything and make other people, whatever their ages, do things their way. Thus, since they are all constantly snuffling and cold of nature, they want everyone to dress as warmly as they do and abstain from a thousand different things they feel to be harmful to them, such as drinking cold liquids in summer. And they say that the liquids each person drinks should be as warm as is his or her particular blood.

---

[4]This passage could be read as a concession to the practice of Joubert's own father, or to that of the royal families he served as court physician. See Joubert's tract *La Santé du prince* (herein translated in appendix C).

[5]We recall that Henri III called upon Joubert to resolve the problem of sterility in the queen, Louise de Lorraine (Amoreux 121).

I agree with this statement, but only with respect to them, for since their blood is cold, as are their bodies, they do not need much coolness. But a young man whose blood boils would never quench his thirst if he drank liquids that were as hot, not even if they were as tepid as temperate blood in the summertime. For thirst is an appetite for cold and moisture and is caused in an unnatural way by anything that is hot or that dries. How then could it be appeased without a moistening coolness? Experience shows most clearly that if one drinks hot liquids, one will only have to drink again, because one's thirst has not been quenched.

To conclude on this matter I will add that if it were healthy to drink liquids as warm as one's blood, then old people would have to drink liquids much cooler than do young people, a completely absurd and ridiculous idea. There is another more common and plausible opinion: it is from those who subscribe to the notion of drinking liquids as cool as those that have been brought up from the cellar or drawn from the barrel or, in the case of water, from a well or a spring. In neither case, however, should they be cooled. One will thus be governed by the disposition of the cellars, caves, wells, and springs, such that whoever has the cool ones will have the best of it and the others will suffer great setbacks in their health when they will not dare to cool the wine, the water, or both.

But (I ask you), what harm can come from the liquid's being cool, whether because of the air around it or because of the water with which it is cooled? If the water is not unhealthy because of its coolness when it is drawn from the well, spring, cistern, or river, it will not worsen the wine that is diluted or cooled with it. I admit that such wine will not be as tasty, but it will not be less wholesome than that which is brought cool from a very cold cellar, inasmuch as the cooling cannot bring to it any unhealthy qualities.

There remains, then, only the coolness that is being so maligned, wherever it comes from. But stop and think! There are cooled wines that are less cool than others that come directly from the barrel, with which nobody finds fault. And why do people not complain even more about drinking certain things ice cold, as is done in winter? Is it possible for liquids to be drunk so cold in summer that they freeze your teeth and often stop you from taking as long a swallow as one would like? Yet you normally never hear anyone speaking against that; on the contrary, most people think it is a bad idea to heat wine or water in the winter. Are these people not acting completely against nature, wishing, in the manner of giants, to work against it? Our bodies are boiling hot, burned, and dried in the summer! Will we therefore not drink abundantly of cool liquids so as to fight off the intemperateness and the inclemency of the air that converts our sweet humors into bitter ones (which are called choler), causing tertian and burning fevers, dysentery, and various other illnesses that thrive in summer? And in winter when we are half-frozen and kept in by the cold, all stiff and snuffling, will we drink ice?

Appetites that are not reflected upon but are spontaneous are in the main governed by nature, which controls them. One must therefore comply with them in a reasonable and subdued way, such as warding off the cold with heat, and heat with its contrary. Otherwise, the seasons of the year will, as a result of the drying of the air, cause us a thousand different troubles, which can be prevented by proper usage of the things God gives us at the proper time and in the proper amount. Is it for nought, or is it rather a great providence of nature, that wells, fountains, and cellars are cooler in summer and warmer in winter? And if one does not have such conveniences oneself, should one not make them up through artifice? Is it for nought that the cool and juicy fruits are produced in summer, when they are necessary for us, and not in winter, when wine begins to gain force, coming propitiously to arm us against the cold? The shade-making bough protects us from the sun in summer; it would not be near as useful in winter. Hence we do not have it naturally. Does the person who does not have shade in summer from groves, arbors, and trellises do evil in re-creating it by means of a bough-covered latticework? Certainly, just as it is beneficial to make use in summer of that which cools and in winter of everything that warms; following natural reason and the advice of the most wise (who are the most knowledgeable), it is therefore also most beneficial to use that which in fact possesses the desired qualities.

But why is it necessary to spend so much time impugning such gross errors and people who do not have sound arguments or, as is the case with those in a true doctrine, at least ones that do not contradict each other. For in like matters such people contradict themselves very awkwardly, as in the question of eating fruit to cool off. Is there a single person who does not find it bad to eat cherries, plums, figs, grapes, melons, and other such fruits while they are still warm from the sun? People cool them, some in a cellar, others in cold water. And why, then, will one not drink cooled liquids to quench one's thirst? There is many an artifice that can be considered suspect, such as putting ice or snow in wine, or cooling bottles in water with saltpeter in it, even though the amount of saltpeter is not enough to hurt you if you were to swallow it. But what harm can there be in cooling bottles in plain water that is good to drink, since this same water is drunk by itself or with wine? Or what danger can come from cooling wine and water in the air of a well? Someone might object here, citing colic, and of course those who are subject to it or who are otherwise troubled by drinking cold liquids should abstain not only from chilled things but also from those that are naturally cold. For it is an obligation and the height of wisdom to avoid something one has in the past discovered to be harmful to one's nature. Otherwise, cheese would have to be generally forbidden because it is harmful for those who form kidney stones, and wine because it is bad for those with gout. Is there anything more unjust and tyrannical than trying to bend to one's own will the appetites or feelings of others who are of a different complexion? Such are those good people who find fault with drinking liquids cool and who advise all to have them only at the temperature of their own blood.

CHAPTER ELEVEN
AGAINST THOSE WHO COMPLAIN OF HOT NIGHTS
IN SUMMER AND YET SLEEP ON A FEATHER MATTRESS
WITH THE WINDOWS CLOSED

We often see people complain in summer about the extreme heat of the nights, more than of the days, in a specific place, such as in the house, and especially in the rooms in which people sleep. These rooms might be considered as ovens, being stuffy for not having been aired out and kept completely opened while the sun was not shining directly in, and for not having been cooled often with very cold water mixed with a little vinegar and with lots of leaves, for those people who have access to them. For if rooms are left in summer as they are in other seasons, one must not be surprised if they become stifling hot. What is worse, most people sleep on feather mattresses, just as they do in winter, not differentiating between beds except for the lighter covers they use in summer.

It serves no purpose telling me that not everyone has the means of owning mattresses separately from their beds, for it would be even better to sleep on straw or on wheat or oat chaff (a very soft material), also called *balousse*.[1] One is a little less comfortable on it than on a feather mattress, but the coolness and enjoyment one has from it offsets the softness considerably, especially since, when on it, one sleeps ever so much more restfully, more pleasantly, and more peacefully. And as in all things it is only a matter of becoming used to it. As long as the mattress is fully packed and the straw well fluffed, one is quite comfortable and quite cool, not to mention the unparalleled pleasure of the sound sleep one enjoys on it.

Another error no less serious is that of keeping the windows closed all night, even when one has the advantage of bed curtains or of a canopy, which protects one from drafts if perchance a wind were to come up while one slept. For as far as simple coldness is concerned, it is not to be feared, because it is never as cold in summer with the windows open as it is in the winter with everything closed, even with linen-covered windows in a matted and tapestried room in which a huge fire has been burning all day. Even in such a room you will need more covers when in bed (if you do not wish to feel the cold) than you will in summer with the windows open. If one is not afraid of such cold in the room in winter, why should it be feared in summer, when it cannot even be properly considered cold but is moderate and temperate? Fearing the cool air of the evening when under the covers and in a curtained bed is wrong, as can easily be understood from the arguments I have made concerning this elsewhere.[2] For there is no quality in the outside air of the evening that must be kept from entering into bedrooms. Indeed, there is nothing but the coolness or cool quality required for pleasant sleep and rest. And who, having to choose in

---

[1] Cotgrave translates Joubert's *balousse* as "the chaffe of oates, or barley."

[2] There is a printer's error in this sentence. Fortunately the text is repeated: *"... & temperé? De craindre le serain sous vn couuert, & temperé? De craindre le serain sous vn couuert, & lict encourtiné, c'est abus...."* Joubert is referring to his discussion of the cool air of evening in his brief tract entitled *Du serain*, published in the 1579 edition of the *Erreurs populaires*, translated herein as "Nightfall, What It Is, and Whether It Falls on Us" in appendix D of the present volume.

summer between two rooms, one very hot and the other very cool, both on the same floor, would not rather choose the cooler? And so, if one can conveniently cool the one that is hot, for example by keeping the windows open from sunset until morning, what harm can come from it? We presuppose that the air in the street is no worse (if not better) than that of the closed and stuffy house.

Those who sleep outdoors, keeping livestock or watching over fruit, and soldiers on campaign, bedding down under the moon and the stars next to a hedge or under a tree, or in small cabins and lodges, so as to be protected only from the dew and the wind, sleep so much more healthily (not to mention with what inestimable pleasure) than do those who close themselves up in houses. I experience a similar thing with my whole family and all who live in my house,[3] having embraced the habit of leaving all the windows of all the rooms open at night most of the summer, and keeping them closed, along with the shutters, during the day. If one is afraid of being surprised in the night by feeling cold one should keep an emergency cover at the foot of the bed. And how many times does it likewise happen in winter that we wake up because of the sudden feeling of cold that comes upon us? This is remedied in the same way without any more thought given to it. But one might reply that it is worse in summer since the pores are more open because of the heat during the day. Well, there is a remedy: putting on more covers as soon as one goes to bed. For it is reasonable to put on more or fewer covers, according to the temperature of the room. Still, there is this pleasure and profit of breathing not stuffy but fresh air, the main thing to be sought after in all this. For we do not want all of the fresh air to touch the rest of our warm bodies, but only the face, around the nose and mouth, where we breathe. Also, the true means of cooling the entire body is by cooling the heart, the lungs, and the brain, all from the inside. For when we are shocked by cold externally, the surface of the skin, by closing up the pores, multiplies the heat and causes greater distress, thirst, unrest, exhaustion, and other troublesome symptoms because of this heat, building up in the entrails and in the joints.

---

[3]Joubert is probably referring to the family domestics.

CHAPTER TWELVE
THAT BLOOD SAUSAGES DO NOT KEEP WELL,
WHENCE THE CUSTOM OF GIVING THEM AS PRESENTS

Blood is considered a bad nutriment from whatever animal it comes and however it is prepared, because, as soon as it is out of its natural site (the veins and the arteries, which alone are able to preserve it in its integrity), it begins to spoil and decay. So whoever wants to make use of it must not wait long, for it always gets worse. Man's appetite has put to his use a lot of foods that are not wholesome. Poverty and want have introduced others that are just as pernicious. Ox blood is certainly one of those we use more out of necessity than out of any craving, in view of its lack of flavor. Sheep blood is much better, since the meat is also more tasty. But if the truth were told, the best is not fit for consumption; and it would be good if they fell from fashion in France, where the blood of such animals is not allowed as food but rather considered as poison or excrement. Goat blood is still worse than sheep blood, and the meat likewise. As far as the blood of male goats is concerned, I do not think it is used except by apothecaries for the dissolving of kidney stones, for which purpose it is found appropriate when properly prepared. The blood of she-goats, considered a delicacy, has always been in demand and highly prized by the ancients (as Homer bears witness).[1] They would mix a lot of grease with it and stuff it into the bowels or the stomach of such animals, which is the origin, I think, of our blood sausage. But we must not allow ourselves to be taken in by the tastes, and even less by the judgment of the people of those olden times, who had as yet no knowledge of finer, and more digestible, kinds of meat, as Galen states.

Today people use such blood. Mixed with parsley or other herbs, along with lard, it is considered to be of a better quality than those mentioned above, to which nothing is added. The blood of lambs and of kids is prepared as just mentioned and is much better because their meat is tastier, kid meat surpassing that of lambs. The same preparation, which is prized above all others of our times, is used for pullets, chickens, and capons. In Italy fowl is not bled; rather, the neck is broken and a large quantity of blood congeals there, making a sort of

---

[1]Joubert's note: Galen, Book 3, *On the Faculty of Nutriments,* chapter 18 [*De alimentorum facultatibus*].

blood sausage that is considered very delicious. And in truth it is much better for it this way than if it had been exposed to the air, for the skin of the neck preserves it and keeps it from decaying.

The ancients made much of the blood of hares or young hares; even in the time of Galen,[2] their blood was the most sought after, and the meat the greatest delicacy, cooked with the liver. The blood of pigs wins the highest honors today, distributed as presents to our closest friends in the form of blood sausage. Common folk have observed this custom for ages without really knowing why it had to be practiced. They see it as a symbol of benevolence and friendship or, because there happens to be a lot of it, wish to share it with others, expecting similar behavior from them. This is why people have plenty of fresh blood sausage around, since each will want to return the favor in kind. The first intention is an honest one, for, in order to make a more decent present of blood sausage, people will add to it a lobe of liver and will hang on some of it a spleen and on the rest of it some filets or some ribs. Less honorable ones are revealed when kidneys or lungs are added. The whole is covered with a wrapping or a crepe cut in as many sections as there will be presents. All these pieces add to the embellishment of our blood sausage, which, in the main, symbolizes (as it were) some heartfelt and tender affection, as does blood. It also represents love, because it comes from the liver, in which Plato places its seat.[3] Thus in sending blood one wishes to show a token of friendship, one that is strongly believed to be healthy and delicious.

Another motive is at work among those who care about maintaining their health and who scrutinize diligently the quality of their food. For blood, whatever its source, cannot remain wholesome for long without being corrupted by air; and for this very reason it is advised that the pork blood (the one considered to be the finest) be put in the bowels, which, because of their thick skin, will better preserve it. Thus the best blood sausages are those made while the blood is still warm. Later

---

[2]Second century A.D.

[3]Joubert is referring to Plato's *Timaeus* (69C–71A). He discusses Plato's division of the soul and the philosopher's placing of all the emotions "in the heart, except for love, which he relegates to the liver so as to put it under the vegetative: whence comes the saying that the liver constrains us to love."

This passage, and a much lengthier discussion of Plato's division of the soul, can be found in Joubert's *TL* (29–35).

it is parboiled, not only to make it keep better but to make it easier to cut. In order better to preserve the sausage, people put along with the blood, salt, thyme, and wild thyme.[4] Some add fennel, while others use rosemary, parsely, hyssop, and other aromatic herbs, except for savory, because common folk believe falsely that it can stop the blood from thickening when cooked, inasmuch as it is given to the sick to dissolve blood clots. Lard is not forgotten but is used in huge quantities, except by stingy women, who are jokingly called good housewives when they have economized on the lard. But if blood sausage is not made with lots of fat, it is not wholesome, especially since it remains a good while in the stomach and is slow to digest because of its harsh and dry qualities. Fat makes it slide through better, making it less dangerous, like other foods that do not stop for a long time in the body.

Whatever the case, it is better to abstain from it completely, or to be very judicious in your use of it, making sure it is no more than one or two days old at the most. This is why the custom of giving them away is very good. For by keeping them a long time, they become so pernicious that they could be deemed poisonous. A woman of Montpellier furnished an example, one might say. That is, she suffocated after eating blood sausage that had been kept too long. She thought she was being thrifty by not giving it away and by not eating any other food as long as the blood sausage lasted. Scarcely had she finished than she died, just as one does when poisoned.

---

[4]Joubert uses the term *serpoulet*. Cotgrave gives the following explanation: "Running Time, wild Time, creeping Time, mother of Time, Puliall mountaine, our Ladies Bedstraw. *Serpolet sauvage*. Wild creeping Time; of two kinds, the one bearing a white, the other a red flower: (*Gerard* shewes us no fewer than then [sic] six kinds of *Serpillum*, all of which as he calls wild Times (though with some small and different additions) so many hold (sayes *Mathiolus*) that euerie *Serpolet* is wild:) Some also tearme Water-mint, and others Balsamint, *Serpolet sauvage*."

CHAPTER THIRTEEN
AGAINST THOSE WHO HAVE AN INORDINATE FEAR
OF BLOODLETTING, AND THINK THAT THE FIRST
USE OF IT SAVES ONE'S LIFE

Inasmuch as blood is the treasure of nature, nutriment of the humors, and the subject of natural heat (which governs the body in all its operations), one does well to revere it and to treat it with great care, for it is necessary for the maintaining of our strength and the preservation of our health. Hence it should not be carelessly squandered by taking poor care of it; rather, two main principles should be observed with respect to it. One, it must be kept free of any impurity; two, there must not be an excessive amount of it, even if it is perfect in every aspect. For if it is corrupted, polluted, and foul, it does more harm than good; if it is too abundant, it puts the vessels in danger of bursting and the natural heat of being dissipated. This is why, when it is copious, one must not fear letting some of it out in order to make room for the new, which is constantly being formed. Likewise, when it is hot and boiling as a result of a fever, if it is not given an opening through which it might spew out (as one does in venting new wine), it puts the patient in grave danger and causes horrendous suffering.

When it is polluted with a large amount of bad humors, and before it becomes completely corrupted, a small amount of it is let out, so that the rest can be more easily cleaned by drugs that separate and draw these humors out of the blood and finally expel them, for which reason they merit the name of purgatives. It is therefore not right simply to decry bloodletting as foreign to nature or to fear it so, as many do (following Erasistratus,[1] who called those who prescribed it bloodthirsty and considered them murderers), since a great number of illnesses springing from the aforementioned causes cannot be cured without recourse to this practice. When a fever is very violent, the face inflamed and the veins swollen, is bloodletting not required? If one is strangled by a quinsy[2] or suffocating from an inflammation of the lung or from a true pleurisy, there is nothing that will bring relief as quickly and interrupt the illness as promptly as an immediate bloodletting,

---

[1]On Erasistratus, see *PE*, bk. 1, chap. 1, n. 9 (284).

[2]Suppurative tonsillitis.

which is generally indicated in all disorders caused by an abundance
and excess of blood, whether good or bad.

I am astonished by some, who will more willingly take twenty
different drugs than endure one bloodletting that is necessary, given its
great ease and simplicity. For one can control perfectly the amount we
wish to let flow; it can be stopped at will and be repeated later so as
not to weaken the patient too much in a single application. This is not
the case with drugs, for often they cause more voiding than is desired
and cannot be stopped when we want. These are considerable draw-
backs, not to mention the nausea, the upset stomach, and the severe
intestinal cramps they usually bring about.

Now, when one is phlebotomized, if the blood coming out is bad,
we must convince ourselves that the best has remained in the body and
rejoice over such a voiding. If the blood coming out is fair, we must
realize that what remains is healthier still and that what was removed
was superfluous. Someone might judge this manner of treating patients
against the rule of nature, which is careful to preserve blood as a
treasure of its very own. To this we reply that it is nature itself which
teaches us that we must use this remedy in several conditions. For the
flow of menstrual blood in females shows us most patently that abundance can be harmful if it is not quickly evacuated. In this, nature
itself orders blood to exit, not once a year but every month. And if
through some hindrance this blood is retained, the woman feels very ill
because of it. It is folly to think that it must be voided as something
entirely useless, foul, and poisonous, since the unborn child is very
aptly nourished by it in the womb of its mother. Otherwise why would
it be suppressed during pregnancy since it could just as well be expelled without ever touching the child? It is through the veins of the
mouth of the uterus that those women who have more blood than the
fruit of their womb can absorb rid themselves of such blood.

Pliny recounts that plants touched with such blood die, that fruit
falls from the trees in which menstruating women have climbed, that
such blood causes ivory to lose its luster and a blade its edge, and that
dogs tasting such blood go mad and if they bite someone afterward the
wound will never heal.[3] Others claim that the blood of lepers is not
much worse than menstrual blood. I do not believe any of this, for
women would have to have suffered far more horrendous illnesses than

---

[3]Joubert's note: Book 7, chapter 15.

those they endure when their menses are blocked; besides, the unborn child would be ill-nourished by such blood. It is therefore more superfluous in quantity than foul in quality, and it is superfluous exclusively because it is unrefined and phlegmatic.

The blood exuding from hemorrhoids is often much worse than menstrual blood, for it is melancholic, the worst of the humors, and, when spilled on the ground, makes it boil as does strong vinegar. But it is rarely concentrated and pure. For all of the grossest blood amasses in the hemorrhoidal veins in order to be voided when nature has thus seen fit, to the great benefit of the entire body. Here then are two sorts of voidings of blood, performed by nature, which show very clearly what must be done when we recognize the need and when nature cannot manage it alone. And if one claims that in these cases the blood is voided because of its foulness alone, one admits by this very claim that bloodletting is helpful when blood is both corrupt and overly abundant. For if it is only corrupt, it is retained in the body to provide the body food and is not voided. But what will you say about the fact that very often, even though blood is not corrupt, nature squirts a portion of it out in order to ease the overly swollen veins and to relieve the body of a heavy burden? This is the relief many feel with a nosebleed. Thus if we wish to hinder nature and break its habit of using the passages of the nose, we must furnish it with another exit on those occasions when we see that it is profuse. For otherwise several disorders will result from the closing off of this exit, such as the bursting of veins in the stomach, in the lungs, or elsewhere, causing the spitting up and vomiting of blood in certain people.

Stop and think! Several illnesses that could become serious are cured by a voluminous flow of blood at the critical moment; and often a headache goes away after a nosebleed. All these examples show clearly that, following nature's lead, physicians (who are but its ministers) must at times reduce the quantity of blood, which invites a variety of illnesses or in fact causes them. Will we be less reasonable than wild animals, which, instructed by nature, know the value of bloodletting? Pliny writes that the hippopotamus, when feeling too full, looks for a recently cut cane shoot and, upon finding a sharp one, pushes its thigh against it so as to open a vein, thus alleviating its body, which, without this practice, would become ill.[4] Goats also, suffering from

---

[4]Joubert's note: Book 8, chapter 26.

clouded vision, wound themselves in the eye with a pointed reed in an attempt to relieve this organ of a quantity of blood, as the same author recounts.[5]

There are many people who are opposed to bloodletting for the simple reason that they have seen people die after being bled. But their argument will seem very weak (or rather ridiculous) if we are convinced (since it is true) that all illnesses cannot be cured no matter who the patient might be, and that those which are absolutely fatal make light of all remedies, including bloodletting, even if it is wisely prescribed and serves no real purpose, as is proven by its effect. But when people try nevertheless to blame an incident of death on phlebotomy because death happened to follow it, similar reasoning can be used against them by saying that people die because they ate, supped, or slept, since they died shortly afterward. If one were to see a man die while he was being bled, there would be strong evidence that such a remedy was not fitting, or that it was poorly administered.

Still, anything we are not sure about must be given the benefit of the doubt, and we must not launch unfounded accusations against a physician who has prescribed bloodletting, even though the illness was not resolved in the patient's favor; rather, we must believe that it was the potency and the magnitude of the disease, and not a strength-annihilating remedy, that precipitated death in the patient. I grant that on several occasions bloodletting is improperly prescribed and that uninformed physicians commit huge blunders in advising it; still, common folk are unable to make judgments in the matter and must refrain from doing so. Otherwise they will do great injustice to the most learned, for they will say the same thing indifferently about all physicians.

I have heard others say they do not want to make a practice of using this type of remedy but wish to keep it for when the need is grave and extreme, such as the imminent danger of death. For they are of the firm belief that the first bloodletting will save their lives unfailingly. It is quite true (and this must be said) that one never dies from the first bloodletting, for if such were the case, one would never be bled again, and hence, such a bloodletting would not be called the first, properly speaking, but the only one, since the first is relative to

---

[5]Joubert's note: Book 8, chapter 50.

the second and others that follow.[6] But that the first bloodletting saves one's life, in that it is somehow more fitting, is a mistake that has been uncovered through long experience, teaching us the very opposite. For people are seen dying everyday from various things that a first bloodletting is unable to remedy; and with phlebotomy thousands of people who have often had recourse to this remedy are cured of the most horrible illnesses. This belief about the first bloodletting is most dangerous and prejudicial, especially since illnesses are slight at the outset; this is why so few sick people are concerned about a cure. Now, those who entertain such a fantasy refuse to undergo bloodletting during the first few days, wishing to hold it in reserve for more severe illnesses and for the extreme necessity. Meanwhile, the opportunity (which Hippocrates rightly calls sudden and ready to be seized)[7] passes us by, and then when the patient, upon feeling the extreme seriousness, begins to comply with the remedy, it is no longer applicable.

On the matter of habit, it is in this case much more unlikely to be harmful than beneficial. For a person accustomed to being bled (provided one's strength is not obviously diminished by it) will endure it much more happily than one who is not, just as ordinary illnesses and ones that people are familiar with are less alarming, in keeping with Hippocrates's aphorism: "Those who are accustomed to hard work, even though they are old and weak, can stand it better than the young and healthy."[8] Thus the first bloodletting must not be so highly valued, and bloodletting in general must not be so suspect in the eyes of common folk when a wise and learned physician prescribes it, since this very remedy is taught to us by nature and is painless, sound, and useful in several different illnesses.

---

[6]Joubert is playing on words: the "premiere" incident of bloodletting would, strictly speaking, be the first in a series; a "vnique" incident would be the sole case.

[7]Joubert's note: *Aphorisms*, 1, Book 1.

[8]Joubert's note: *Aphorisms*, 49, Book 2.

CHAPTER FOURTEEN
THAT BLOODLETTING CAN BE USED
ON PREGNANT WOMEN, CHILDREN, AND THE ELDERLY

At some time in the past common folk have learned from physicians that it is dangerous to bleed pregnant women, children, and the elderly. If the physician now wants to do bloodletting, it is considered something new, foolhardy, and hazardous; and if the patient should happen to die, this remedy will not only be blamed, but blamed bitterly, even though the disease, and not the remedy, caused the patient to die. If the patient gets better, then it is (to hear them talk) more a case of luck than of proper treatment. We should not be surprised at this, since our forefathers shared this same belief and passed it on to common folk.

I say "our forefathers," meaning the physicians of the last two or three hundred years. They understood that Hippocrates and the other ancients had taught that it was a grave mistake in such cases, and that although bloodletting seemed necessary they did not dare prescribe it. But if they had read carefully the books written by those who are much closer to the first physicians and who lived halfway between Hippocrates and ourselves, the Greek and Roman physicians, whose knowledge was rare and whose methodic experience was consummate, they would have understood much better the advice of our good authors, who had the custom of writing roughly in but a few words their rules. For in an attempt to say that the strength of the patient is utmost in the practice of bloodletting, they said that the elderly and children should not be subjected to it and even limited its use to those who could stand it, patients between sixteen and sixty years of age. For those younger or older do not normally have the required conditions. The prescription is given generally and may be dispensed with and disregarded in a particular case without contradicting the intentions of these authors, as when one comes across (a frequent occurrence) a child with a good constitution, healthy and plump, strong and vigorous, or a strong old man, both in need of bloodletting because of their diseases.

Galen leads us to believe one should pay less attention to a person's age than to a person's strength, which can be determined by a strong, powerful, and regular pulse, a most trustworthy sign and one that never fails to indicate with certainty one's strength. And for this reason, on those septuagenarians who have such a pulse he allows bloodletting to be performed if the illness requires it, because (he says) there are some very sanguine and robust people at seventy, just as there are others at sixty who could never stand bloodletting.[1] As for children, he never allowed them to be phlebotomized, not out of fear for their weakness (for they have more vital and natural strength than they will have at twenty or thirty years of age), but because of the rapid dissipation of their substance, which is as yet composed of a soft, young, thin, and very soluble material. Nevertheless, it has been discovered that bloodletting is often effective in treating them, even those under six years of age, as several people have reported and as we have happily discovered ourselves. Avenzoar writes that he bled his son when he was not yet three years old and that he [the child] felt very good afterward.[2] And why should they be entirely deprived of it, since, even while still at their mothers' breasts, they sometimes have nosebleeds without suffering any harm? If nature in its own movements sometimes allows for discharges of blood in children, will not the physician, who is but its minister and imitator, dare to use the practice? A small child will produce more blood when punched in the nose than we draw from the arm each time, for one must pay close attention to the amount voided and take care not to extract too much.

And so one can rightfully absolve our Galen when he forbids the practice to be used on children, for in his time they took large amounts of blood, as much as four pounds of blood, it appears; he says he has seen up to six pounds taken from a patient who experienced great relief from it.[3] Today it is considered a lot if one draws three or four saucers of blood[4] (which are ten to twelve ounces) from a young man

---

[1]Joubert's note: *Book of Curing through Phlebotomy [De cognoscendis curandisque animi morbis]*.

[2]Avenzoar was an Arab physician of eleventh-century Spain. His principal work was *Teiseer*, a source for the *lapidaires*.

[3]Joubert uses the term "liure" in the medical sense; Cotgrave sheds some light on the amount of blood in question: "*La livre Medicinale*. The physitians pound; containes 12 ounces; but they be diuided into 96 drammes, they into 288 scruples, those into 576 *Oboles*, they into 1728 *Siliques*, and they into 6912 graines."

[4]Joubert uses the term *palete*. Cotgrave gives the double medical sense of the word: "*Palette: f.* A Lingell, Tenon, Slice, or flat toole wherewith Chirurgians lay salue on plaisters; also, the saucer, or porringer wherinto they receiue bloud out of an opened veine; also, a battle-doore."

who is strong; and from children, a proportionately smaller amount. Still, we insist that such children be huskily framed, as mentioned above, and that their illnesses call for it urgently.

As for a pregnant woman, Hippocrates has written that bloodletting does not put her own health at risk but might cause an abortion even if the child is well developed, because it will be deprived of its food.[5] This is why he says it is impossible for the child to be healthy if the mother has her flowers in normal quantities during pregnancy.[6] But when one sees an excessive repletion, caused by too much idleness, an abundance of food, and a natural heaviness, threatening to stifle the child or forcing it out of a proper position (as happens to a few women who, for lack of being bled, begin doing harm to their children in the third or fourth month), why will one not dare to draw out some of the blood, which is too abundant and unhealthy. If the same abundance, or even a much smaller one, becomes far too hot because of a burning fever and begins to boil, almost causing the veins to burst, will we not dare (out of concern for the pregnancy) void a small amount of blood and tap the vein when the woman with child is burning with fever? Hippocrates says that an acute disorder such as the one I have mentioned is fatal in pregnant women.[7] He says this because, even when one refrains from administering phlebotomy in such a case, an abortion will be the result, as stated above. Now, losing one is less bad than losing two; most often, however, both can be saved, thank God.

And how could the child in the burning embers of its mother be healthy? What nutriment can boiling blood give to it? It is crucial to use all means to extinguish this raging fire in order to provide relief both for the mother and the child. Hippocrates allows us to purge a pregnant woman from the fourth month to the seventh, something all physicians observe.[8] If, then, pregnant women can without any danger endure purgation, which racks, upsets, and causes the body to shudder incomparably more than does phlebotomy (especially the strong drugs used by Hippocrates), why will we not dare make use of bloodletting when it is called for, especially since it is one of the surest and least

---

[5]Joubert's note: *Aphorisms,* 31, Book 5.

[6]Joubert's note: *Aphorisms,* 61, Book 5.

[7]Joubert's note: *Aphorisms,* 30, Book 5.

[8]Joubert's note: *Aphorisms,* 1, Book 4, and *Aphorisms,* 29, Book 5.

painful remedies? For one only draws the amount of blood one wishes and no more, since it is in our power to stop it at each drop, something we cannot do with the action of drugs when they cause more voiding than we would wish.

But what can be said about the fact that several women go on having their flowers during the entire pregnancy without the children being any the worse for it? Moreover, we often see that a pregnant woman will bleed from the nose or from a wound without aborting or suffering any other ills. These are things that happen every day, leading us to conclude that bloodletting is not as harmful to pregnant women as previously believed. Still, lest one think this idea is new and shared by people of today, Celsus (who lived in the time of Augustus more than fifteen hundred years ago) has most fittingly pointed out that one has only to take into account the condition of those one is to bleed, saying: "Drawing blood from large women who are not pregnant and from the young is an old practice; doing the same to children, to the elderly, and to pregnant women is something new. For the ancients considered the very young and the very old unable to withstand such a remedy and were convinced that women would abort if thus treated during pregnancy. For some time now experience has shown that these rules are not all inclusive and without exception, but that a few observations must be added in which the judgment of the healer is taken into consideration. For it is not a matter of looking at age, nor of pregnancy, but solely of one's condition. Thus if a young person feels weak or if a woman who is not pregnant has little strength, one does wrong to draw blood, because the energy that is left languishes and dies as a result. But a very strong child, a very tough old man, and a lusty pregnant woman can surely recover from it. Still, in such a case, an ignorant physician can easily make a mistake, because there is not as much energy in these age groups and because a pregnant woman needs her strength after recovering, not only for herself but for her child. Thus the principal thing in the practice is thought and prudence, and above all not simply counting years or only looking at the pregnancy but, rather, assessing the strength and understanding whether it will be able to work toward the sustaining of the child, the old person, or the woman bearing another body in her own."[9]

---

[9]Joubert's note: Book 2, chapter 10 [for a discussion of Celsus, see *PE*, bk. 1, chap. 1, n. 8 (284)].

From these wise observations one can easily understand the error into which our forefathers had fallen for nearly three hundred years, right up to our own time, during which the sciences have regained their former dignity through the opening of good books, which ignorance had been keeping hidden. And we are able to say, as did Celsus, that our ancestors have indiscriminately deprived pregnant women, children, and the elderly of bloodletting. Since that time, experience, guided by reason, has made known to the more worthy minds of this age that one can indeed practice bloodletting when the illness calls for it, and that the patient can withstand it. Thus, let common folk, who are ill informed, henceforth cease their false calumniation of good and wise physicians, who with great care and sound deliberation have recourse to this remedy when it is needed.

CHAPTER FIFTEEN
AGAINST THOSE WHO USE BLOODLETTING
RASHLY AND TOO OFTEN

What I have set forth in the preceding chapter could support the error of those who use bloodletting too quickly and too indiscriminately. I see several of them who at the slightest discomfort want to be bled. There are overconfident barbers who, without the guidance of a physician, apply this remedy for everything. It is most effective when one knows how to make use of it, but only a physician (including under this name the learned surgeon) should have the right to administer it. For the strength of the patient and the extent of the illness, present or future, which are the two determining conditions for bloodletting, must be gauged. But it does much harm to bleed injudiciously and needlessly, because when the necessity arises one can no longer have recourse to this remedy, with the body more exhausted than it should be and weakened by the squandering of its humors, which are spilled and lost in considerable quantities when a lot of blood is voided. What happens then is that, since the body is chilled, the natural functions are poorly executed. This is why Galen was right in saying that it is not expedient to bleed several times a year.

Celsus, speaking generally, gives the advice that one must not use up remedies meant for sickness when one is in good health.[1] Likewise, in times of peace one must not waste stocks and munitions set aside for war for fear of not having any when the need arises. Blood is the treasure of nature, and it must not be spilled except for protecting what remains, such as when the disease is so serious and impetuous that it could cause everything to be lost. In a similar fashion, merchants, in the extreme fury of a tempest and a storm threatening to sink the vessel, have no qualms about throwing their riches overboard in an attempt to lighten the ship and save lives. It is not allowed to use bloodletting when the extent of the illness, present or future (as we have said), does not call for it, and when the condition of the patient is not resistant enough to sustain the body after phlebotomy. If either of these two is lacking, bloodletting is a bad choice, especially since the sole repletion and abundance of blood (unless threatening because of some unfortunate accident) do not constitute a sufficient reason for using this remedy. For in a body that is otherwise healthy, fasting, purging, frequent baths, vigorous massage, or simple exercise can be effective enough, as Galen has well shown.[2] Bleeding a person simply because of excessive heat in the liver is not always appropriate because there are many heat-caused illnesses in which the application of cooling remedies are much more effective than phlebotomy.

Besides the two conditions mentioned above (which are the only ones that justify bloodletting), there are several particular considerations, constituting special circumstances for us, to be included under the heading of the strength of the person one wishes to bleed. These must be diligently observed, and one must not draw blood indiscriminately from anyone, in any region, in any season, something common folk do not understand. Skinny people with large veins have much more blood than do fat people, who, consequently, cannot withstand bloodletting as easily. In cold regions people are heavy eaters and drinkers (mainly meat and wine) and are copiously nourished; it thus is the case that they engender a lot of blood and are able to withstand bloodletting more than people from regions having an opposite climate.

---

[1]Joubert's note: In the book, *On Scarification*, Book 1, chapter 1 [Joubert is referring to the *De medicina*; for the passage from Celsus, see *PE*, bk 1, chap. 18, n. 4 (292)].

[2]Joubert's note: *Method*, Book 2, chapter 6 [*De methodo medendi libri XIV*].

For heat dissolves the integrity of our strength and makes the body languid, aside from the fact that it dissipates our substance and is not conducive to the production of a lot of humors. This is why people from hotter regions are small and thin and are unable (without seriously compromising their health) to withstand bloodletting, either frequently or in large voidings.

On the question of season of the year, Hippocrates teaches us that if bloodletting is used preventively, one must bleed patients in the spring, because the blood is then abundant and the strength of that patient at its maximum because of the temperate air.[3] But if one must practice bloodletting in another season, it is no cause for concern, provided one is careful to take modest amounts, especially in summer. This is a matter in which the empirics err grossly: they indiscriminately and prodigally bleed people during burning fevers, which are rampant in the canicular period. Furthermore, I will add this in conclusion: much more discretion and ability are needed in properly prescribing bloodletting than in purgation, because purgation weakens the body less when the potency of the drug and the strength of the patient are sufficiently known and the humors properly readied for it. For the complications that can result from purgation are not as serious as they are from bloodletting. Hence it must be diligently prescribed and prudently administered, as a more serious remedy than purgation. For Galen forbids its use on children but allows them to be given prescribed drugs. It therefore must not be used so commonly, as I see several people doing, having themselves bled as if with a light heart. And magistrates ought to forbid barbers from administering bloodletting without a physician's prescription.

---

[3]Joubert's note: *Aphorisms,* 55, Book 7.

CHAPTER SIXTEEN
THAT PURGATION CAN BE APPROPRIATE IN ANY SEASON, EVEN DURING THE DOG DAYS

Common folk, having often heard physicians speak of the dog days as inappropriate, troublesome, and dangerous for purgation, in accord with the opinion of the ancient physicians, are absolutely convinced it is a bad practice to administer any drug whatsoever during this season, even though certain ones might be otherwise necessary. Our predecessors have not done well to put forth such reasons, among which important distinctions need to be made. For these idiots, having thus learned the rule purely and simply as it was pronounced before them, without knowing how to put limits on it, are trying today to debate with physicians about not purging during the dog days, or they at least find it very odd and begin murmuring about it if a physician attempts it.

In order to save them from this error, it will be necessary for us to interpret the aphorism from Hippocrates that is at the foundation of these remarks. He says that the administration of laxatives is troublesome before, during, and after the dog days,[1] meaning by this that there are other times that are more appropriate and that this one is the worst. Anybody hearing these words in a sane manner will not immediately conclude that purging is so condemned and banned during this season that it may never be prescribed under any circumstances, even when needed, but that it is highly fraught with danger, that it brings more complications than when used before or after the dog days, and that it is due to the fiercely hot air. For during the dog days our bodies burn and melt with heat. Purging drugs are so potent (especially those used by the ancient physicians, which were extremely violent) that it is impossible to take them without suffering a great deal of discomfort and pain, aside from the danger that there is of enkindling an even more searing fire.

This is why it comes about that, because they are improperly treated during this season, several people become feverish during this season, as Galen says. Moreover, our strength, already beaten down and weakened by the heat in the air, becomes even more feeble under

---

[1]Joubert's note: *Aphorisms*, 5, Book 4.

the effect of the drugs,[2] such that we can say that this season is not an appropriate one in which to purge our bodies and that purgation should not be attempted unless the illness forces us to do so. For whoever might have to take medicine once a year (as is the case with those who usually, after the accumulation of a large quantity of pernicious humors, fall victim to some illness) would do badly to choose or to await the dog days.

Spring is the most appropriate season for it, or else autumn, depending upon whether these customary illnesses come around in winter or in summer. When it is done as a precaution (that is, in order to prevent illness) and not as a cure for an existing illness, we void such matter much earlier and choose the month, the day, and the time that most suits us: that is, when the sky is clear and calm, the air temperate, and the weather cool. But when one is in fact ill and purgation is required, nothing must be put off nor anything considered other than the strength of the patient and the type of medicine to use.

The patient's strength is at its greatest during the first few days of the illness; the opportunity for our remedies is very narrow, and it must be met head on (as the proverb goes).[3] Those who wait until the next day thinking about it often arrive too late, only making the disorder worse and causing a lot of damage. And so if necessity requires and calls for immediate purgation, we must not be concerned about the weather except in our choice of drugs. For if it is in summer the drug must be more gentle, and especially if the air is burning hot during the dog days. Winter is more accepting of the strong ones, and temperate seasons necessitate the use of average ones. With this restriction we make our drugs correspond to each season of the year, all for the benefit of the patient. Thus the warning of Hippocrates, which will always be true, must no longer be misinterpreted: namely, that during the dog days our bodies are less able to withstand being purged than during other times of the year, and hence the drugs provoking it must be very gentle when the type of illness necessitates purgation.

Stop and think! If I need to void a choleric humor causing a tertian fever or a very dangerous burning fever, and if this happens during the

---

[2]Joubert's note: At the beginning of the above aphorism.

[3]Joubert's expression is very figurative: "... & il la faut prendre par le front (comme on dit en commun proverbe) où elle a des cheueux." Literally, "it must be taken by the forehead (as one says in the popular proverb), where it has hair."

dog days, will I be required to wait for a better time of the year? If the humor is not purged, the illness will twist the body into a rage and will batter down the patient's natural strength (already considerably weakened by the season) in such a way that it will be unable to void any of this foul matter, which in the end will overwhelm the patient. Will we let the patient die for lack of a little assistance, recalling the inappropriateness of [purging during] the dog days. Again, if it were an illness that could be dragged along until after the dog days, there would be some justification for forcing a delay. But when it is a question of either healing or letting the patient die within this time, if purgation seems to be appropriate, there must be no more concern expressed over it; and if the patient dies, it is from the violence of the illness and not because of the remedy.

[On the other hand], anyone prescribing drugs as strong as those used during the times of the year most conducive to supporting laxatives, drugs that attack from all sides and uproot the matter they are sent after, would do so totally in vain, and the damage such action would cause would be completely out of proportion with the desired effect. For Hippocrates views suspiciously the use of medicine during the dog days because of its violent action, for the poor man had only at his disposal those drugs that today we are fearful of using even in winter and on very robust patients. Anyone who takes the trouble to interpret his aphorism in the light of the drugs he was using would still have to hold this same conclusion, that no purging whatsoever must be prescribed during the dog days. For our bodies have little by little become so fragile and weak that we are but children compared to the men of time past. Which of us could endure a bloodletting of six pounds of blood at a time, as Galen witnessed in those of his time? And these people were already no longer as robust as those of Hippocrates's time. Their drugs were so potent by comparison that they horrify us just hearing about them, let alone accommodating them to the dog days. And yet they do not forbid their use entirely, for they merely say that purgation during such a time of the year was troublesome. If they had had access to our cassia, senna, rhubarb, manna, rose syrup, and other light medicines that are harmless, they would not have found it bad to purge during periods of great heat when the particular illnesses call and beg for it.

It must therefore be said, concluding with the truth, that for two reasons the advice given by Hippocrates is not applicable to those who purge today during the dog days, since he does not absolutely forbid laxative medicine but only points out that it must be used carefully, and since we do not use his drugs, for we admit that it would be bad to give them to our patients on dog days.

I will add this for the sake of women, who have more control over this than men (attempting to inform physicians that they must not purge during the dog days): a piece of very helpful advice concerning the health of their husbands. It is that carnal copulation is no less dangerous during the dog days than is purgation. Moreover, the games of love must be entirely suspended where medicine is involved. For one purges for the sake of regaining health, and Dame Venus ruins it. Celsus says that in summer (if it is possible) one must practice complete abstinence, and the common proverb supports this opinion, saying that in summertime one should wet the beak and keep the member dry. Others claim that during the months that do not contain an r, women are out and wine is in.[4] But I am not so strict: I only set aside certain days as dangerous for such business. These are the dog days mentioned above, which deplete the body considerably, tiring and debilitating it a great deal, without its having to work still more for women's appetites. The dog days begin around the twentieth of July and last forty days. They are the Lent or the quarantine of married people, who should during this time abstain totally from the workings of the flesh. This is what women should mainly be busying themselves with (refusing themselves, if they are able to do so), and not contradicting physicians on the subject of purgation or of any other remedies they know how to accommodate to the season, if they have the slightest intelligence.

---

[4] The months whose spelling contains at least one "r" are the same in French as in English. The popular saying Joubert gives contains a rhyme that is lost in translation: "... tous les mois qui n'ont point de R, laisse la femme & prens le verre"; literally, "[during] all the months that have no r, leave your woman and raise your glass."

CHAPTER SEVENTEEN
HOW ONE SHOULD CONDUCT ONESELF ON DAYS WHEN
MEDICINE IS BEING TAKEN. WHETHER ONE MAY
SLEEP AFTERWARD. CONCERNING THE TIME OF DAY FOR
ADMINISTERING A LAXATIVE BROTH. CONCERNING THE
MEALS THAT SHOULD BE TAKEN ON SUCH DAYS.
AND WHY ONE SHOULD NOT GO OUT OF ONE'S ROOM

It seems to me that it would be a good thing to instruct common folk on how they should conduct themselves on the days they take medicine, especially when they are in a neutral state, not sick in bed yet fully under the care of the physician, who in such a case must lead them step by step as he knows is needed, according to the nature of the illness and the condition of the patients. This being the case, I do not want to meddle in the affairs of another.[1] I mean to speak only to those who are attended only by their ordinary servants and who do not know how to take care of themselves or manage on their own when they must take or have already taken medicine.

Such people should know that they ought to have had a light supper the night before, so that the next morning, after having slept soundly, their stomachs are empty. Otherwise, the potency of the medicine, diluted by the as yet undigested food, is weakened and broken. This is why there is the common expression that the day one takes medicine is a day of feasting, because one must fast the day before. In order to swallow it more easily and hardly notice its bad taste, it is a good idea to chew beforehand on some lemon or orange peel or a few cloves. This way, with the mouth distracted and warmed, it will not notice the taste of the remedy as much. And so as not to smell its horrible odor, the glass or goblet must be covered with a cloth soaked in some good rose vinegar, and it would be even better if it were perfumed with musk, if one has the means to do so, and if the patient is not a woman victimized by her womb.

To avoid vomiting, nothing surpasses rinsing out the mouth with some diluted wine or other sweet liquid and then taking a swallow of the wine or of some barley broth, tisane, hydromel, or soup. For this rinses the throat and the esophagus (the canal for food and drink from

---

[1]Joubert's expression is more metaphorical: "*... je ne veux mettre ma faucille en la moisson d'autruy*" ("I do not want to put my sickle in another's harvest").

the mouth to the stomach), in which the traces and sensation of the medicine remain for a long time and are conveyed to the mouth, whence the disgust and the vomiting, especially if the upper sphincter of the stomach (commonly called the heart)[2] is not washed clean of the odious quality of the medicine, for then it will resort to vomiting.

This is the practice I adopt with those who are afraid of throwing up their medicine as they usually have in the past. And I can assure everyone that I have scarcely seen one in a hundred who has vomited following the above procedure. It matters little which liquid is given them, provided it is compatible with the medicine, such as the ones mentioned above, in which it would not be difficult to dissolve a laxative so as to make it more pleasant for the patient to take. There are other remedies to hinder vomiting, such as chewing on an apple, a pear, or some other fruit, and swallowing a little of the juice; sniffing vinegar; soaking the hands in a basin of cold water or covering them with a cloth moistened with diluted vinegar, which is called *oxycrat*;[3] refraining from speaking, spitting, coughing, or otherwise moving the body, and remaining still for a time, then walking about. One of the best remedies is also wrapping the neck in a very hot cloth.

And so this is how to avoid vomiting, which is quite horrible, not only because one suffers the double distaste of taking the medicine and then of throwing it up, but also because one has to start all over again if one has not kept it down for at least an hour or thereabouts. Once this amount of time has gone by, it is no longer necessary to stop the patient from vomiting, since the medicine will not have much more effect than if it were kept for a longer time; at this point vomiting rids the patient of a lot of excrement, which is thus quickly voided, causing considerable relief. And so forcing the patient to keep all of this foul matter inside often provokes worse complications: weakening of the pulse, fainting, cold sweats, severely upset stomach [to the point of] feeling as though it will burst. Since this matter amassed in the stomach is inclined to go up, let it exit in that direction; it would be good riddance. And even if the medicine coming with it has done nothing else, it is far from a total loss. But (as I have said) the medicine will

---

[2]This term is still used in modern French to express the idea of being sick to one's stomach: *avoir mal au coeur*.

[3]Cotgrave gives no single-word translation of this term. Joubert already used it above (chap. 1, n. 3, p. 29). It has no English form.

not fail at the same time to drive out the other humors the other way. For its potency and vapors, spreading throughout the body, perform the main, if not entire, task.

As for sleeping afterward, I am never opposed to it but rather am convinced of its benefits both by reason and by experience. Among those who forbid it, some are afraid that the medicine, activated by the body's natural heat (which is increased internally by sleeping), might become stronger and more violent. And why do they then not prescribe a weaker dose, so that with the sleep (most pleasant to those who take medicine, and especially rhubarb) it will become more vigorous and perform the task expected of it? The others fear, on the contrary, that the medicine will lose its strength, weakened by this same natural heat. And why do they not prescribe a stronger dose, since they think it will lose its strength as the patient sleeps? Or why do all not agree to allow, or even to prescribe, the medicine in the form of pills? It is claimed that, because they melt and their potency is enhanced by the body's natural heat, pills work faster and better.

And is it not just as well that the effect of a potion, a gobbet,[4] or a laxative tablet be quickly excited, so that it will act without delay rather than overwhelming the stomach and the entire body with its presence? Some are afraid because the vapors of the drug enter the brain, which is what induces patients to sleep so strongly that they can scarcely keep awake; they are horribly upset when they are stopped from dozing off. And how can this vapor be harmful? On the contrary, it is most beneficial when we wish to purge the brain. For this vapor makes its way in and pulls or drives out the humors we wish to remove. I agree that when the drug begins to have its effect the patient must no longer be allowed to sleep, unless one wishes to stop its operation, as is sometimes necessary, for sleeping puts a stop to all voidings except sweating. Hippocrates noted this well: "When you wish hellebore to purge more, move the body, and when you wish the purgation to cease, stop the patient from moving and encourage sleep."[5]

There are some who dare claim that through sleep drugs are converted into food (which would cause us to be foiled in our intent),

---

[4] I have used Cotgrave's translation ("gobbet") of Joubert's term *bolus*; the drug was applied to a small piece of food.

[5] Joubert's note: *Aphorisms*, 15, Book 4.

especially if they are weak, such as cassia, manna, tamarinds, senna, rhubarb, and so forth. Oh, such huge amounts of food for dinner! Is it possible for drugs to become food, seeing as they are foreign to our nature and nowise similar in substance to be able to undergo such metamorphosis? These people fail to realize that it was a trick on the part of our ancestors to convince common folk that medicine sometimes turned into food, so that if the drug had the desired effect the patient would not be worried, distraught, and saddened, as if it were supposed to cause damage. For it is the most beautiful and enticing excuse in the world to say that the medicine (which was not potent enough to have any effect) turned into food. Besides, I do not agree that the stomach is more apt at digesting when one sleeps, as I have sufficiently proved in my *Paradoxes*.[6]

But I am forgetting my purpose, for it would seem I am angry with physicians, whom it is not my intention to address in this treatise but, rather, all sorts of other kinds of people, even apothecaries, who, in spite of our warnings, go so far sometimes as to dare tell the patients we are treating that they must not sleep after taking their medicines. This is why I am often forced to write at the end of my prescriptions, *et superdormiat*, that is, "let the patient sleep afterwards." Someone could indeed reply to what I have just said and argue against me that one can be nourished by poison, as we read of an old woman in the city of Athens, fed hemlock since childhood, and of the young Indian woman fed *napel* since childhood and sent to Alexander the Great.[7] And how much more easily converted into food will a purging remedy be, which is classified only halfway between poisons and the human body, as Galen has pointed out in the fifth book of his *On the Virtue of Simple Remedies*.[8]

It is easy to reply to such an objection;[9] it is that poison can never be a nutriment that might be converted into a body substance. The body, however, can well become accustomed to its quality, which

---

[6]Joubert's note: Decade I, Paradox 3 [on Joubert's *Paradoxes*, see *PE*, bk. 1, chap. 2, n. 12 (286)].

[7]For a discussion of this poison, see *PE*, bk. 2, chap. 13, "Whether It Is Possible to Poison a Man through the Venereal Act" (125-29).

[8]Joubert is referring to the *Ars medicinalis*.

[9]Joubert's note: Response.

slowly imprints itself into the spirits, humors, and solid tissues. In the same way, one can become accustomed to the cold, or to the heat of the sun, to moisture, to wind, to work, to any disorder, going about it little by little so as not to be shocked by it. Thus several people are so accustomed to discomfort and to a few illnesses that they no longer even feel them, so long as the pain or the person do not go to extremes.[10] Hence some become so accustomed to clysters, to drugs, and other remedies, that in the end they are no longer affected by them, or very little, except for becoming more resistant to them. For the quality of gradual accustoming over time does not bring about any emotion, movement, or change in the body. But that such poisons here discussed come to be converted into bodily substance (which is the same as saying that they are nourishment) is something not to be at all believed.

On the matter of broth taken before dinner, it is called a lavative,[11] which signifying its use, which is to wash and rinse out the stomach and the bowels, ridding them of any traces of the medicine. This is why it must not be taken so long as the medicine is still in the stomach. For by diluting it, just as when one puts a lot of water in a small amount of wine, the medicine would lose its potency and would never be able to accomplish the desired operation. Now, limiting the amount of time the medicine stays in the stomach is impossible, since the same thing in the same person will sometimes go faster, sometimes slower, according to the particular circumstances. And how much greater diversity indeed must be expected from different drugs in different bodies! Still, one cannot say exactly that broth is to be taken so many minutes or hours after the medicine, as is done among common folk; rather, the time between must be set by an estimation of when the medicine (or most of it) has gone through the stomach. This

---

[10]Joubert's phrase is much more theoretical: *"... si l'obiect ou suiet n'est excessif"* ("... if the object or the subject is not excessive").

[11]Cotgrave does not give the English term, which was probably not in common usage later in the seventeenth century. The *Oxford English Dictionary* shows the word in its medical sense: "A draught to wash down food or medicine," citing James Hart's *Kliniké, or The Diet of the Diseased* (1633): "Now and then they will afford themselves a cup of good liquor, as a lavative, to wash downe this rubbish" (I, viii, 30); and later, "As for the lavative, ordinarily given after purgations ... it is hard to determine the particular houre" (III, xv, 288).

is when it no longer leaves a taste in the mouth by its vapors and when the stomach feels empty after some movement in the bowels, which have voided much more than usual, as is the case with medicine, and after a fair amount of time has passed since taking it. And so, at whatever time this may be, and not sooner, broth must be taken. From the time this broth is taken (which is to rinse, as the term suggests, and clear out the remaining traces of the medicine, more than to nourish, although it does serve that purpose somewhat) until the next meal, one must impose a delay so that the broth can act in the stomach, for it is mainly a question of rinsing and cleaning it out, so that when nourishment arrives it will find the stomach clean and not befouled by medicine, which would pollute the food. Thus eating must be put off until this washing and rinsing is completed, so that the meal will not encounter this broth. Otherwise, it would be as if a wine pot were rinsed and the rinse water were left in it before filling it with good wine.

Now, this broth, whether given in large or small amounts, does not remain in the stomach for more than two hours, just as is the case with the slightest thing one might swallow. This is why I cannot approve of allowing a meal to be taken one-half or a full hour after the lavative. It is true that it is not possible to determine exactly the time to be observed between the broth and the meal, no more than that between the medicine and the broth, but by an estimation one can more or less set the time. One sign is that a long time after taking the broth the stomach feels empty, as when one is hungry. Then the patient must eat, whatever time it might be, the later the better. For a drug taken at five or six in the morning is scarcely out of the stomach by nine or ten. At that time the broth must be taken, which will remain in the stomach for two or three hours, such that mealtime will be about noon or one o'clock. And it is not to be feared that in the meantime the patient who is being purged will experience weakness. For if the body had needed nourishment, it would have taken enough from the broth so as to be able to make it until mealtime. Besides, it is necessary to allow the medicine time to do its work and not to impede nature, which is cooperating (indeed, which is doing the main task) in any purgation. For if the patient eats before the execution is nearly completed, nature, preferring food, will pay little attention to the medicine, which, finding itself acting on its own, is not able to do much.

Indeed, eating is one of the means Mesua teaches us for stopping the action of a drug when it is too violent.[12] This is attributed to mechoachan and is conceded to it in particular;[13] but it is common to all laxatives that their operation is weakened or interrupted if something is eaten or drunk that might come upon them. I will also add the following reason: the stomach loathes and scorns food as long as there remains any trace of medicine, and if the stomach is forced to accept food before it is thoroughly rinsed, rested, and restored, it will not make good use of the food but, rather, will find in it more trouble than sustenance. For this very reason the meal must be very light, because the stomach, all upset by the medicine's passing through it, is not digesting normally. And because medicine heats and dries to a certain extent (which frequently causes one to be thirsty), moistening and cooling agents must be administered in much the same way as with fevers. Thus boiled meat will be better than roasted, along with a soup of lettuce, purslane, sorrel, borage, and so forth. It is also necessary to dilute one's wine, which must be a dull red and fairly aged, and to abstain from any soft and overripe fruits, for fear that runny bowels might follow a purgation. But for dessert a tart pear is allowed, cooked and covered with some tender fennel or, even better, a quince or quince marmalade, so as to tighten and draw up by means of their astringency the tissues that have been slackened by the passing of the medicine and the humors.

As for supper, I do not find that it serves much of a purpose on such a day, so interrupted and with the stomach out of sorts, such that meals cannot be taken at their usual times, unless the medicine was taken two to three hours after midnight the day before, which is not an inopportune time to do so, provided one had not had any supper the evening before. For it could thus be the case that one would be ready

---

[12]Mesua (Iahia ibn-Masawayh) was a Persian Christian physician of the ninth century. He wrote thirty books of *Demonstrations* on various subjects (pharmacopoeia, fevers, food, catarrhs, baths, diarrhea). Several editions of his works appeared in Italy in the late fifteenth and early sixteenth century. His life and *Canons* were published together with Nicolaus Prepositus's *Antidotarium* in 1523 in Lyon, the city in which his three-volume *De re medica* was published in 1548 and his *Receptarium antidotarii* in 1550.

[13]Mechoacan is a variety of weak jalap, the purgative tuberous root of the Mexican *Exogonium jalapa*, named after the town Jalapa, in which it was first discovered.

to have dinner at ten or eleven o'clock and supper between six and seven. There would also be more of a chance of sleeping right after taking the medicine, which is what one would want to do, until the next morning. But since most sick people and others who must take medicine prefer that the apothecary himself bring them their medicines, and since it is too inconvenient for the apothecary to go out before dawn or early in the morning without a pressing reason, this time of day has been chosen as the most agreed upon. Hence it is around the time of the equinox (at which time we suppose that, speaking of the very day itself, it is the most fitting day for purgations that are freely provoked and not forced) that daybreak is at five, and one cannot have dinner before eleven o'clock or noon, according to the calculations I have made. I therefore heartily advise that on that particular day one sups on no more than a strained meat broth, or barley soup made with meat bullion or almond extract, or only toasted bread and sugar. This can be eaten six or seven hours after the noon meal, and then an hour or two later one can go to bed and sleep as soundly as if one had just had a big supper. And if one is thirsty, one can drink a little diluted wine. That is the regimen I prescribe for those who are in my care on those days when medicine is taken, if they wish to follow my instructions, as well as for myself and my family and relatives. It is the true *regimen artis,* which we put at the bottom of our prescriptions. As for the other word, *custodia,* I shall now explain it.

Common folk think that we order people to stay in their rooms solely because the outside air can harm a patient who has taken medicine. This is indeed one of the reasons, but there are others that I shall mention in a moment. As for the air, this point must be noted, whether the weather is variable or stable. For if the air is the same temperature both inside and outside the room (as it most likely is during temperate seasons), how can the outside air be more harmful than that in the room? When the air in the streets is windy, rainy, or colder or warmer than the inside air, which we require to be temperate, either of itself or by artificial means, then there truly is good reason to order the patient who has taken medicine not to go out of the house. For the cold, the wind, or the rain, shocking the pores and penetrating into the body, agitated, opened, and weakened because of the medicine, does it great injury. Heat, likewise, encountering a body that is vulnerable and overheated as a result of medicine can cause fever, severe thirst, weakness, exhaustion, and other troublesome symptoms. The patient must be kept in temperate air of the kind that those who have all the comforts are able to maintain all the time. But if the air is, of itself, everywhere moderate, both inside and outside the house, it cannot harm the patient, and the windows may in this regard be kept open.

But there is another reason for keeping patients indoors: it is that the darkness assists in the purgation insofar as the humors move inward more readily, toward the center of the body in darkness, and are conversely encouraged by brightness and light to move outward. Hence if it is a bright day, and especially if the windows are open and the patient has a pleasant view or is able to look at bright colors, paintings, and other artifacts in the room, this can discreetly thwart the operation of the drug. Thus it is better to keep everything closed, even the windows, and to light a candle, accept to remain for the day in a darkened room, and have no visits, so as to be free of any constraints or any excessive excitement. For that also thwarts the drug's operation or renders it less effective.

The other reasons for not going out of one's room are, first of all,[14] if one goes into town one might at some point have to have a bowel movement, and one will not have the convenience to do so; moreover, excrement that is churning about and held back by force causes a lot of complications, besides the stomachache and the horrid cramps. Second,[15] going into town, along with the hurrying it involves, heats the body unduly and puts it in danger of provoking a fever, since at any rate the body is naturally made hotter and drier by the medicine. Third,[16] if one has business to see to (which cannot honestly be avoided as long as one is able to go out), the mind is taxed and has greater need of relaxation when the body is in distress. These are the points that we must consider. And it is still not enough to rest and keep quiet the day on which one has taken medicine; one must continue to do so until after dinner the next day and must retire early, that is, before sunset.

I was a little prolix in discussing the regimen of the art, which must be observed, we say, when medicine is taken. Since this is most often put under the supervision of apothecaries, to whom our prescriptions

---

[14]Joubert's note: 1 [these numbers appear marginally].

[15]Joubert's note: 2.

[16]Joubert's note: 3.

are addressed for execution, and since most of them understand poorly the directions, it follows that common folk are the more poorly served. Women who treat or care for those who take medicine are even more ignorant. Hence I was obliged to instruct common folk so that each might understand how one should care for oneself. For medicine is a serious matter and can do much harm or much good, depending on whether it is put to good or bad use. One must not forget the cramps that drugs often cause, which we treat with warm cloths applied on the stomach. It is windiness or huge amounts of phlegm that cause these pains, that is, the windiness stirred up by the turbulent matter, and which fill and stretch the bowels just as with colic. The large amounts of phlegm cannot enter into the openings and extremities of the mesaraic veins in the bowels (as they should, if they come from elsewhere) without causing a few violent wringings. We often witness very thick phlegms voided during the last bowel movements, which come neither from the stomach nor from the bowels. For they could not have remained there so long without the medicine's taking hold of them and carrying them out. They therefore come from farther up and must necessarily pass through the small ends of the mesaraic veins, causing no small pain, although they are not as large when they pass through the veins as they are when we see them in the basin. For they are thin upon coming out and later draw up into a larger mass. The warm cloths melt and soften these gross humors and make them flow more gently; the heat also reduces and calms the windiness. In this way the sharp cramps causing the patient such discomfort cease.

CHAPTER EIGHTEEN
WHY IT HAPPENS FREQUENTLY THAT PATIENTS
WHO RECEIVE THE MOST CARE MOST OFTEN DIE

One sees it often to be the case that it is the husband whose wife constantly cherishes and outrageously spoils him who will die sooner (everything else being equal in matters of illnesses, age, condition, and strength of the patient, the climate, the region, the required conveniences, and other particularities) than the husband whose wife would very much like to be a widow. Likewise, the wife whose husband is so in love with her that he seems besotted will die sooner than one whose husband would rather have her in the earth than in the meadow. It is the same with fathers and mothers in regard to their children. For they often lose those they love the most. I am not saying that this is usually the case, but it does happen very often, to the point that common folk complain about it, as if excessive love (and sometimes inordinate) were the cause of death. This is not something I wish to find fault with, knowing that God can be offended and become angry with that extreme affection that takes hold of impassioned people and turns them away from His service (which requires their whole hearts, their every thought, and their whole understanding) and hinders them from humbly accepting His holy will. And so He will often take away from us what is most dear to us in this world, such as an only son, well born and full of hope, so that we will be less happy in this valley of misery and will desire the enjoyment of the object worthy of the excellence of our souls.

Speaking, however, on a more human level, and according to common sense, I do dare to say that the excessive love one has for those who are close, combined with indiscretion and ignorance, often causes the death of those who are loved the most tenderly. For the care and the total responsibility of those who are not loved as much are usually left to physicians and to people attentive to their care, people often called and employed more for the sake of getting rid of the burden than out of any affection, so as to avoid the criticism of having left one's husband, wife, child, or close relative to die without proper care. Now for people like this the physician is free to act in accordance with what is required without having anyone contradict him or check on his procedures, and he practices just as he wishes, for which he receives much more honor than thanks.

But when it is someone who is loved immensely, sometimes too indiscreetly, their common-folk parents, kinsmen, or friends (most of whom are presumptuous, overconfident, and think they know more than Master Mouche)[1] want to understand and know everything prescribed for the patient. They contest, bicker, and bargain over everything, maintaining the physician in fear and distress, arguing with him about each point, either because it is excessive or insufficient. They wish to have their own way in the quantity and even the type of food,

---

[1]Master Mouche (*Maistre mousche*), Cotgrave informs us, was "(the name of a cunning Jugler; hence also) a craftie fellow, subtill companion, slye mate."

in the time and number of meals or in the eating of broth, in the order of foods, in the temperature of the room, in the amount of covers, and in other aspects of the regimen. They blame any accidents that happen, even those that occur frequently, on the poor physician's procedures; and they are so maniacal in scrupling the remedies that the fearful physician dares prescribe only half of what he would normally in order to cure the patient. For in spite of his duties and good procedures some sudden and unexpected serious complication will arrive (as many often do, impossible to predict) or death will occur. Anything unfortunate that happens will be attributed to the physician, and he will be roundly blamed or calumniated if he did anything contrary to the advice of common folk or the attendants. For people have tyrannously usurped the place of physicians, to whom they should be totally disposed, accommodating, obedient, and submissive for the good of the patient; people should in no way be defiant or give the physician reason to fear them but rather should leave them full liberty and sovereign authority. Otherwise, the most worthy physician in the world is but half a physician and can do nothing outstanding because he has lost his boldness, which is an absolute requirement for combatting sickness. And so, forced to bend, comply, and be subject to those who domineer in everything or who hurl out jabbing remarks, the physician dares not press on (let alone constrain or convince), guided by reason to do what he thinks best. Thus many die because of this poor business, most contrarily to the wishes of those who love them inordinately.

Is it not a great pity that ignorant common folk keep the physician (who holds to his honor and reputation more than anything in the world, else he is unworthy of his profession) in such a state of subjection and servitude that he lacks daring and is fearful, even when treating those he holds dear, because of doubts and anxiety? For if his wife, child, or other relative is looked after and treated by him in a way other than that which the idiots presume to know and understand, he will be suspected either of not loving his family very much or of being ill-informed, adventurous, and fearless, to such an extent that even in his own mind, if he were to believe common folk, he would not be a good physician. Now would this not amount to huge disorder and horrible confusion if the one who ought to be obeyed, even admired, without the slightest defiance, either because of his prowess or his ability, were obliged to subject himself to the whims of the most ignorant people in the world, and that such a predicament be to the detriment and harm of poor sick people, who would be much better cared for and much more skillfully treated if the attendants were more careful about the physician's wishes: I mean doing no more or no less than the physician orders.

CHAPTER NINETEEN
AGAINST THOSE WHO MAINTAIN THAT DEATH NEVER COMES WITHOUT REGRET

This remark is too general and is for the most part false. For those who die of extreme old age, and like a candle going out because its wick has no more tallow or wax, die without regret over any procedure practiced in their regimen or treatment. For one must understand what is meant by regret in this instance. Likewise those who are fatally wounded and who are considered dead from the moment they suffer their injuries. For since one abandons any hope of their recovering, one therefore has no regret over one's role in the matter.

There remain those who are considered curable right from the beginning, who, when they end up dying (sometimes as though it were secretly), cause great regret among their friends, who are unable to be consoled.

Now, regret can be of two types, and each one is understandable but not at all common or in every case is not sincere insofar as physicians are concerned, as those who use this word so often would wish. The first kind is that due to the grave mistakes the ill commit, or their friends, when they fail to provide properly and without delay for a good and faithful physician along with everything else required for the recovery of health at the onset of illness. Sometimes the help will be at hand and it will be scorned, just as the illness itself is scorned, which, as it gets worse and finally leads to a death that no one can forestall, causes an extreme regret. In other cases a thousand useless remedies are applied either through ignorance or to comply with the patient's wishes, all of which are very costly and cause huge regret when one learns afterward that this most obviously was the cause of death.

One could not begin to explain the vast diversity of errors committed by patients or by those who care for them, which end up causing

regret over the ensuing death. It is sufficient to have shown that because of these three instances, that of extreme old age, that of people
saddened by an unexpected death, and that of errors committed by
common folk, there will not always be regret over the procedures
practiced by the physician, which is the other type of regret, that occa-
sioned by patients who were thought to be curable. I do not wish to
maintain here that no one dies because of a mistake on the part of a
physician. For I would be doing injury to the more worthy, learned,
and well trained if I considered all those who grant themselves our
status all likewise irreprehensible. Furthermore, I know very well that
ignorant and careless physicians commit such gross errors that the
cemeteries look like hunchbacks because of them; as the ancient author
says, the earth covers the errors of physicians.[1] But it is certain that
the more knowledgeable, prudent, and diligent are very often calumniated and unfairly suspected or accused of the deaths of people they
treated. For although I confess that some patients die from a disease
that was not, or did not seem to be fatal, at the onset, the physician
must nonetheless not be held accountable for it so long as he was not
negligent and went about treatment diligently with proper investigation
and due observation, especially since there is such a vast diversity
among bodies and illnesses that human weakness cannot always manage to comprehend instantly either the nature or the extent of them.
And when God wants to call someone to Himself, He removes all
means of keeping the patient alive, such that one will not even have
the idea of calling upon the help of a physician in time opportune, or
the physician will not be able to properly recognize the illness and the
condition of the patient, or the remedies will not be as effective in this
case as they usually are.

One must therefore not throw the blame on the physician when
someone happens to die for whom one had high hopes from the beginning, nor should one have regrets over his procedures (provided he is

---

[1]Joubert is probably referring to the Greek compiler Stobaeus, whose *Florilegium
Monacense* (217) contains a saying attributed to Nicocles, translated into English as
follows in the 1688 edition of *Wit's Commonwealth*: "Physicians are happy men
because the sun makes manifest what good success soever happeneth in their cures,
and the earth burieth what fault soever they commit."

knowledgeable and skillful, an upright and diligent man as concerned about the patient as he should be) but should accept in a Christian manner that God has thus ruled in the matter according to His will, which alone is just. Whenever one does regret something, one should bear it humanely as an accident and attempt to learn from it so as to avoid it in the future. For this is the way things are in all things, even for the most perspicacious and prudent, to whom many good undertakings finish badly without its being their fault in any way, unless it be that of not being able to divine what the human mind cannot understand through ordinary and legitimate means.

CHAPTER TWENTY
AGAINST THOSE WHO IN ORDER TO HAVE LOOSE BOWELS WALK BAREFOOT ON COLD SURFACES OR DRINK LOTS OF OIL, AND WHAT CONSTITUTES HAVING A HEALTHY STOMACH

It is evident and certain that cold applied to the feet causes the bowels to move. The reason is that the brain, source of all the nerves, gets chilled and catches cold when the extremities of the body, parts full of nerves, are chilled. And this is because of the continuity that exists between such parts and the brain, by means of these nerves. Now, the brain transmits its chill to the stomach and to the entire lower abdomen, to which it is strongly linked by the sixth couple [branching] of nerves. And so what ensues is that the intestines, likewise chilled, do not retain the food long enough for proper mixing and digestion. Hence indigestion follows and a weakness of the stomach, which causes the bowels to run.

And is this healthy? Not so very much. It would be much better to remain constipated, or else to cool ever so slightly the kidneys and the liver with external applications so that the fecal matter does not become foul, which makes it difficult to be voided properly. For this some ordinary rose ointment is enough, and the purple that I describe in my *Dispensatory* is even better.[1]

But to provoke a weakness of the stomach by application of cold to the feet is most ill-advised because the stomach, the bowels, and other parts of the lower abdomen are weakened by it. And, in fact, it is a base trick and a schoolboy's prank used to make one sick so that one can have a reason to be sent home to one's mother for a few days. This type of diarrhea, when the true cause is known, is cured by a good beating. And if one is afraid to uncover the bottom for fear of causing the anus to catch cold or of forcing still more of the fecal matter to the area through which it has been flowing, then the back must be thoroughly whipped, serving as a good revulsion.[2] Still, a whip on the buttocks heats up these parts so well that the chill is driven out quite effectively.

Others drink a dishful of mild olive oil at dinner; still others have a very rich broth or eat a lot of butter. This upsets the stomach with too much laxity, causing it to become weak and not to digest well. For its strength lies in restriction, so as to squeeze the food, which it must embrace and touch from all sides, otherwise there is a fluctuation, making the sound "glug-glug" in the stomach and causing the digestion or churning to be less effective. A medium laxity is the most fitting for the bowels, which perform their function poorly when they retain the excrement for too long a time. Then there follows nausea, dull headaches, depression, and unprovoked wearisomeness. Hence it would be better for those who complain about constipation if this oil, this rich broth, or this copious amount of butter were injected into the bowels with a clyster so as not to have to pass through the stomach. For (as we have said) astriction is good in the stomach, and medium laxity in the bowels. This is something that can be happily achieved through diverse means, such as having an astringent fruit at the end of each meal, or having someone administer a highly mollifying clyster. Such a one would be composed of a dishful of very fatty mutton broth, with

---

[1]Joubert uses the word *dispensaire*. He is referring to his *Pharmacopaea*, published first in Latin in Lyon in 1579 through the intermediary of his student Jean-Paul Zangmaistre, who gave a French translation of the work two years later.

[2]Cotgrave translates Joubert's term *reuulsion* both generally and in the medical sense: "A revulsion, a pulling up, or plucking away; also, the drawing, or forcing of humors from one part of the bodie into another."

a half dishful of very mild oil, or a quarter of a pound of fresh butter, two or three egg yolks, and a dram of salt.[3] This clyster is easy to retain, and if one is a little patient, it can remain in the bowels for over an hour, provided it was taken lying down on the left side (as it must always be the case), and after seven or eight minutes from that position one then turns over on the stomach and remains there for another seven or eight minutes, then again on the right side, and finally on one's back, seven or eight minutes each time. This makes it go through a complete revolution in the bowels and causes the clyster to penetrate throughout the colon and remain there, where it will finally loosen the large and foul excrements. Besides this specific action, the clyster will moisten, soften, and lubricate the bowels so that there will not be any constipation for three or four days.

There remains to determine what constitutes having good bowel movements: whether it means having them softer or harder. They are called soft when they are loose, runny, and turn out matter that is not well bound together; or, conversely, tight. If they are in between, this is commonly called "prize bowels,"[4] and I think that such a condition is properly called good bowel movements, since every good thing consists in being in the mean. But just as of the two vices, which keep to the extremes, one is closer to virtue than the other (as prodigality seems closer to generosity than does avariciousness); similarly, loose bowels are said to be better than constipated ones and are especially more natural, beneficial, and desirable in small children and in anyone who eats a lot. This is why wet nurses say that the child has good bowel movements when it excretes very soft stool, and that children who have loose bowels are much more healthy than the others. Those who are constipated do not live as long and are subject to several illnesses unless they change from this condition, either on their own or through art. And it often happens that (according to Hippocrates's aphorism)[5] those who have moist bowels in their youth have tight ones in their old age, and vice versa. But the most common condition is for old people to be constipated, making them subject to hemorrhoids very

---

[3]Cotgrave confirms both the general and the apothecaries' value of a *dragme*: "A dramme; the eighth part of an ounce, or three scruples; also, a handfull of."

[4]I have thus translated Joubert's expression *benefice de vantre*.

[5]Joubert's note: *Aphorisms*, 20, Book 2.

often, as are pregnant women. The aforementioned clyster will help deter such unpleasant and harmful indispositions in many patients. But pregnant women, if they are the slightest bit subject to overexcitement, must not make use of it, unless it be in extremely small quantities. For in softening the bowels, it could also soften the uterus and dissolve the ligaments, to the child's detriment.

CHAPTER TWENTY-ONE
WHETHER OR NOT OYSTERS AND TRUFFLES
MAKE A MAN MORE LUSTY IN THE VENEREAL ACT

As for oysters on the half-shell, which are the most highly prized, and to which this remark mainly applies, one must consider the water contained in the shell and the type of oyster that is eaten. The water comes from the sea, drawn in by the creature for its nourishment or for some enjoyment, which, inasmuch as it is salty, spurs one a bit in love, just as salt does and all that is salty. Hence shepherds sometimes have their flocks eat salt not only to prod their appetites but also to make them fecund. And poets teach us in this respect that Venus was engendered from the foam of the sea. Moreover, it must be understood that the flesh of oysters has a salty juice, as is witnessed by Galen,[1] by virtue of which also it is able to excite.

But all that counts for little in making a man lusty, and less so (if there is no other element involved) than do anchovies or salted pilchards or a ham. And I think that there is nothing more in oysters that drives men to the venereal act than (perhaps) the windiness they cause, resulting from the pituitousness into which such food converts itself for the most part. They cannot therefore produce much of an effect in love's games, as they would if a lot of semen were engendered from oysters, which is what common folk think and believe firmly. But this is a mistake that is too obvious. For nothing makes semen other than highly nourishing foods, which are turned into wholesome blood. This

---

[1]Joubert's note: Book 3, *On the Faculty of Nourishment* [*De alimentorum facultatibus*; Joubert makes use of Galen's own technique of deductive reasoning so well employed in this work; Galen states (II, viii) that foods that are by nature colder produce more phlegm, consistently referred to as being cold and moist].

is something oysters will not do, but, rather, a good capon will, as will other delicacies: lamb, veal, doves, omelets, fresh pigeons, good bread, good wine, and so forth, in reasonable quantities.

I understand that in Venice people eat oysters just before going to bed so as to be more lusty in their love making; in this they are clearly mistaken. For it would be necessary at the very least that such food be digested and converted into semen before beginning their games, which is impossible for oysters eaten after supper, which take three or four days. For they first must be converted into blood, and the spermatic vessels must then draw it from the liver or from the vena cava, after it has been through many a passage. Then it must spend some time in the testicles or next to them in the spermatic vessels, also called prepara-tories.[2] Thus the oysters will not be making the fellow more lusty on that particular night. For they do not have the exciting effect of can-tharides and other similar drugs that spur people in the games of Ve-nus. And if they are to serve a few days later, after having converted themselves into a lot of sperm (as common folk believe), it would be better to eat them along with other food, and especially at the noon meal, as do most people in our part of the country. For food taken separately on an empty stomach maintains its qualites, virtues, and faculties much better, as can easily be understood. But far be it from oysters to engender a lot of semen (which is a condition proper to very substantial foods); they produce, rather, nothing but coarse and viscous phlegm, as Galen points out in all his books dealing with food, and in particular in the third one, *On the Faculty of Food*,[3] in which he says that oysters are more of a laxative than a food.

I know people will counter, citing experience and common practice in this sphere, to whom I say, if they are more inclined to indulge in coitus and sexual congress because of eating oysters, it is due solely to the heavy vapors and windiness that make the male member stand up, but without much efficaciousness for lack of supporting munitions. The customary herbs would do as much for people if eaten in sufficient quantity, and even better would be certain vegetables, peas, beans, earth nuts, kidney beans, and so forth, which, besides windiness, also provide more nourishment for the body, something oysters will not do.

---

[2] Joubert uses the term *preparans*.

[3] Joubert's note: Chapter 33 [*De alimentorum facultatibus*].

And still more, chestnuts, which make both men and women more lecherous; this is why there are more wet nurses from the mountains than from elsewhere, precisely because of such food. Common folk think oysters are hot and are effective enough in provoking lustiness. But they are sadly mistaken, for they are clearly cold and felt to be as much in the stomach, even when they are eaten raw and without pepper, which is their true condiment or seasoning.

The same is true of truffles, which are also mistakenly thought to be hot and thus apropos for the venereal act. If one is only seeking to become heated, why not use, rather, some good spices or some hippocras, mustard, or garlic, which are clearly unsurpassed in generating heat (the same is true of very vaporous, subtle, and penetrating wine), and forget about oysters and truffles, which must be heated by means of the addition of pepper?

I shall not linger here on the grossest of errors (might I even dare say stupidities, since it is not even founded on common or animal sense?) committed by those who maintain that pepper cools! Yes, about as much as fire. Do you not feel a terrible fire in the mouth and throat when you have taken a little too much? Is that fire cold? If we want to talk like that and change completely the meaning of words for things, then we will also say that cold actually burns. For I know only too well that it is said loosely, especially since it does sometimes produce an effect similar to that of fire because of the way it seems afterward. If, therefore, pepper is the true corrective of oysters and truffles (which everybody will readily grant), and if pepper is very hot according to the perception of the senses—which must be trusted unquestionably—it necessarily follows that oysters and truffles are cold. I spoke of oysters in the sense Galen does. Here is what he says concerning truffles: "They have no outstanding qualities, and yet those who eat them do so for the seasoning that accompanies them, just as one eats other insipid and bland things that are called watery. All of these foods share the common trait of giving no worthwhile nourishment to the body but are on the contrary chilly and loathsome in their own way, namely, more loathsome than truffles, and by nature proportionately more moist and wet than gourds and other vegetables."[4] Truffles are thus a long way from producing a large quantity of sperm or from

---

4Joubert's note: Book 2 of *On the Faculty of Foods*, Chapter 68 [*De alimentorum facultatibus*].

spurring people to the venereal act by virtue of the heat they contain if they are compared to gourds. This reminds me of what the Parasite says in the Italian comedy entitled *Calandra*: "Love is like truffles, which make that thing become erect in the young and belts to tighten in the old."[5] And in fact they are able to engender and produce nothing more than wind and coarse vapors, the same as oysters. This can indeed make people lecherous, but in no way fecund.

My fear is that sterility would more likely come from it, just as it is true that the more lecherous one is the fewer children one has. I could go on at length about the virtues of oysters and truffles, but I reserve this for my *Matinées de l'Ile d'Adam*, in which I treat at length the qualities and virtues of all the foods eaten in France, and the way to make healthy use of them, a work needed as much as any that has yet come to light in the maintenance of good health and in the healing of several illnesses.[6] I am giving it this title because I started and wrote most of it on the Ile d'Adam at the home of Monsieur de Montmorency, Peer and First Marshal of France.[7] May God grant me the grace to be able to finish the little that remains to be done so as to satisfy several people who never cease asking physicians while they are at the table: "Is this bad or unhealthy? What does this do? What does that do?" To such an extent that the poor physician, who often is very hungry but interrupted and distracted over and over in providing answers to these questions, gets up from the table only half fed. From

---

[5]The play from which Joubert cites the Italian (*"L'amore è simile à le tartuffe, lequali fanno à i giouani rizzar quella cosa: & à i vecchi tirar corregie"*), *Calandria*, was written by Cardinal Bibbiena (Bernardo Dovizi, 1470–1520). The title was taken from the main character, Calandro; it was the first Italian play to imitate and comply with classical traditions and unities. Although the subject matter of the play was very licentious, it was staged for the first time in Urbino in 1508 and again in 1513, and even in the Vatican in 1518. It was first printed in Siena in 1521 and then in Venice in 1522. Some twenty-five years later, at the height of the vogue of things Italian in France, it was staged in Lyon at the court of France before Henri II and Catherine de Medici in 1548.

[6]This work by Joubert was never published and has unfortunately been lost. See Amoreux 105.

[7]Laurent Joubert's previously unpublished epitaph of François de Montmorency has been recently reproduced in an article by Gregory de Rocher and Geraldine Bailey, "L'Épitaphe de François de Montmorency par Laurent Joubert," *Bibliothèque d'Humanisme et Renaissance* 55.1 (1993): 77–80.

now on it will be possible to tell these inquisitive people (I except great lords and others who have physicians nearby for their health) to read the *Matinées de l'Ile d'Adam*, which will satisfy all their curiosity. I call them inquisitive, for most of those who ask such questions do not take the trouble to note what the physician tells them but, rather, enjoy the banter, both talking and listening to the physician, who would be as happy dispensing with all of this as was the monk when similarly interrogated. But he got out of this unpleasant circumstance very politely, answering only in monosyllables: "yes, no, white, black, green, gray, brown, long, short, good, stop, dry, soft, cold, hot, nought, well, late, far," and so forth.[8] One particular gentleman got out of it as well when someone wanted to ask him about the nature of oysters. The gentleman had decided to amuse himself by acting as server to the guests he had invited to dinner. After all had been served, he was very hungry and was about to begin, when one of them started going on about the oysters (which they all had on their plates), how their shell closed and aligned so perfectly, closed so tightly, yet opened so easily when fire was applied, whether oysters were truly a fish or an animal, how it lived and what it ate, where its mouth was, whether it was alive as long as its shell remained closed and, consequently, whether we eat them alive and whether they go into our stomachs alive when we swallow them whole, what happens to them then, and so forth. The gentleman was the only one to answer him, since he bore the principal responsibility of conversing with his guests. But when he thought this was starting to become excessive and realized that, because of his guest's drunkeness, each question gave rise to another such that the gentleman was unable to eat, he finally said to the guest: "Goodness, my dear sir, I don't know the first thing about all that; I've never been an oyster."

---

[8]Joubert is referring to the fifty-eighth story ("Du moyne qui respondoit tout par monossylabes rymez") of Bonaventure des Périers's *Nouvelles recreations et joyeux devis* (Lyon, 1558).

TO MONSIEUR FRANÇOIS JOUBERT
CHEVALIER OF THE HOLY SEPULCHER OF JERUSALEM,
COUNSELOR AND PRINCIPAL MASTER OF REQUESTS
IN THE PALACE OF THE KING OF NAVARRE,
CHIEF JUSTICE OF VALENCE
FROM
CHRISTOPHLE DE BEAUCHASTEL,
HIS MOST HUMBLE NEPHEW
GREETINGS

Monsieur,

Since Monsieur Barthélemy Cabrol has indeed dared have printed
and published on the sly a number of chapters from the *Popular Errors
and Common Expressions* set down by Monsieur Joubert (your very
dear brother and my most esteemed uncle), and since he had nonetheless informed me of his intentions, I decided to send him on my own
four additional chapters (so as to make a foursome) I found among the
drafts written by the author. They treat four subjects discussed differently than they are in the first book of the first part. I do not know
whether they were written before or afterward, but it seems to me they
will be judged to be as good or better than the ones the author himself
has had published. Besides, variety is a most pleasant thing. Food may
be prepared in any of several ways, and in each be found quite delightful. Moreover, having seen the catalog that Monsieur Cabrol was
having printed for the *Popular Errors and Common Expressions*,[1] and
which was sent to Monsieur Joubert, I decided to do likewise and
publish a gathering of some others that I had at hand, most of which
have been furnished by Monsieur Jean Momin,[2] doctor of medicine of
the University of Montpellier, a most studious individual. I know that
many of them have been discussed by Monsieur Joubert, who, in
addition, has in complete readiness the five other parts of his work he
has promised us, divided into thirty books. But I do not know when
they will be available. In the meanwhile we can enjoy seeing what
different people have sent him from all over the world, and everyone

---

[1]Beauchastel inverts the two parts of the title in this phrase.

[2]On Jean Momin, see the introduction to *PE* (xxi).

will be encouraged to do likewise, according to his exhortation contained in the First Part, "To the Broad-minded and Studious Reader."[3] And if by chance someone wanted to treat one of these subjects, he is requested to abstain from discussing at the very least the topics that have already been promised to Joubert.

Monsieur Cabrol sent a letter to Monseigneur de Villeroy[4] so that my sire and uncle would not be saddened and angered by his undertaking. In the same spirit I am writing you, whom he honors and respects most highly both because you are his older brother and because of the unparalleled virtues that you possess, if not because you are the most worthy inheritor of the principal wealth of your paternal and maternal estates, Joubert and Genas.

Please take up, then, and maintain the defense of my present enterprise, and if there is any unpleasantness because of it, I beg you to see to my reconciliation, since I am sure it will be most easy for you to do. I for my part pray God that He multiply His graces in your regard, as well as your own prosperity.

From Paris this fifteenth day of February, 1579.

---

[3]For the translation of this letter, see *PE* (24–25).

[4]This letter is translated herein, pp. 4–6.

CHAPTER TWENTY-TWO
AGAINST THOSE WHO MEASURE THE ABILITY
OF A PHYSICIAN BY THE SUCCESS HE ENJOYS, WHICH IS
OFTEN DUE TO LUCK MORE THAN TO KNOWLEDGE[1]

There is no profession more subject to calumny than that of the physician because of the great worth of life and health, valued above all other things in the world. There is therefore no profession in which more people want to meddle, in which there are more busybodies, and about which everyone wishes to know more so as to determine the talent of its professors. Now the most unfair of all allegations is about the success, which often is the result of luck or chance, not of the ability or good procedures of the particular physician. For sometimes we see a sick person recover to whom were given all the wrong things, proving it was the strength of the patient that resisted both the illness and the failures of the physician, just as sometimes the patients escape terrible harm after making some grave mistake but were nonetheless able to overcome it. Moreover, there are physicians so blessed that they frequently meet patients who are curable and are not called upon to treat those who are about to die. This is most fortunate but not usually the case for any general allegations.

And so one must agree that it is care and diligence, accompanied with honesty, prudence, and fidelity. For good and poor success make no distinction between the knowledgeable and the ignorant physician, since the best physician in the world can have bad luck even after having done everthing expected of him. But if he is extremely lucky (which means he is never called in mortal illnesses), then so many frequent good outcomes will be seen that a determination of his talent is possible. In such a matter, when some knowledgeable physician is scorned because he failed to comply with someone's idea or opinion and when an ignorant or worthless one is bragged about for having had better luck in an identical or similar case, I tend to say that the mistakes of a wise doctor make for better stories than the great accomplishments of an ignorant one. And yet the ignorant one preaches about his accomplishments constantly, for they can be easily remembered, and his blunders are innumerable. Of the knowledgeable one, on the other hand, the detractors will always be repeating the mistakes, be

---

[1]This chapter appears in a longer, more elegant version in *PE* (63–65).

they actual (for good old Homer dozes off at times) or fabricated. Also, his heroic cures are countless. Ungrateful common folk forget rather easily the benefits they receive often and retain in memory the most insignificant mistakes.

But in order to reveal very clearly the blunder of judging the ability of a physician on the basis of his success, I need no other argument than the fact that one and the same person will be called a good and a bad physician (a contrary and therefore impossible thing) in this instance. For of a similar illness, suffered at the same time and under the same circumstances, one of two patients will die and the other one will recover, both treated by the same physician, because the illness will be more vehement and the strength weaker in one than in the other, or the same orders will not have been followed in both cases. One therefore cannot determine the ability of a physician by his success, which is all too often more due to luck than to knowledge.

CHAPTER TWENTY-THREE
THAT LAYMEN HAVE LITTLE RESPECT FOR A PHYSICIAN
WHO DOES NOT TREAT ACCORDING TO THEIR DIAGNOSIS;
THAT THE LAST-USED REMEDIES GATHER ALL THE GLORY;
AND HAPPY THE PHYSICIAN WHO ARRIVES
AS THE ILLNESS IS WEAKENING[1]

Just as there is no one more unjust and unreasonable than the ignorant, there is likewise no one more ungrateful and unappreciative. For ignorance blinds one to such an extent that one is insensitive to the value of what is received and feels bound to do just the opposite. In the curing of illnesses common folk (incompetent judges that they are) consider it for little or nothing if we do not cure patients who are in a hopeless condition, or even if we make them recover sooner and easier than they had anticipated. Otherwise they say it is all nature's doing, that youth was on the side of the patients, that it was the good soups, broths, and other foods, or the good care of the attendants that made them get better.

---

[1]This chapter appeared in a greatly expanded version in *PE* (53–56).

In short, the physician will not get one iota of credit but rather will be said to have done more harm than good; and it will often be said that if one had done nothing at all the patient would have recovered sooner, and other similar absurdities that common folk go muttering about. But if the patient is considered to be as good as dead and is then healed, even if the physician did not proceed correctly (provided, however, he continued his visits and always did a little something, whether good or bad, without abandoning the patient completely), he is thought to have done very well, to have brought about a remarkable cure, even a miracle, no less than if he had raised the patient from the dead or absolved him from death, into whose clutches he had already been condemned.

The same is true of violent headaches, earaches, sore eyes, colic, nephritis, gout, and other similar maladies. If the drugs prescribed do not immediately remove or alleviate the pain, the physician is not at all respected, and people will say that in the end the illness went away just as it came, and that the drugs served no purpose whatsoever, even though they were what calmed the pain, but not as soon as one would have liked. For drugs, like every other thing in nature, require time to have their effect. Is there anything in the world as active as fire? Yet, if you wish it to consume and reduce to ashes a huge green log or to melt copper in an instant, you would be unreasonable. And who will say while the fire is working that it is doing nothing? This is why common folk want us to change prescriptions every hour, as if the one being administered were doing nothing. To this the physician must not agree if the drug is appropriate and properly administered, according to the aphorism of Hippocrates, which says that if the remedy does not work as planned, a person who does everything with a plan must not go from remedy to remedy, as long as what seemed appropriate from the beginning is still effective.[2] Nevertheless, in an effort to calm and amuse the patient one can perfectly well prescribe another form of the same remedy and, giving the same quality or type of drug, change frequently the form and preparation.

And here is where another error is uncovered: attributing the recovery to the last drug administered, since it in no way differed from the others in potency, and since all the previous ones played an important part. As when after a hundred blows with an ax a tree falls, it is not

---

[2]Joubert's note: *Aphorisms* 52, Book 2.

the hundredth stroke that did it all, but each of the preceding ninety-nine that did its fair portion. Common folk would wish (and if they are not to be blamed for wishing or desiring, how wrong they are to pester the physician) that just as one breaks a spring or cuts a string one should also be able thus to slice through a disease, which is sometimes as tough and deep-rooted as an old oak tree that will absorb a thousand blows before falling. But little by little, all things are accomplished, and much more surely than through great violence, just as water, which is gentle, wears away and breaks through stone by constantly dripping on it. This calls to mind the common expression: "Happy the physician who arrives as the illness is on the decline." For it is impossible for patients to die of a waning disease, since they had the strength to put up resistance to the onslaught of the illness, as Galen has taught us. Hence those who appear at the tail end of the illness, where there is no longer much challenge, have very little to do. And yet they acquire (fraudulently) a reputation for saving patients' lives, and the other physicians are said to have done nothing worthwhile. This brings us back to our contention that common folk consider a cure worthless if it was done against their opinion. For in the throes of the illness everything is so exaggerated because of worry, sleepless nights, hallucinations, unquenchable thirst, and other such symptoms that common folk expect nothing less than death. If a physician arrives at this point and the patient dies, the ones preceding him are excused or suspected. If the patient gets better (as when after a battery of symptoms, the illness begins to wane, if it is curable), it is the last physician who saved him. And this is how those who have taken the greatest pains in treating the illness are compensated with ingratitude. In this I still excuse the ignorant common folk but not the presumptuous and vain physicians who arrogantly and impudently appropriate for themselves the glory of the healing, even though (if they are not ignorant and gullible) they know full well that it is not rightfully theirs. For arriving at the end, they only gather the fruit of another's labor or of some freak feat of nature.

CHAPTER TWENTY-FOUR
CONCERNING THE IMPORTUNATE AND THE DISTRUSTFUL, WHO CALUMNIATE THE PROCEDURES OF THE PHYSICIAN. CONCERNING THE OVERCONFIDENT AND THE PRESUMPTUOUS, WHO ARE DANGEROUS AROUND A SICK PERSON[1]

The physician suffers no lack of work when, besides the illness he must combat, he finds reticence on the part of the patient or the attendants, or both. For just as he is about to confront the enemy, which he puts before him, he is assailed or distracted from behind and from all sides by the importunity of those who see everything in a bad light and who blame the symptoms, along with the tenacity of the illness, on the physician. For if the fits of fever are more severe after bloodletting or purgation, they murmur or complain that such remedies are to blame. They do not realize that every illness increases in strength up to a certain point, after which, if the illness is curable, it begins its decline. Furthermore, they do not understand that the fits of fever would be even more violent and have a longer increment if such evacuations had been omitted. Nor do they realize that illnesses recur for various reasons, that sometimes they go into remission only to return to wage a more fierce war than before, depending upon how the humors move about and rebel, secretly opposing one another. Sometimes it will happen through misfortune that the drug will be followed by a bloody bowel movement. This condition was already ripe but will be attributed to the drug, which is not at fault. Sometimes a headache will develop, along with vomiting, thirst, stomach cramps, restlessness, insomnia, and other distressing symptoms that were not present at the onset of the illness, since as is most often the case illnesses in their slow beginnings are simple and light.

What will those people say who are suspicious about everything and see everything as provoking in some strange way various symptoms?

---

[1] Of the four chapters appearing in some form, both in *Popular Errors* and in *The Second Part of the Popular Errors*, this chapter resembles its counterpart the least, of which the title was as follows: "Against those who scorn physicians for diagnosing illnesses incorrectly; against those who wish death upon physicians who diagnose their illness as fatal; and whether it is proper for a physician to abandon the patient he judges certain to die." See *PE* (12, 58–63).

They will say this happened after the clyster or after the compress, the unction, the powder, the potion, and the other remedies that will have been prescribed. It is quite true that it did happen afterward, but not that the preceding application was the cause of the development of the condition. Else I will similarly say that the symptom came about after the patient had some broth, or slept, or spoke to someone, and so forth. Only the physician, expert and subtle in the search for causes, and diligent observer of the effects occurring in the course of illnesses, can truly tell where these symptoms originate and whether they are to be attributed to the nature and essence of the disease or to the error of the patient and the attendants or to external factors.

Meanwhile the physician is responsible for everything, and if he is not the object of complaints or blame it is for fear of vexing him, seeing as he is needed. But people do not stop murmuring or expressing regrets about everything. It is the greatest torment imaginable for a physician to be constantly argued with and questioned: "What's this caused by? What's that caused by? He wasn't suffering from that yesterday; it was after such and such a remedy. I told you that would cause him serious complications," and other similar stinging and bitter remarks, most difficult for the good-hearted physician to bear or to swallow when he is trying faithfully to help the patient, when he has all his thoughts stretched and taut like the strings of a pair of virginals,[2] struggling to discover and integrate the means of overcoming the illness in the most expeditious, the surest way possible, and with the least suffering. And what will be the purpose (I ask you) of thus pestering him every moment, of putting everything in doubt and suspicion, other than, in a spirit of defiance, willfulness, or hautiness, making him lose the courage and boldness he must indeed have at his disposal, supported and encouraged by all the attendants, who should not be astonished by any complication whatsoever, so long as the physician, more experienced in the matter, puts their minds at ease.

I will still grant, however, that the physician himself is often at a loss in this, since the diagnosis of illnesses is difficult and uncertain, according to the declaration of the great father Hippocrates.[3] For (as

---

[2]Joubert uses the term *espinette*, which Cotgrave translates as a "paire of Virginalls." Cotgrave also translates *espinette organisée* as "Virginall and wind Instrument ioyned together; a set of Pipes added to a Virginall."

[3]Joubert's note: *Aphorisms,* Book 1, 1.

Celsus has very well demonstrated): "Medicine is a conjectural art, and the reason for the conjecture is that although medicine often serves us well, it sometimes deceives us. But if only a few times and rarely, in a thousand cases, we are mistaken, this is not serious, since it serves us well and is fortunate in helping countless people. What I say applies not only in what is dangerous but also in what is health confirming. For often one's hopes are dashed, and someone dies when the physician was the most sure of a recovery, and things used for treatment sometimes make the illness worse, something human ignorance cannot avoid in such a diversity of diseases. There is nonetheless a credibility in the medical arts in that it most often is successful, and for the great majority of people."[4]

It must be taken for granted that as long as it pleases God (in whose hands the principal things must be entrusted, if not everything), we are able to predict the future on the basis of the present and the past, because of which we are either hopeful or doubtful about the curing of the sick. But there happen along cases so strange and unexpected that the most experienced physicians in the world would not be able to anticipate them. And what would you do then? Nobody could possibly account for it in view of the hundred thousand possible outcomes that we observe in various illnesses. For nature has within it secret movements, and there are sometimes errors resulting from its impotency that offer us no noticeable warning before the actual revelation of the disorder. Then ignorant common folk, full of suspicion, relate it to something that was resolved in a positive way. And then you have another case of heaping blame on the physician.

This case should be seen in quite a different light, and judged most soundly. In spite of good procedures countless accidents can happen,

---

[4]Joubert's note: Book 2, chapter 2 [the celebrated passage from Celsus reads as follows: "... *conjecturalem artem esse medicinam, rationemque conjecturae telem esse, ut quum saepius aliquando responderit, iterdum tamen fallat. Si quid itaque vix in millesimo corpore aliquando decipit, id notam non habet, quum per innumerabiles homines respondeat. Idque non in iis tantum, quae pestifera sunt, dico; sed in iis quoque, quae salutaria. Si quidem etiam spes interdum frustratur, et moritur aliquis, de quo medicus securus primo fuit: quaeque medendi causa reperta sunt, non numquam in pejus alicui convertunt. Neque id evitare humana imbecillitas in tanta varietate corporum potest. Sed est tamen medicinae fides, quae multo saepius, perque multo plures aegros prodest. Neque tamen ignorare oportet, in acutis morbis fallaces magis notas esse et salutis et mortis"* (De medicina, VIII, II, iv, 11.18-31)].

and such is of the nature of illnesses, constantly initiating new attacks and assaults from the side we least expect. Sometimes we think it is finished, and we must start all over again. Illnesses are not enemies that can be seen with the eyes, and whose every design can be understood so as to be able to crush them or prevent them. It is already a lot to be able still to repair the damage they do and finally to make them give way. In the meanwhile thousands and thousands of complications or annoyances can arise that trouble and compromise the cure. Things must be taken in good faith, and without persecuting the physician (who is as sorry over it as anybody), [and there must be] trust that no other remedy could be prescribed than the one being used.

We have attacked the importunate and the distrusting, who never cease supervising the actions of physicians and troubling them by casting doubt on what they do. Now we will talk about the overconfident, the foolhardy, and the presumptuous, who think they know quite a bit about medicine and illnesses, either through observation or through experience, or, for a few, after doing some studies. These are very dangerous people and they exasperate to no end a good physician. Simple people who are ignorant and not overconfident only undertake what is asked of them for the patient, no more and no less, moved by a wise fear of doing something wrong. On the other hand, those who think they know everything and yet have not the slightest foundation are always doing things unseasonably and value nothing other than what they think is right, finding that the physician is very skilled if he agrees with their ideas. If not, he is considered austere, venturous, churlish, and unfriendly by nature. Terence speaks of such people with much precision, saying there is nothing more wicked or unjust than an ignorant man, for he considers nothing to be well done unless he has done it himself.[5]

Thus the only kind of people needed around sick people, in order to serve them, treat them, and care for them, or guide them in their affairs, are well-trained physicians, along with assistants who know nothing except how to execute promptly what is asked of them and who have the ability to understand. For those who know only half-truths or think they know without any foundation are exceptionally dangerous. They are neither hot nor cold but are lukewarm and hence

---

[5]The reference to Terence is from *The Brothers*: *"homine imperito numquam quicquam iniustiust, / qui nisi quod ipse fecit nil rectum putat"* (I, 1. 98).

should be vomited, that is, thrown out of the patient's room.[1] Now, I approve of ignorant people for the caring of the ill, not insofar as they are dull and stupid, but because they understand nothing more than the service required, such as preparing soups exactly as the physician orders, cooking food, making the bed, helping the patient in and out of bed, using with discretion all things prescribed, as will be explained to them by the apothecary, following the orders of the physician. They are able to recall very precisely what happened, either at night or during the day, observing everything very carefully. I also find it very good that they present a few uncertain points to the physician, pointing out to him what he is less likely to know about, since he is not always present and at hand. For having other pursuits keeps him often on the road.

CHAPTER TWENTY-FIVE
THAT IT DOES NOT USUALLY PROFIT PATIENTS
TO HAVE SEVERAL PHYSICIANS[2]

Common folk are gravely mistaken in thinking that the more physicians they have the better treatment they will receive, just as in war the larger number of men you have makes for a greater force. It is true that several people are of the same conviction, but since it is very difficult to find people who have the same opinion in all areas, a multitude is most often harmful, as the good emperor found to be the case, who said on his deathbed: "The participation of too many physicians is what killed me."[3]

I find it very good that at the first sign of a major difficulty one calls upon the advice of a number of learned and experienced people;

---

[1]The reference is to the New Testament, Apocalypse [Revelations] 3:15-17.

[2]A longer and more elegant form of this chapter appeared in the first part of the *Popular Errors* with the following title: "That it does not usually profit patients to have several physicians, but that one physician must be most assiduous in treating them" *PE* (12, 70–72).

[3]The phrase is attributed to the Emperor Hadrian and was frequently cited during the Renaissance: Cornelius Agrippa, for example (*De vanitate scientiarum,* lxxxiii); and Montaigne (*Essais,* II, xxxvii).

but in the execution of the duties of diagnosis and treatment of a sick person, normally there should be only one superintendent of all the details, who, because of his prudence and discretion, adds, decreases, varies, speeds up, slows down, regulates, decides upon, and orders each and every aspect. Otherwise, one does not make much progress, if one person depends upon another or is in conflict with another over something that does not even merit talking about. During such delays a thousand crucial opportunities come by and are lost, at the loss of the patient, who counts on the discretion of those caring for him.

Another big disadvantage with a group is that when physicians are not expressly at the home of a patient and in charge but visit the patient somewhere in the city, since these physicians are on the move, it is unlikely that they will be able to meet at the same time, and if one waits for another, he wastes time that could be needed for other patients. If he does not wait for him, there will not be any discussion or consulting, as the relatives of the patient wish. This is extremely inconvenient for patients and even for physicians. This is why I usually say that a patient who is intent upon being poorly served will have several physicians.

Here is how one ought to proceed. At the very beginning call a small number of them to consult and decide what must be done in order to put the patient on the path of recovery. Then retain the one who seems the most pleasant of them and grant to him alone full discretion in everything. Then if some new complication arises, or if the illness is stubborn, or if the possibility arises for considering other remedies, call the council together once again, which will be from then on the duty of the physician in charge.

MEDLEY
OF OTHER COMMON EXPRESSIONS
AND POPULAR ERRORS

[The seventy expressions already published in the 1578 edition appear once again at this point. Since the only difference between this list as it appears in the Micard edition (1587) and that of the first edition of *Les Erreurs populaires* (1578) is very minor, I am not reproducing the "Medley" in this volume. The minor variation is in the first expression only and is as follows: "Why it is said that marriages in the month of May are unhappy" (1587), as opposed to "Why it is said that many marriages are unlucky" (1578). A translation of the "Medley" appears in *PE* (16-19).]

A GATHERING OF COMMON EXPRESSIONS AND ERRORS
WITH A FEW PROBLEMS SENT BY VARIOUS INDIVIDUALS
TO MONSIEUR JOUBERT

[1.] Village barbers do not want any women's shirts for the purpose of making lint, dressings, pessaries, compresses, and bandages; nor do they want any linen, or any linen stuffing, for the dressing of wounds, ulcers, contusions, and fractures.

2. People who have carbuncles are warned not to pass over any water, neither on a bridge nor in a boat, nor in any other fashion.

3. Why does one's voice become rough from being seen first by a wolf?

4. Why is it that salted meat or fish soaked in sea water is better and more quickly desalted than if soaked in fresh water?

5. Does fish fat bother the stomach more than all other kinds of fat?

6. Once a fish is out of water, it must never be put back in.

7. Dogs go mad from fasting.

8. How is it that by staying up at night one goes mad, if one has the slightest inclination toward madness?

9. Why is it that the more one sleeps the more one wants to sleep, and vice versa?

10. After food and drink, of healthy sleep you'll not have a wink. [*Apres le boire & le repas, le dormir sain ne trouueras.*]

11. How can one have a liver that is hot and a stomach that is cold?

12. Is it true that the younger pigs and lambs are the less good they are to eat, and the opposite with kids and calves?

13. Ewe's wool gathered from the mouth of a wolf generates scads of lice.

14. Why is it that one feels cold and pain more in the ends of the fingers than in other parts of the body?

15. That meat from an animal killed with a single blow is more tender than [that of an animal] killed otherwise.

16. Against those who claim that sick people recover sooner if left to live and do as they please.

17. Why is it that a healthy body cannot with its touch heal a sick one in the same way a sick one can infect a healthy one?

18. Why do people say that those who are cool in summer are very healthy, and that the opposite is true for those who are hot in winter?

19. Must a sickness run its course?

20. Why is the change from hot to cold more dangerous than the change from cold to hot?

21. Why is it not good for small children to look at bright light too long?

22. Why it is said of people who chatter that their feet are hot.

23. It is said that small ears are the sign of a good mind, and also of mischievousness, especially in women.

24. Those who have foreheads with large and prominent veins that swell readily are mischievous.

25. Whether one should drink most [of one's wine] at the beginning of the meal, and whether it should be more or less diluted than what is drunk afterward.

26. Why is it that capons contract gout both more and sooner than roosters; and is castration a remedy for gout?

27. How is straw able to preserve snow and ice, seeing that it makes fruit and cheese ripen?

28. That the first and last chills are the most dangerous.

29. Why is it that the sun of the month of March [causes one to be] more rheumatic than [that] of any other season; and why does one sneeze more in the sun than next to a fire?

30. That a sick person should sleep whenever possible if unable to do so at the appropriate time.

31. That sick people must be believed when they say they are sleepy, thirsty, or in pain.

32. Is it right to say, "What you wore in winter must not be taken off in summer"?

33. There are four bad poisons: peaches, figs, melons, and mushrooms.

34. Why do people say, "Whoever has a fever in the month of May will stay healthy and happy the rest of the year"?

35. Whoever is born on a Sunday will never die of the plague, even if he catches it.

36. People say that most hens and hares are leprous.

37. He is as healthy as a fish and has a stomach as hot as a quail's. He will kill all he sees and eat all he kills and be no more the worse for it.

38. Whether foul-smelling breath can kill a child in the womb, and whether a stinkbug can cause a marriage to end in divorce.

39. Whether it is possible for the hair and the fingernails of a dead person to grow.

40. Is it true that as long as one has relapses, one is still growing?

41. Bad luck for a week, bad luck for a year, bad luck forever.

42. Foolish for a week, foolish for a year, foolish forever.

43. Eggs within the hour, bread within the day, meat within a year, fish within ten.

44. Is it possible to catch the pox by sitting on the privy seat just after it was used by someone with the pox?

45. Whether it is healthier to warm the linens of the sick with a fire made from vine shoots and to perfume them with bran.

46. Whether vision is harmed by parsley and improved by the juice of green grapes.

47. How one can be nourished by clysters.

48. Hippocras drunk in the evening makes the voice raspy and some-times causes quinsy.[1]

---

[1] On quinsy, see *PE*, bk. 1, chap. 5, n. 1 (287).

49. Hyacinth makes one have pleasant dreams, and when an emerald is given to the wife by the husband, it will break the moment she breaks from her marriage.

50. Everything is beautiful about something new; everything is good about something seasoned.

51. An illness never comes unaccompanied, and illness on top of illness does not make for good health.

52. Drugs should come late in the treatment of a deeply rooted disease.

53. Why is it that wine taken internally is harmful to the parts that have nerves but is good for them when used externally?

54. How every poisonous animal carries its own antidote; and why, if the animal dies, so too does its venom.[2]

55. Why people say that since the invention of cutting hair and of wearing slippers, physicians do not travel around much any more on mules.

56. What is the use of taking steel for pale colors; and why do hens that drink water from the forge end up without milt, as the sheep do that graze on the tamarisk near a certain river?

57. Is it true that one must always drink when one is thirsty, and eat when one is hungry, and sleep when one is sleepy, and that one must not stop oneself from eating except to extremes?

58. Why is it said that if a child can get through the first nine days it is out of danger, and why can it be ascertained from this that he was brought to term and was on time?

59. Are there some illnesses of which, after a certain number of days have gone by, the patient cannot die?

---

[2]See Cabrol's "Catalog," no. 98, in the section immediately following.

60. Whether soup that is cold or eaten at the end of the meal is more fattening.

61. In a well-tempered body, does the desire for food and for sleep always come at the same time of day, as is the case with usually waking up at the same time?

62. Why is it that some people who get up early in the morning have a headache for the rest of the day?

63. Why one must not drink or eat after strenuous exercise or when one is sweating.

64. That recovery is often attributed to a change in the air, when it is often no less due to a change in the water.

65. Why do people say that ashes are medicine, and that moldy bread makes one's vision sharper?

66. Whether eating garlic makes one engender male children, and whether it is good for the plague, in which case it is called the theriaca of country folk.

67. Whether a woman's flowers, whether red or white, are increased when she wears a white shirt, and conversely, whether one must change clothes often when one has the mange or the plague.

68. Whether a woman's white flowers are contagious, such that a man can catch a burning piss from them.

69. Why is a person who has fallen from a height wrapped in a sheepskin torn from the animal on the spot; and does a mummy stop blood from clotting in the stomach, which is also said of rennet?

70. Why are men more hot for love in the winter and women more so in the summer?

71. Whether sleeping with an old woman makes a young man sterile.

72. Why is it that the man tires quickly in love's skirmishes but never the woman, and that one rooster is enough for thirteen hens but one woman for fourteen men?

73. Is a piece of toast, a crust of bread, or a drink of cool water after a meal good for a headache?

74. That food well chewed is half-digested.

75. Why do people say [it is better to have] a young barber and an old physician?

76. Handsome at twenty, strong at thirty, wise at forty, rich at fifty, old at sixty.

77. Is it good for children to eat a lot of bread without meat?

78. That water mixed with honey, known as hydromel, is as nourishing [nutritious] as wine.

79. That our whole life is nothing but an illness.

80. That the venereal act is not necessary for the preservation of health.

81. That a black tongue at the onset of an illness is not always a bad sign.

82. Against those who say that a seven-month fetus does not have any fingernails.

83. That extremely cold and clear water is more dangerous than it is praiseworthy.

84. Whether a frost is a good and wholesome thing, both for the healthy and the sick.

85. After a fig, a glass of water; after a melon, a glass of wine.

86. A peacock can be kept for one year.

87. Is it true that if a woman conceives during a waxing moon it will be a boy, and if during a waning moon, a girl?

88. That one must not be apprehensive about everything that can happen, even though what happens to someone might happen to everyone.

89. Is it true that nothing is wholesome that is not wholesome all year long?

90. Concerning those who are buried alive because they are thought to be dead.

91. Is it true that a dog's tongue has medicinal value in curing lesions?

92. Catholicon,[3] holy water of medicine and of taverns.

93. Who hold their urine longer, men or women, and why?

94. Why is it that children's lower teeth appear before the upper ones?

95. What does it mean to make medicine limp along?

96. Whether it is right to say, "Wash your hands often, your feet rarely, and your head never."

97. When one has the plague, one must not blow on one's soup; and it is better to speak more often to God than to men.

98. What is not healthy is hardly wise, for illness forces many an imperfection on people.

---

[3]Cotgrave defines this term as "a certaine composition in Physicke, so tearmed, because it purges all kind of humors."

99. Why people say of those whose stomachs growl that they have frogs inside.[4]

100. Is it bad to heat the stomach after a meal, as if it might hinder or slow down digestion?

101. Whether it is better to study in the evening after supper, or in the morning, and for what kind of people.

102. If a man wishes to eat only once a day, at what time should he have his meal?

103. Whether drinking water is good for the liver and the eyes, and whether it is harmful for the stomach and the womb.

104. Is it true that a quartan fever goes away with excesses and drunkenness, and that it never announces its coming, and that a man is the stronger the rest of his life for having had it?

105. How is it that if one misses one's meal at the usual time, one loses one's appetite?

106. Whether one can piss wine from too much drinking, or blood from too much embracing.

107. That wine drunk without moderation shortens one's life span, just as does quicklime put at the base of a tree.

108. Whether light from an oil lamp is better for studying than that of a candle.

109. Whether it is good for a man with scurvy to get up in the morning and go walking.

110. Whether one should eat little, drink little, and do a lot of exercise in the house on rainy days.

---

[4]This is still the familiar French expression for a noisy stomach.

111. Is it true that those who do not eat a lot are not vigorous in their work?

112. Whether wheat bread obstructs; whether rye bread loosens the bowels and heals hemorrhoids; whether barley or millet bread constipates; whether homemade bread is more wholesome than the baker's; and whether a little bran in the bread makes the bowels move.

113. Why those who have bad lungs or a bad liver have a preference for wine that is not diluted; and why some people wet the bed if they put water in their wine.

114. Why is it that muscatel [*vin musquat*] makes one drunk faster and for a longer time if one adds water to it?

115. Is it good to take a hefty drink of undiluted wine upon sitting down at the table, before eating, in order to loosen the bowels?

116. Why do more people die during the night than during the day?

117. Why is it that the dew of the moon [causes one to be] more rheumatic than [does] that of the sun, and that the morning is cooler than the night, even when night is still the farthest from the sun?

118. Why do people say that gout is the illness of the rich and the mange that of the poor; and yet is it not the beggars who get the most pleasure out of scratching themselves?

119. Why are lepers more lusty than healthy people and less susceptible to catching lice, fevers, the plague, and other contagious illnesses?

120. Whether those whom the Gascons call "Capots"[5] are truly lepers, and where they come from.

121. Whether one can be a leper without having the sores on the face, which are considered the unequivocal signs of the disease.

---

[5]Cotgrave translates this term as "a White Leaper."

122. Why is the great pox on the decline and more easily healed now than it used to be?

123. Why is it that those who suffer from the gout, the pox, and a broken bone feel a coming change in the weather?

124. Why is it that in regions where good wines are produced, people drink less of it than elsewhere?

125. Why do people say that the Spaniard eats, the German drinks, and the Frenchman does what others do and is called the monkey of other countries?

126. That going to bed after eating milk curds is like taking poison, and [that going to bed] after drunkenness is like taking medicine, especially if the drunkard has vomited, or if a bucket of water has been thrown on his shameful parts.

127. Is it within the power of a woman to become sick and to recover whenever she wishes, according to the old saying?

128. Why do people say, "Garlic and onions for the Gascons, tripe and blood sausage for the Limousines"? And [why people say] that a Limousine is a great bread-eater, an inhabitant of Bordeaux a great meat-eater, a Spaniard a great salad-eater, an Italian a great sauce-eater, and an inhabitant of the Cévennes a great chestnut-eater.

129. Why is it that there are so many people with gout in Bordeaux, so many people with hernias in Montpellier, so many people with goiters in Savoy, so many mad people in Béarn, so many fools in the outskirts of Montpellier (where they are called dolts),[6] so many epileptics in Tuscany, especially in Florence, so many people with the king's evil [*les escrouëlles*] in Spain, so many people with phthisis in Portugal, and so many lepers in the Limousine region?

---

[6]Cotgrave gives an interesting list of terms to translate *bauch* (also spelled *bauc*): "A sot, asse, doult, dull-pated noddipeake, heavie-headed cokes, grosse-headed coxcombe."

130. Why it is that keeping the head covered too much makes the hair turn white, and whether cold on the head causes a loss of memory.

131. Is it true that frequent coitus and taking medicine often make people age?

132. How is children's urine good for a cold?

133. Whether a venom can be engendered in our bodies, and whether the incubus is a spirit.

134. Must the practice of bleeding people once a year as a preventive measure be continued every year thereafter, lest they fall ill?

135. Whether it is good for people who are fat, plump, and sleepy to get angry often, and for those who are impudent to be sad, and whether the company of women is of any use to the melancholic.

136. Why is it that a contagious illness passes from an older person to a younger one, rather than vice versa?

137. Is it better to let a man live as he sees fit, even if it is bad, than to make him change all of a sudden?

138. Whether it is true that well water is warmer in winter and colder in summer, or whether it simply seems so.

139. Whether it is good to allow children to go bare-headed, and whether it was wise to do what they did in England in the past in plunging them in cold water.

140. Is it true that what is pleasant to the taste is good for the stomach?

141. Why is it that women talk more than men and are usually more beautiful?

142. Is it true that women are less ingenious and less energetic than men and are more avaricious and stubborn?

143. Is it fair to say, "Wing of a partridge, thigh of a capon; tail of a fish, head of a salmon"?

144. Why did a great physician once say that partridges engender lice?

145. That the meat closest to the bone is the best; and that a roast is usually tougher than a broth [see no. 199].

146. That sugar given to children stops them from catching worms, but that if they already have them, it makes them worse.

147. Sugar never ruins a sauce.

148. Why do people fear that, by screaming too much, children get hernias, especially if they are males?

149. Whether it is a good sign if the child wants to suckle when it pisses a lot.

150. Is it true that midwives are able to form a child's limbs as they are being born; and that they are able to make them stupid by pressing on the cranium or make them faint often and vomit by squeezing the stomach sphincter?

151. Is it true that tight swaddling clothes stop children from growing; and that one should pull over its eyes the hat of a child that holds its head down, so that it will form the habit of holding its head up?

152. Is it true that cold meat stimulates the appetite, and that hot soup at the beginning of a meal ruins it; that undiluted wine makes one eat less, and that water on the other hand makes people ravenous?

153. Why do people say of a person who feels a coming change in the weather, "He has an almanac in his head"?

154. Is it true that tying the garters very tight makes the blood rise to the head and the face turn red?

155. That phlegmatic people live a long time but are susceptible to a lot of diseases, and vice versa for the choleric.

156. Should one eat foods that are easier to digest at the beginning of a meal, except when the stomach is full of bile?

157. Is it true that a choleric person will be poisoned more easily than some other kind?

158. Why is it that eight-month fetuses do not live?

159. Why is it that a man is stronger when angry or frenetic than when calm and reasonable?

160. Why do people say, "Swine wine, lion wine, and monkey wine"?[7]

161. Is fish more tasty cooked in butter or in oil?

162. Why do people have so many covers when they sleep, and why do they say, "Velvet robe, bench belly"?

163. Why do people like to have different kinds of food but do not tire of bread?

164. Why do people say, "Different bread, the usual wine"?

165. Why do people say, "Bread a day old, flour a month old, and wine a year old"?

166. Why is it that a quince eaten at the beginning of a meal constipates and at the end of a meal makes the bowels move?

---

[7]Cotgrave gives over fifty expressions containing the word *wine*. He defines the three expressions as follows: "*Vin de porceau*. Which makes the drunkard to sleepe, vomit, and tumble him in his vomit ... *Vin de Lion*. Strong, and headie wine; or, such wine as makes the drinker a swaggerer ... *Vin de singe*. Wine which makes the drinker (or drunkard) pleasant, wanton, or toyish."

167. Why do people say, "Between two small men there is a bragger, and between two bruisers a clown"?

168. Why people say that those who eat while standing or while walking eat more, and whether the custom of the ancients, who ate lying on a bed or on the ground, was praiseworthy.

169. How is it that lettuce seeds eaten with an egg three mornings in a row makes a woman have an abundant supply of milk?

170. Why is it that a relapse is more dangerous than the first stage of the disease?

171. Why is it that tertian fevers usually cause one to be constipated?

172. Why is it that the very young and the very old are more susceptible to illnesses than others?

173. Why do birds drink so little and wolves eat so much?

174. Why are all children born with large heads and flat faces?

175. Why are those who go around with their belts tight at the waist more prone to lechery?

176. If our bones are without feeling, why do we feel such pain in our teeth?

177. Why is it that animals procreated from different species, such as mules, are sterile?

178. What role can the forehead play in headaches?

179. Why do males grow more often inside the womb and females outside?

180. Why does every animal refuse coitus during gestation and at certain other times, while women do not?

181. Why is it not good to talk a lot while eating?

182. How does panada[8] help loose bowels?

183. Is man inferior to animals in that he knows by instinct of no remedies for his illnesses, as do the other animals?

184. Why is it that sweet wine is called old wives' wine?[9]

185. Why do people say, "A clerk's lunch, a lawyer's dinner, an old wife's snack, a merchant's supper, and a wet nurse's late-night dinner"?

186. Why do people say that the melancholic person eats, the choleric drinks, and the phlegmatic sleeps?

187. Why is it that children eat a lot, drink little, and do not cease to trot about?

188. Why is it that when one drinks wine one feels it immediately in a wound or in one's gout, even though it is still in the stomach?

189. That it is not so astonishing to see an ostrich digest iron since hens are able to do the same.

190. That laughter and being cheerful stop one from aging.

191. Why is it that our teeth hurt if a plate or some other thing is scraped with a knife?

192. Why is it that swimming in rivers causes one to become ravenous?

---

[8]Cotgrave translates Joubert's term *panade* as follows: "A Panado; crummes of bread (and currans) moistened, or brewed with water."

[9]Cotgrave translates Joubert's expression *vin de commeres* as "palate wine, sweet and pleasant wine."

193. Why is it said of people whose feet stink that they are in good health?

194. Why do those who have large livers eat a lot, and those who have large hearts are bashful and have faint pulses?

195. Does drinking water at bedtime make one fall asleep?

196. Why are widows and nuns more susceptible to suffocation of the womb than married women, and does the sniffing of foul odors do any good in recovering from this condition?

197. Why is it that children are more susceptible to the mange, to worms, and to epilepsy; young people, to fevers and hemorrhages; old people, to coughing and the gout; and women, to stomachaches and headaches?

198. Is it true that those who blow their noses hard are more healthy than those who spit a lot?

199. Is it true that the best meat is closest to the bone; and that in the fish the best is near the tail, in a partridge, the wing, in a capon, the thigh, and in a woodcock, the shit? [see no. 145].

200. Thighs are good when wings are eaten.

201. Whether twins are the result of one act of coitus or of several (according to Hippocrates) through superfetation; and whether there can be a five-month fetus, just as some grain is sown in the earth earlier than others.

202. Is it better in times of the plague for there to be a wind or for it to be calm?

203. Why is it so bad to sleep during the day or in the evening or immediately after a meal?

204. Why do fat people and skinny people have smellier pubes than others?

205. Why is it that those who drink water and who stay up and work eat more, and that those who drink wine hardly eat at all?

206. Why will one sooner do without food than without water?

207. Why do people say that dancing comes from the belly?

208. Can a physician heal the passions of the mind, given the fact that he treats only the body?

209. Why is it that some people sleep and move their legs while sleeping; and why does a child often have a fright when sleeping?

210. Why do people say of a man who is magnanimous and generous that he has a great heart, given the fact that those who have small hearts are the most hardy?

211. Why is it sometimes said that some people's eyes are bigger than their stomachs?

212. Why do people say, "Pears cause stones, walnuts ruin the voice, wine makes blood, water makes one thin, happiness makes one fat, and sleep nourishes"?

213. Is it not important to cure the mange children catch on their scalps?

214. Whether one should let a cold run its course.

215. Is it true that pale women enjoy coitus more than those with a ruddy complexion, and skinny ones more than fat ones, and that small women are more fecund than tall ones, and skinny ones more than fat ones?

216. Why is it that one says, "Shitty Parisian, farty Champenois, pissy little girl, bleary-eyed old man, crappy child"?

217. Why are old people so fussy and always only praising the old days?

218. Why is it that fish begin to go bad in the head, and other animals in the stomach?

219. Should one eat a lot in times of the plague, or should one lose weight?

220. Why does a small crumb of bread put in milk make it sour?

221. Whether it is true that one of the worms that glow in the night in summer will stop milk from curdling if it gets into the house.

222. Is it true that man drinks more than all the other animals, and that his stool is much smellier because of the diversity of his food?

223. Is it true that animals that eat the meat of their own kind become leprous, and that if men did likewise the same would happen to them?

224. Is it good to wear one's belt tightly in order to avoid feeling so hungry, and to eat paper so as not to quell one's thirst?

225. Why do people say that in times of war one must neither eat nor sow mint?

226. Why do birds speak rather than other animals?

227. Why are breezes bad for the chest and southerly winds bad for the head?

228. Why new wine makes one so drunk, and how its vapors can suffocate a person when it is fermenting violently.

229. Is it true that oil is better at the beginning [of a meal], wine at the middle, and honey at the end?

230. Is it a better sign during a fever if the worms come out alive or dead?

231. Why man is more susceptible to illness than the other animals, and why he does not live as long as a raven, a crow, a deer, etc.

232. Why is it that animals feel a coming change in the weather sooner than do men, and plants sooner than do animals?

233. Why is it that the longer urine is held the more it smells, and vice versa with stool?

234. Why is it that lepers are not as susceptible as others to fevers, do not catch the plague as quickly, and do not have as many lice as other people?

235. Do the other animals dream, as man does?

236. Do dreams come from what we have previously seen and heard, or from what we desire, or from the condition of our humors, or from divine inspiration?

237. Is it true that undiluted wine goes bad more often?

238. Why is it that those who have a mutilated limb become fatter in the other parts of the body?

239. Is it better to eat less and more often, rather than in some other way?

240. Is it better to drink less and frequently, as do the Germans, or in large quantities, as do the French? And is it better to put water in the wine or to drink the wine first and the water afterward, in the Greek fashion?

241. Fire, love, and a cough are easily recognized.

242. Why do people say, "Whoever wishes me ill makes me blanch, and whoever wishes me well makes me blush"?

243. Is it right to say, "Dress warm, eat scrimpingly"?

244. That the sepulcher, the vulva, dry earth, the sea, and fire never say, "Enough!"

245. What it means to say, "For a single pleasure a thousand sorrows." And whether the consolation of the wretched is to have company ["misery loves company"].

246. Why do people say, "He lies like a tooth-puller"?

247. Why do people say, "From the confessor, the physician, and the lawyer nothing should be kept"?

248. Why do people say, "Healthy as a fish"?

249. Why is it that children, old people, and the ill are unable to reproduce?

250. Is it true that man is a little world, and that all the animals are inside him, both in form and in behavior, as can be seen in his physiognomy?

251. Is it true that men have the same character as the horses of their region?

252. Why do people say that a lot of children is the wealth of the poor?

253. Why are women wider from the waist down and men from the waist up? And why do almost all women wear no garters?

254. Why is it that holding one's breath makes one's hearing sharper, and closing one eye makes one's vision better in the other?

255. Is it true that diluted wine makes one vomit?

256. Why is it that, except for cows, males are larger then females and have deeper voices?

257. That animals have nocturnal emissions.

258. That twins are usually not nearly as strong as other children.

259. Why do old people hold a thing far from their eyes when they want to look at it?

260. Why do people say, "Salute a bearded woman from afar and with three stones in your hand"?

261. Why is it that love makes a coward brave, a melancholic joyful, and a dullard articulate?

262. Why does white wine make one piss more than does another kind?

263. Why is it that after one eats salad or soft fruits, wine has a bad taste?

264. Is it true that those who like vinegar and salt a lot are in bad health and have diseased livers?

265. Is it true that eating pigeons makes one talk big?

266. Why do people say, "When you speak of the wolf, you see his tail"?

267. Whether drinking before eating is unhealthy.

268. That there is no better cosmetic than being healthy.[10]

269. That vinegar is the death of a choleric disposition and the life of a melancholic one.

270. That a well from which water is drawn often gives better water.

271. Why is it that bastards are most often more intelligent than legitimate children, and also stronger, meaner, and very often left-handed?

---

[10]Joubert's term is *embonpoint*, which literally means "plumpness" but which must be seen in its historical context, as Cotgrave can bear witness: "Fullnesse, plumpnesse, healthfull estate, good liking, sound disposition, of the bodie."

272. Why do people say that a woman has the face of an angel, the mind of a devil, and the eye of a basilisk?

273. Does food that is too refined corrupt a good mind?

274. Is the blood of a bull poisonous?

275. That the odor alone of a drug can purge a person sufficiently.

276. Why is it that children learn things by heart quickly but do not retain them for long, and old people vice versa?

277. Why is it that children like bits of bacon and old people do not?

278. Why is it that one who has good judgment does not have a good memory, and vice versa?

279. Is it true that the bite of every animal, including man, is venomous, and why does a person bitten by a rabid dog seem to see the dog's reflection in water?

280. What good does it do to put butter and batting on the bottom of children's feet to stop them from catching cold, and to put coral rosaries on their arms and around their necks to protect them from venoms?

281. How does aconite drive venom from the body, but why, if there is no venom, will it act as poison?[11]

282. Why does one hear better at night than during the day?

283. Why are sea animals healthier than land animals?

284. That animals are all physicians.

---

[11]Joubert mentions aconite in *PE*, bk. 2, chap. 13 (126). Cotgrave defines the term *aconitum* as "a most venemous hearbe; of two principall kinds, *viz.* Libbards-bane, and Wolfe-bane."

285. What is the meaning of "The stomach has no ears"?

286. Whether it is true that one must put no salt in the soup of sick people if they have a fever, nor any herbs if they have a runny stool; and whether it is allowed to add a little pork or beef to take away the bad taste.

287. Why is it that castrated animals have more tender and flavorful meat?

288. Why women are more choleric than men, and more so when sick than when healthy.

289. Why it is that hemlock cannot be harmful if one drinks wine afterward, and whether it is more poisonous if mixed with wine.

290. Why is it that the bodies of people who were killed by lightning keep for a long time without decomposing?

291. Why does one change color in the face more than in the other parts of the body?

292. Should one force oneself to eat if one is not hungry?

293. Why is it difficult for women to get drunk and easy for old people?

294. Whether grapes are better fresh or after having been dried.

295. Why is it that certain people have a bowel movement only after eating?

296. Which is more necessary for human life, water or fire?

297. Why is water better when it comes from springs facing the east?

298. How can the urine of bats and the stool of swallows cause one to lose one's sight?

299. Whether freshly picked fruit causes one to dream, and beans also.

300. How clothes keep one cool in summer and warm in winter. And how one's breath can both cool and warm.

301. Whether a healthy man has need of a physician.

302. Why does one eat more in autumn than in other seasons?

303. Why is it that those who sail vomit?

304. How the odor of roses can cure a headache and the smell of flowers can keep one from getting drunk.

305. Which is better after a meal, a walk or a nap?

306. Does the child breathe in the womb of the mother?

307. Is it true that sadness stops a woman from conceiving?

308. Is it healthier to live inside or outside the city?

309. Whether wine should be followed by more wine.

310. Is it right to say that one must live according to reason and not one's appetite?

311. Why does one get tired sooner walking on a flat and straight road than on a varied one?

312. Why is it that animals are susceptible to but a few diseases (as dogs are to rabies, goats to the mange, swine to leprosy) and man to a thousand kinds of illnesses?

313. Why do women fear so much having cold water splashed in their faces?

314. Is it possible to pass something through one's bowels as soon as one swallows it, and to piss a liquid as one is drinking it?

315. When one has been burned, is it good to bring fire near the area affected?

316. Why is well water more likely to cause colic than water from a spring?

317. Why does man have a larger brain than that of any other animal?

318. Is it true that a woman is in greater danger when she aborts than when she carries to term?

319. Why do people say, "He's as thirsty as a dead man" and "He drinks like a templar"?

320. Why is it that dogs always have a cold nose?

321. Is it true that by eating bread crusts and sinews or sinewy parts one will become strong?

322. Is it true that wine makes good blood, and good blood makes for sharp intelligence?

323. Why do people say, "Food that is well prepared never hurt anyone"?

324. Why do people say, "The beans are flowering, he must be very much afraid"?

325. What is the origin of the expression "He's talkative; his feet are hot"?

326. Is it true that raw chestnuts give one lice?

327. Why do people say, "Never does one eat cheese without being ashamed of it or hurt by it"?[12]

---

[12]In French this expression is a rhyming couplet.

328. Why do people say, "A fresh-water physician"?[1]

329. Whether it is good to sleep after having milk, barley soup, broth, bouillon or a preparative, and other things one eats in the morning.

330. Is it right to say, "More rhubarb and fewer diets"?

331. Why do people say that shit sustains one?

332. Why do people say of people who have green eyes that everything good is distasteful to them?

333. Is it healthier to get up in the morning or to sleep in?

CATALOG OF SEVERAL DIFFERENT POPULAR ERRORS AND SAYINGS GATHERED FROM SEVERAL PEOPLE AND GIVEN TO MONSIEUR JOUBERT BY MONSIEUR BARTHÉLEMY CABROL

1. Soup before and soup after makes a man live for a hundred years, or thereabouts.[2]

2. When the leaf rises and falls, man too falls and falls again.[3]

3. What does not keep forever does not keep well.

4. Gluttons dig their graves with their own teeth.

---

[1]Cotgrave gives a rather long explanation of this expression: "An unskilfull, or unexperienced Phisition, a duncicall dog-leach; one that hath not trauelled farre for the (little) skill he hath: (*Asclepiades*, a better Orator then Phisition (as *Plinie* reports) was the first that allowed a Patient to drinke cold water; and thereupon caused himselfe to be tearmed, The fresh-water Phisition.)"

[2]In French the expression is an octosyllabic rhyming couplet.

[3]Imperfect rhyming couplet.

5. One must die with one's blood.

6. Drinking after having one's soup troubles one's vision.

7. [Whether] it is proper to give a drink to those who have hot lungs for fear the heat might remain in the tankard.

8. Easy come, easy go. It's better to have cheese than broth.

9. A man with gout is a sign of money.

10. If the blood is thin, more of it must be drawn.

11. Minced meat, jellies, and partridges have red stomachs.

12. People with weak constitutions are the ass's bridge of health.

13. A skinny woman is a tavern of blood.

14. Thick evening dew engenders catarrhs.

15. There is nothing like an old spinster for making a lot of children.

16. Neither when cold nor hot, attempt bloodletting one must not.

17. Sleeping after their pablum, children will get fat; and sleeping after having nursed makes children wake up in the morning; and sleeping after taking their milk is the ideal.

18. A milk enema is in no way harmful.

19. The day on which one's medicine is to be taken is a great feast because it is necessary to fast the day before.

20. A raw egg cleans out the heart.

21. Cake, a weight on the stomach; and vinegar, enemy of nature.

22. When the stool is runny, one should only drink water.

23. Whoever drinks verjuice[4] will piss vinegar.

24. When one is sick to one's stomach, one should sleep.[5]

25. Keep your feet warm, and your head; for the rest, live like an animal.

26. Illnesses whose names end in *ique* make a mockery of physicians.[6]

27. Whether it is true that a leper has no feeling, and that he has a lot of blood.

28. Whether it is true that the very deep and rigid curtsies,[7] along with the squeezing of the body, are the cause of many girls' being hunchbacked, and that children are more often hunchbacked on the right side because of wet nurses.

29. That it is not good to keep children bound and wrapped tight in their swaddling clothes for a long time, and especially not in summer; that such a practice can make them susceptible to kidney stones and other diseases.

30. That the impatience of sick people sometimes makes the illnesses become long and sometimes makes them fatal.

---

[4]Cotgrave translates the term *verjus* of this expression as follows: "Veriuyce; especially that which is made of sowre, and unripe grapes; also, the grapes whereof it is made."

[5]Literally, "nausea wants to sleep."

[6]Cotgrave, as is often the case, sheds much light not only on the word *nique* but on the entire expression as well: "*Nique. faire la nique,* To mock by nodding, or lifting up of the chinne; or more properly, to threaten or defie, by putting the thumbe naile into the mouth, and with a ierke (from th'upper teeth) make it to knacke. *Les maux terminez en ique font au medecin la nique: Prov.* Such be *Hydropique, Hectique, Paralitique, Apoplectique, Lethargique,* &c, because they are hardly, or neuer, cured."

[7]Cabrol's text uses *reuerences fort basses*; Cotgrave translates *"Faire la reuerence á"* as "to arise, giue place, make courtesie, vaile bonnet, unto; to solicite with cap and knee."

31. Why it is that the preservation of fish is more troublesome than that of meat.

32. Why do people say, "Apostemes[8] are decoctions"?[9]

33. Whether it is right to say that putting on a clean shirt every day makes one thinner, and that the spinning done by women and the use of walnut oil [make one thinner].

34. Whether it is true that cutting and shaving one's hair frequently makes it turn white and makes one's whiskers become thicker.

35. Against those who claim that the heart grows by a dram[10] each year until the fiftieth and then it shrinks.

36. Whether it is true that in male twins one is unable to reproduce and, similarly, in female twins one is unable to conceive; and whether twins are unable to produce other twins.

37. Is it true that children born in the seventh month or at any other time before their term are always sick and in danger of death until they complete the time they were supposed to spend in the womb?

38. Is it true that seventh-month children are born without fingernails, [as are] those whose mothers ate a lot of salt while pregnant?[11]

39. Whether combing one's hair on Friday causes a headache; and whether it is bad luck to put on a clean shirt on that day.

---

[8]On apostemes, see *PE,* bk. 4, chap. 11, n. 4 (314).

[9]Cabrol's term is *apozemes*; Cotgrave gives the following translation: "A decoction, of water with diuers sorts of hearbes and spices, used instead of a syrop." The sense of the expression is that abscesses function as a drawing agent, attracting the poisons in the body.

[10]On the word *dram*, see n. 3 of chap. 14 above ("That bloodletting can be used on pregnant women, children, and the elderly").

[11]See no. 82 in "Gathering," the section immediately preceding.

40. Friday is the most beautiful or the most ugly day of the entire week, and never was there a Saturday when one did not see the sun.

41. Why is it that a piece of iron or glass put among burning coals stops one from becoming heavy-headed?

42. Why is it that all children are dwarfs, that is, short-armed and short-legged in proportion to their bodies?

43. Why is it that a cough becomes worse if one touches the forward part of the ear canal, and that sneezing becomes worse if one pricks one's nose?

44. Why do those who recover from long illnesses seem larger, even if they ate very little?

45. Against those who think that it is a sign of health to be cold after a meal.

46. How having one's body tightly bound can cause obstructions.

47. Why it is that an iron spoon will stop peas and rice from cooking?

48. Which is more nourishing, cold meat or hot meat?

49. Is it possible to hear the cries of a child inside its mother's belly?

50. Why is milk that curdles in the stomach considered bad, since curdled milk and cheese are easily digested?

51. Is it true that one hour of sleep before midnight is better than three after midnight?

52. Whoever wants to be old for a long time has to begin very early.

53. In perilous diseases he who does nothing does enough.

54. Medicine and war are practiced according to circumstances.

55. Why do people say that water-drinkers never need anyone else's feet?

56. Why do people say that wine is the yeast of melancholy?

57. Wanting to recover is a part of health.

58. Where there is both youth and wealth, there is illness aplenty.

59. Is it true that during a general famine people are hungrier than in normal times, even though food is not especially lacking?

60. Against those who allow and prescribe the venereal act to treat gallstones, kidney stones, and other back pains.

61. Whether it is right to say that water must not be poured in the room of a person thought to have kidney stones.

62. How a woman can live without a womb as well as a man [can] without a penis and testicles.

63. Concerning the serious abuses committed in the absurd usage of the so-called mummy.

64. That myrobolans[12] are not of such excellent virtue as thought by common folk.

65. Whether it is good for children to begin eating [at a] very early [age] bread, pablum, soup, meat, and other solid foods.

66. Which roasted meat is more wholesome and more tasty, larded, stringed, flamed, or greased?

67. Why is it that water-drinkers are great eaters?

---

[12]Cotgrave defines the *myrobalan* [alternate spellings: *myrabolan; mirabolan*] as follows: "An East-Indian Plumme called, the Myrobalan Plumme, whereof there be diuers kinds distinguished by severall names (as *Bellerics, Chebules, Emblics, &c.*)."

68. Whether it is possible to determine through its color, smell, consistency, or other manifest qualities if *terra melia* or *terra sigillata* is genuine and potent.[13]

69. Is it true what several women claim, that bloodletting at the buttock makes the skin rougher and of poor color?

70. That it does not necessarily follow that if the liver is hot the stomach will be cold, and that one often accuses wrongly the liver of being inordinately hot.

71. Against those who consider it to be a sign of excellent health if one does not spit or blow one's nose.

72. Which is better when one has a cold and congestion, sleeping with the head high or low?

73. The error of those who say that the physician must give his all to the patient, and that the patient owes the physician nothing but a little money.

74. Why do people say that a good physician is a bad man and that a good man is a bad physician?

75. Why is it that people's wounds, lesions, and other afflictions heal quickly when the spots on their dressings and other linen are easily removed with lye?

76. Since food and drink go down the same passageway into the same receptacle and will thus have the same reason or basis for tasting the same, why it is that people usually prefer their soup hot and their

---

[13]Cabrol's text gives *"terre lemnie & sellee"* but should perhaps read *"terre melie,"* as given by Cotgrave, along with *"melienne"* and defined as follows: "A rough, and ash-coloured earth, which being tasted of, bites, and dryes, the tongue like Allum; and is used for the cleansing of the bodies outside, whereto it giues a liuelie, and gracious hue." Cotgrave also mentions "terre seelée" but only briefly: "The medicinable earth called, *Terra sigillata.*"

drinks cool; and yet as concerns meats and fruits, why some like them hot while others like them cold.

77. How can saltpeter cool water, given the fact that it is hot and easily converts into fire?

78. Why is it that one's appetite is so great when one is at sea?

79. Whether it is true that a laxative clyster can excite one to coitus, as several say they have sometimes felt to be the case.

80. How can virgins be susceptible to illnesses of the womb, even before puberty?

81. That many people take better care of their horses than of themselves, whence the soundness of the expression "Whosoever wishes to live a healthy life should give himself the same treatment as he does his horse."

82. Whether the pale skin of girls is contagious, and whether it can be caught by sleeping or bathing together.

83. That a weak and cold stomach will accept pure water better than it will young or sour wine.

84. Why do people say that of all foods mutton makes us grow old and cheese keeps us from aging?

85. Whether it is true that sour or unripe grape juice applied to the eye clears one's vision.[14]

86. That it is correct to say that one must touch the eyes and nose of a sick person only with the elbow.

87. Against those who believe that a toothache will return with worse pain than before if the extracted tooth is thrown in the fire or if hot coals or ashes are put on blood that came out of the socket.

---

[14]See n. 3 of no. 23 above.

88. That greasy foods do not make one put on weight, as is commonly thought.

89. Why is it that the broth of a black hen is whiter, and the milk of a black goat is better?

90. Why are fair people more fragile?

91. Which is healthier for you, oil or butter?

92. Why people say that fire is always good; and whether it is healthy to heat with fire.

93. Why do people say to drink hard before a journey[15] and that the horses go better when the riders have drunk a good bit?

94. Why do people say that one thinks more when fasting than after having eaten and [more when] dead than alive?

95. Whether one is considered a good fellow if one always has a hollow leg for one's friends.[16]

96. Whether it is true that coitus is dangerous if it is done with a woman in her flowers.

97. Is it true that fat people and hunchbacks do not live as long as other people, and nor do those who have spaces between their teeth and pointed knees?

98. Is it true that when the animal dies its venom is no longer poisonous?[17]

---

[15]I have used Cotgrave's translation for Cabrol's expression, *faire iambes de vin.*

[16]The French expression is more direct than the English counterpart: *auoir tousiours vn boyau vuide pour ses amis*: "to always have an empty bowel for one's friends."

[17]See "Gathering," no. 54, in the section immediately preceding.

99. Why is it that small children usually have more violent tempers than adults and often are more witty?

100. Whether the smoke of an extinguished candle or lamp can cause leprosy, and whether it can cause a woman to miscarry.

101. Why is it that the water in a well is improved if some small fish are thrown in it?

102. Whether it is possible for a man to perform the venereal act in a cold or hot bath and for a woman to conceive from a bath in which a man has ejaculated sperm.

103. Is it a good sign if a sick person loses a lot of weight, from the very beginning of the illness?

104. Can one tell if a man is a virgin?

105. Is it true that if a woman carries a child to the baptismal font, either that child or the one she is carrying in her womb will die?

106. Whether a woman who has given birth to twins can heal dislocations, as they say; and whether the seventh male child is able to cure the king's evil as long as he remains a virgin.

107. Why is it that some are in better health in winter and others in summer, and that people gain weight in winter?

108. Why is it that one sings better after having drunk?

109. Whether it is true that the plague is caught or transmitted by money and by bread.

110. Whosoever eats, shits, and sleeps well does not need to fear death.

111. Concerning Polish people, who, even at death's door, get out of bed and get dressed when it is time for the physician to visit them.

112. Whether swollen or split lips mean that the illness is going away.

113. Why is it that people usually look at the discharge from their noses but not at their other excrements, except perhaps for an occasional melancholic person?

114. Where should one crack an egg, at the point, on the bottom, or in the middle?

115. Should one drink once each time one eats an egg, or more than once?

116. Is it healthier to have one's hair cut on the first Tuesday of March, or on some other day of this same month, or of some other month?

117. Whosoever does any less is unfaithful to his friend.

118. One does not usually get drunk with one's own wine.

119. Who eats little eats enough, and who eats enough eats little.

120. How can one have a cold in the eyes, the nose, the throat, and the ears?

121. Whether it is true that those who have been cut open to repair a hernia can never reproduce afterward.

122. Why do people say, "If a man cannot eat let him drink"?

123. Is it true that natural baths are worthless or harmful to those who have had the pox?

CATALAN[1]

1. He who eats pork eats his own death *[Qvi mingeo porc, mingeo sa mort]*.

2. A gift and a capon are always in season *[Dono e capon, es touiours de seson]*.

3. He who does not have a tough stomach cannot sleep soundly *[Qui non ha lou ventre dur, non pot dormir segur]*.

4. Between shit and piss is the handsome son being developed *[Entre la merdo, & lou pis, se nourris lou bel fils]*.

5. Never make a Kiou [anus?] with your mouth *[Non faïs iamais Kiou, de ta bouco]*.

6. He does enough who does little *[Assais fay, qui ren non fay]*.

7. No flower, no seed *[Qui non flouris, non grano]*.

8. He who goes to bed thirsty will rise in good health *[Qui se vay dormir en sed, se leuo en santad]*.

9. In June and in July neither hay [fennel] nor little tails *[En Iun, & en Iullet, ne fenno ne caulet]*.

SPANISH

1. The first olive is golden, the second is of silver, the third is leaden, the fourth is of iron *[Vna azeintuna es de oro, la dos es de plata, la terzera de plomo, la quarta de hierro]*.

---

[1]I wish to express my indebtedness to my colleague, Professor Spurgeon Baldwin, for his gracious assistance in translating the Catalan expressions.

ITALIAN[2]

1. A salad that is well salted [seasoned] has little vinegar and a lot of oil *[Salata ben salata, poco aceto, & ben ogliata]*.

2. Dress warm, eat sparingly, drink a lot, and you will live *[Vesti caldo, mangia poco, beue assai, & viueray]*.

3. Staying up under the moon and sleeping under the sun neither adds to nor takes away from honor *[Vegliar à la Luna, & dormir al Sole, non fa ne prone honore]*.

4. Throughout the entire month of April do not uncover yourself *[Per tutto April, no te discuprir]*.

5. Like Saint Luke, put your hand in your mouth *[Da Sancto Luca, metti la man in boccà]*.

6. Good wine captures the mind and frees the tongue *[Bon vino, cattiua testa, & fauola longa]*.

7. Wine from a bottle is good in the morning but spoiled in the evening *[Vin di fiasco, la matina bouno, la sera guasto]*.

8. Fish spoils water, meat seasons it *[El pesce guasta l'acqua, la carne l'acconcia]*.

9. He who is unable to govern himself for one year is doomed to have five years without enjoyment afterward *[Chi non se gouuerna vn anno, é cinque anni dapoi senza allegressa]*.

10. He who dines badly digests worse *[Chi mal cena, peggio inghiotisse]*.

11. He who does not do as the goose does has a sad and short life *[Chi non fa come fa l'occa, la sua vita è triste & poca]*.

---

[2]I wish to express my indebtedness to my colleagues, Professors Barbara and Maurizio Godorecci, for their gracious assistance in translating the Italian expressions.

12. Cheese, pears, and bread are the food of a wretch; cheese, bread, and pears are the food of a gentleman *[Frommaggio, pere, & pan, sonno pasto da vilan: frommaggio, pan, & pere, son pasto da cauagliere]*.

13. It takes a madman and a wiseman to slice some cheese *[Bisogna vn matto, e vn sauio, a tagliar del frommaggio]*.

14. Eating stale bread dries up the voice *[El pan sutto, fa diuentar muto]*.

15. Judge wine by its flavor, bread by its color *[El vino à la sauor, & il pan al color]*.

16. He who eats the cabbage and leaves the broth takes the bad and leaves the good *[Chi mangia el cauolo, e lascia il brodo, piglia il cattiuo, e lascia il buono]*.

17. Soup brings about three good things: it makes for good digestion, for sleep, and for rosy cheeks *[Tre cose buone fa la zouppa: fa patire, fa dormire, & fa la gangia rossa]*.

18. He who would be healthy for a week should wash his hair; for a month, should slaughter a pig; for a year, should take a wife; forever after, should become a priest *[Chi vuol esser bene vna settimana, lauise la testa: chi vn mese, amazzi el porco: chi vn anno, tolga moglie: chi sempre mai, si faccia prete]*.

19. For a fatal illness neither a physician nor drugs are of any use *[A mal mortal ne medico, ne medicina val]*.

20. There is a remedy for each and every thing except death *[Ad ogni cosa remedio, excetto la morte]*.

21. He who goes slowly goes in good health, and he who is healthy will go for a long time *[Chi va piano, va sano: & chi e sano, va lontano]*.

22. [Keep] the [injured] hand [in a sling] over the heart, the [injured] leg on the bed *[La mano al petto, la gamba al letto]*.

23. The principal worry of an old man is not being able to have soft shit *[El maggior fastidio ch'habbia vn vecchio, è di non cagar tenero]*.

24. He who goes to bed without any supper tosses about all night long *[Chi va al letto senza cena, tutta la notte si dimena]*.

25. A good meal, a poor one, and a mediocre one keep a man healthy *[Vn pasto buono, vn triste, e vn mezano, mantiene l'huome sano]*.

26. Whoever overdoes it will be scooping beans, and whoever does not will not have any children *[Chi fa quel fatto troppo, scola i fageoli: & chi nol fa, non ha figliuoli]*.

27. He who does it when he can does not do it when he wants; and he who does it a lot does it poorly *[Chi lo fa quanto eì puol, nol fa quando eì vuol: & chi piu lo fa, manco lo fa]*.

28. He who eats meat and remains idle has a more miserable life for it *[Chi mangia carne e pasce, la vita gli rincresce]*.

29. Bitter wine is to be respected *[Vino amaro, tien lo caro]*.

30. One does not age while at the table *[A tauola non s'incuecchia]*.

LATIN[3]

1. From bread that is baked twice, from an unskilled physician, from lightning and tempests, defend us, Lord *[A pane biscocto, à medico indocto, à fulgure & tempestate, defende nos Domine]*.

2. White cheese is not to be praised, nor is Greek cheese, nor a cylindrical one *[Caseus laudatur non albus, nec argus, nec Magdalenus]*.

---

[3]I wish to express my indebtedness to my colleague, Professor Michael Hendry, for his gracious assistance in translating the Latin expressions.

3. Wings are bad, lame fowl is dangerous; the tail is suspicious; the neck is good without the feathers *[Ala mala, coxa[1] noxa, cropion dubium, collum remota pelle bonum]*.

4. Wine that is mixed with water and drunk too fast causes leprosy *[Vinum lymphatum, citò potatum, generat lepram]*.

5. The best medicine is to use no medicine *[Summa medicina est, nunquam uti medicina]*.

6. From cheese [make] a dessert, from bread a slaughter *[De caseo barcam, de pane bartolaeam]*.

TO THE MOST VIRTUOUS AND VENERABLE LORD, MONSIEUR ESTIENNE DE RATE, ROYAL AND GENERAL COUNSELOR IN THE COUR DES AIDES IN MONTPELLIER[2]

FROM JEAN IMBERT, FELLOW APOTHECARY, GREETINGS

Monsieur, I have acted like the monkey of the physician from Montpellier, of which Monsieur Joubert told the story in his *Treatise on Laughter*.[3] This monkey, seeing that all the servants of the physi-

---

[1]Light has recently been shed on the colloquial term coxus: "... *coxus* 'lame', a word known only from glosses and Spanish *cojo*, Portuguese *coxo*" (Edward Courtney, *The Fragmentary Latin Poets* [Oxford: Clarendon Press, 1993], 278). A shorter version of this expression is found in French in Rabelais's *Ancien Prologue du Quart Livre* and in Latin in the prologue to the *Cinquiesme Livre*.

[2]Since there is no English equivalent for this body I have kept the French. Cotgrave gives the following explanation: "A Soueraigne Court, wherein all causes that concerne the Aides, Tailles, &c, are heard, and determined: (Some report, that King Iohn, others that Charles the fifth, about the year 1380, erected that which is at Paris; Charles the seuenth erected another at Montpelier, *Anno* 1437. There be others also, at Roan, and at Montserrat in Auvergne; and one at Bourdeaux, the which was first at Perigueux.)"

[3]*TL*, bk. 3, chap. 14 (127).

cian who was at death's door were beginning to lay hands on his money and furniture, takes possession of the doctoral bonnet. Thus, when I saw that Monsieur Cabrol on the one hand and Monsieur Beauchastel on the other were having printed on the sly (as they themselves openly admit) a few chapters and lists of popular sayings from the *Popular Errors* of Monsieur Joubert, I thought I would do likewise with a few small notebooks I was able to get hold of dealing with metaphorical and poetic remedies, and those which he calls extravagant.

I have always been very curious about them, and he did me the honor of sending them to me some time ago. I found among them a booklet of certain popular sayings and expressions concerning illnesses and other matters of the medical arts and in which he traces all the sources of these phrases. There are also a few wild notions in which common folk are in error. I am publishing all of it, knowing that the slightly beaten cry out as much as those who are roundly beaten. Three will be as easily forgiven as two. We will all three be accorded the same pardon. As for me, I have no doubt about it at all, knowing that you, sir, are in Monsieur Joubert's good graces and are his especial friend and faithful servant, as is proclaimed everywhere publicly and privately. Hence I give to you and dedicate to you my part of the spoils, begging you, Monsieur, to accept it cordially and to believe that I am convinced I have sent it to the person able to restore me to favor, should it be necessary, all the while recommending myself to yours.

From Paris, this twentieth of February, 1579.

SUMMARY OF WHAT IS TREATED
IN THE FOLLOWING SECTIONS

AN EXPLANATION OF SOME POPULAR TERMS AND PHRASES
MAINLY CONCERNING ILLNESSES[1]

1. Flowers, flow, menstrual flow, months, menses, loss, period, smock, "must be having," case, ill, bad week, cardinal, marquis.
2. To abort, to foil, to wound, *dessarrier,* to spoil.
3. Deflowered, devirginated, devirgined.
4. Decircumcised.
5. Suffocation of the womb.
6. Dysentery, bloody flow, *seintegue,* bloody stool.
7. Nephretic, phrenetic; windy, nephretic, and stone colic.
8. Colic, *masclon,* stomach colic.
9. Gout, decline, cold, catarrh, natural gout.
10. Sciatica.
11. Quinsy, the Adam's apple.
12. *Noli me tangere.*
13. Nosebleed.
14. Migraine.
15. Lunatic, and to be frantic.
16. The falling sickness, earth sickness, Saint John's illness, *mau de las passeras,* high sickness.
17. *Mau-loubet.*
18. Plague-sore, *la ghiandozza.*
19. Throttle.
20. Be gone! To faint, spasm, fainting.
21. To dine, to drink, to take a repast, to have a snack, to have supper, to give the lie to.
22. To sleep in.
23. To treat a patient.

---

[1] All of these expressions, as well as those in the rest of the summary, are explained in the notes in the corresponding sections that follow.

METAPHORICAL AND EXTRAVAGANT REMEDIES

1. To increase semen and fecundity.
2. To deliver more easily and to avoid miscarriage.
3. To break up stones in the body.
4. Something bad for one's memory.

SUPERSTITIOUS, VAIN, AND CEREMONIOUS REMEDIES

1. To stop any type of bleeding.
2. For jaundice.
3. For gout with cramps.
4. To speed up teething in small children.
5. To stop vomiting at sea.
6. To make a woman's milk dry up.
7. For any type of fever.
8. For a quartan fever.
9. To make warts go away.
10. To cure the dropsy.
11. For colic.
12. For suffocation of the womb.
13. Conjuring the womb.

FABULOUS STORIES

1. About the viper.
2. About the beaver, also called the water-horse.[2]
3. About the salamander.
4. About the bear.

---

[2]Cotgrave's translation.

TWO OF MONSIEUR JOUBERT'S PARADOXES,
TRANSLATED BY HIS SON ISAAC

1. Whether one can determine that certain poisons must not be given on certain days and that they will cause death within a certain lapse of time.

2. That there is a reason why a few people can live several days and even years without eating.

AN EXPLANATION OF SOME POPULAR TERMS AND PHRASES MAINLY CONCERNING ILLNESSES

1. Flowers, flow, menstrual flow, months, menses, loss, period,[1] smock,[2] "must be having,"[3] case,[4] ill,[5] bad week,[6] cardinal,[7] marquis.[8]

A woman's flowers[9] are so called after the similitude they share with plants, which usually flower before producing their fruit. For women who are to carry fruit (thus do we commonly call the child that is in the womb in the case of a pregnancy) must have such an abundant supply of blood that it sometimes spills over, thus indicating that another body could well be nourished by it. When this flow is perceived, a woman is said to have her flowers and could well produce fruit if she happens to conjoin. Conversely, it is said of those who do not have this spotting (and who are consequently sterile) *qui non flouris, non grane.*[10] For likewise, those plants that never flower, such as ferns and grasses, never have grains or seeds, which is why they are called *agones* by the Greeks. Perhaps one calls them flowers also because of

---

[1]Joubert's term is *Rhodais*; it was a euphemism for a woman's period, as Cotgrave attests: "The name of a good towne in *Languedoc. Elle est de Rhodais.* She hath her flowers." The current French spelling for the city is Rodez.

[2]Another euphemism for a woman's period, according to Cotgrave: *"Avoir sa chemise.* A woman to haue her flowers (for *tachée de sang* is understood.)"

[3]Still another euphemism for the above condition.

[4]An equivocal term, as Cotgrave demonstrates: "A Case, cause, matter, thing; also, a crime, offence; fact; also, esteeme, account, reckoning of; also, the priuities (of man, or woman.)"

[5]Still another popular euphemism for a woman's period, as Cotgrave attests: *"Elle est malade.* Said of a woman that hath her flowers."

[6]Yet another common euphemism, as Cotgrave attests: *"Elle a sa male semaine.* She hath her flowers."

[7]Euphemism, as Cotgrave attests: *"Elle a son Cardinal.* She hath her flowers."

[8]Euphemism, as Cotgrave attests: *"Elle a son marquis.* Saied of a woman that hath her flowers."

[9]Joubert's note: Flowers.

[10]Catalan in the text: No flowers, no seed.

a corruption of the word *flow*.[11] For the blood flows and spills out. But one also calls it the flow of a woman and *menstrual flow*,[12] because it flows each month if the woman is in good health. For this very reason it is also indeed called the *months* of a woman,[13] or the menses, with the word *purgations* understood. There are some who call this *loss*,[14] since it is blood that is being lost and bringing no profit whatsoever. The common folk of Languedoc say jokingly, "She is from Rhodais"[15] (which is the principal town in the region of Rouergue), meaning that a woman is having this loss. And I think that it is a word come down from the Greek *rhein*, which means "to flow." For the same reason, the rose is called *rhodon*, because of the heavy odor that flows out from it. Or perhaps one says she is from Rhodais because the soil in the area of this city is usually red.

One says more politely, "She has her smock," with the words *stained with blood* understood.[16] Likewise, she has what a woman *must be having*.[17] For this is natural for a woman, and she cannot be in good health or carry children if she does not have these natural and spontaneous purgations. Others say, "She's having *her case*."[18] Still others say, "She's sick,"[19] even though this ordinary flow, when it is moderate, is not classified among the diseases nor even among the unnatural conditions. But because women feel more angry during these purgations than before or afterward, they say politely (in order to cover up this infirmity or natural necessity) that they are sick. For that very time they say they are having their *bad week*.[20] Since it goes by weeks, as does the moon, for several women such purgations scarcely

---

[11]Joubert's note: Flow.

[12]Joubert's note: Menstrual flow.

[13]Joubert's note: Months.

[14]Joubert's note: Loss.

[15]Joubert's note: Rhodais [spelled Rodez in modern French].

[16]Joubert's note: Smock.

[17]Joubert's note: Must be having.

[18]Joubert's note: Her case.

[19]Joubert's note: Sick.

[20]Joubert's note: Bad week.

last less than a week. For this very reason people say, "She's having her *time*,"[21] instead of saying, "She's at the moment of her purgations." Others say, "having her *Cardinal*,"[22] because of the color red, and others "her *Marquis*,"[23] because the purgations stain their smocks and sheets.

2. To abort, to foil,[24] to wound, *dessarrier*,[25] to spoil.[26]

To abort comes from the Latin word *aborter[e]*,[27] which means "to prevent the birth or the maturation period set by nature," or to deprive the child of its *ortus* and legitimate birth. Our common folk say *miscarry* and *cast* for the disorder resulting from a blow, such as in the case of a fall or being struck with a rod, a stone, or other blunt instrument. And since such is the most common cause of an abortion, people say *miscarry* for abortion.[28] It is for the same reason that people say in France *to wound*,[29] for it seems that a woman is wounded and crushed when she aborts, especially since she has a lot of pain and loses a lot of blood through some means against nature. In other regions people say *dessarrier*,[30] as if it were a matter of unbinding the

---

[21]Joubert's note: Time.

[22]Joubert's note: Cardinal.

[23]Joubert's note: Marquis.

[24]Joubert's term is *affouler*, which Cotgrave explains at length: "as *Affoler*; And (particularly) a woman to miscarrie, cast her child, or be deliuered before her time, by the violence of blowes (or a fall) receiued."

[25]According to Cotgrave, the following is the only meaning of this verb: "A woman to cast her child."

[26]Joubert's term is *gaster*; Cotgrave gives it the same translation he gives for *dessarrier*.

[27]It is strange that Joubert gives this vulgar Latin form; he wrote extensively in Latin and would have known the classical form of the verb: *aborior, abortus, aboriri*.

[28]Joubert's note: Miscarry.

[29]Joubert's note: To wound.

[30]Joubert's note: *Dessarrier*.

belly,[31] which had been bound, closed, and taut; now it loosens and opens at the wrong time. Others say *to spoil*,[32] as in the case of any other thing that goes bad.

3. Deflowered, devirginated, devirgined.[33]

Plants are said to be deflowered, [as are] girls who are devirginated too young. Plants are *forced*,[34] either when their flowers or fruit are picked at the wrong time, or when they are forced with dung, lime, or hot water to flower before they are in season. Hence they end their lives early and do not keep their greenness, vigor, and strength. They are thus truly forced and, one might say, *degreened* or deprived of their greenness. Likewise, *desantorat*[35] comes from the Greek word *anthos*, which means "flower," as if one meant to say *desanthorat*, deprived of its flower and as such will bear no fruit. Hence people say *to deflower* a girl,[36] which means "to take away her virginity," especially when her age is not yet fitting. Hence she is afterward not as useful in marriage, as I have shown at the end of the second chapter of the second book of the *Popular Errors*. Thus fruit picked before its maturity does not last as long, has a shorter life span, and withers sooner than do the others. Some call this *desourat*,[37] which is like saying to anticipate the *[h]our*, that is, to pick before the proper hour.

---

[31]Joubert plays on the graphic similarities between *dessarrier* and the French *desserrer*, meaning "to loosen or to untighten."

[32]Joubert's note: To spoil.

[33]I have thus attempted to translate the three terms given by Joubert, *"Des-verdiat, des-antourat, des-ourat,"* the last two of which are translated by Cotgrave, respectively: "Deflowered, as a virgine that hath leachered: ¶ *Langued*."; "Deflowered before her time. ¶ *Langued*."

[34]Joubert's note: Forced [I have thus rendered Joubert's term *desuerdiat*, which literally means "degreen," as is seen in his explanation].

[35]Joubert's note: *Desantorat*.

[36]Joubert's note: To deflower.

[37]Joubert's note: *Desourat*.

4. Decircumcised.[38]

This term applies to a Jew or a Turk who has left his religion: afterward his people call him *decircumcised*,[39] as we call such people *fallen away*, but this is in another sense and for another reason. For Jews and Turks, having been circumcised, have the heads of their virile members covered again when they later leave their group and no longer wish to bear its mark. It is a surgical procedure taught by Paul of Aegina[40] and other good Greek and Arab authors to feign a foreskin. It is necessary to practice an incision in the skin of the male member all the way around at the base. When the continuity of the skin is thus broken, the skin is pulled little by little toward the end (much as one removes the bark from a willow shoot in order to make a tube) until the head of the member is covered. Then at the base, where an equal amount of skin is lacking, one allows scar tissue to take its place. This is how one is *sliced again*, that is, one more time, or cut twice. For one is sliced again in order to cover up the missing foreskin. In Latin the term is *recutit*,[41] because one has recovered one's skin, which is called *foreskin*.

5. Suffocation of the womb.[42]

This is what physicians call "suffocation of the womb": when the womb or matrix (which is also called "mother" inasmuch as it produces children, just as the earth is called the common mother of all) swells up with some wind or vapor and presses against the neighboring organs so much that the bowels, pushing in turn against the diaphragm and the chest, bring about a suffocation. This results in the swelling of the woman's throat, sometimes obviously bigger around, other times not externally visible, which causes her to suffocate and stop breathing for a time, accompanied by a loss of speech. At times she loses all

---

[38]Cotgrave gives a mistranslation ("circumcised") and attributes the term to Rabelais. Literally, the term means "sliced again"; the sense is made clear in Joubert's explanation.

[39]Joubert's note: Decircumcised.

[40]On Paul of Aegina, see *PE*, bk. 3, chap. 5, n. 2 (306).

[41]Joubert's note: *Recutit* [literally, "reskinned"].

[42]Joubert's term is *mal de maire*, alternately spelled *mere*.

feeling and movement, as in the case of apoplexy. Some women, on the other hand, scream and laugh and talk incessantly.

6. Dysentery, bloody flow,[43] *seintegue*,[44] bloody stool.[45]

Dysentery[46] is a pain in the belly resulting from the excoriation of the inside of the bowels to such a degree that scrapings and blood, and sometimes mire and pus, will exit. The pain is most severe and drives one to return often to stool, where one is able to do nothing or very little. Hence the patient strains violently, and for that reason this disorder is called *eprensas* in Dauphiné,[47] and in Gascony *espremason*.[48] In Languedoc it is called *seintegne*,[49] from the Greek word *dysentere*, which literally signifies "difficulty in the bowel," that is, that the bowels are having difficulty, pain, and trouble in their action. The Italians call this disorder *cagasangue*[50] and use it as an imprecation, as they do with *cancaro* and *ghiandozza*, that is, a chancre and the plague, as do the French with the quartan fever.

7. Nephritic, phrenetic; windy, nephritic, and stone colic.[51]

Nephritic is a pain in the kidneys.[52] For in Greek the word for kidney is *nephros*. Some use the equivocal term *phrenetic* (which means "hallucination and madness," resulting from the inflammation of the brain) for *nephretic*. This pain in the kidneys usually precedes the

---

[43]Joubert's term is *eprensas*; Cotgrave gives *eprenas*, "The bloudie flix, and bellie ache, that come by the ulceration, or excoriation of the bowels. ¶ Dauph."

[44]Joubert's term, which he later spells *seintegne*, claiming it to be from the Languedoc dialect and derived from the Greek *dysentere*.

[45]Cotgrave translates the term as "The bloudie flix."

[46]Joubert's note: Dysentery.

[47]Joubert's note: *Eprensas*.

[48]Joubert's note: *Espremazon* [spelled with a *z* in the marginal note].

[49]Joubert's note: *Seintegne*.

[50]Joubert's note: *Cagasangue*.

[51]Joubert explains these terms in the following section.

[52]Joubert's note: Nephritic.

passing of stones (called calculi) or heavy sand and stones, produced in the kidneys. Several people, using the word *colic* incorrectly,[53] make the distinction that one is windy and the other nephritic or renal. The term *windy colic* is quite appropriate (although it is never caused by wind alone),[54] but not the term *nephritic colic*.[55] For these are terms based upon aspects rather than the cause of the disorder, that is, colic is a disorder of the bowel, and nephritic, of the kidney. Thus to speak of a nephritic colic is like speaking of a bowel disorder in the kidney. Others speak of a stone colic,[56] intending to express with the word *colic* any pain in the belly, whatever its specific location. It is quite true that there are colic pains (that is, in the bowel called the *colon*) caused by stones formed in the bowel, mentioned by the ancients and also seen in our own times. But those who use these terms understand them differently, for by the expression *stone colic* they mean the pain caused by the stone that is in the kidney.

8. Colic, *masclon*,[57] stomach colic.

One of the largest bowels is called the *colon*, and because it is the one that, above all the others, is the most susceptible to pain, any pain in the belly, even if not originating in the colon, is commonly called *colic*.[58] In some regions it is called *masclon*[59] because males (who are called *mascles*) are more subject to it than females, who, on the other hand, are subject to suffocation of the womb, which is their form of colic in common parlance. For, as they see it, all pain in the belly in women is in the womb, and in men, in the bowel. People also use the improper term *stomach colic*,[60] because the pain is in the stomach and similar to that in the colon, its next-door neighbor.

---

[53]Joubert's note: Colic.

[54]Joubert's note: Windy colic.

[55]Joubert's note: Nephritic colic.

[56]Joubert's note: Stone colic.

[57]Cotgrave translates this term as "The Cholicke of the stomacke."

[58]Joubert's note: Colic.

[59]Joubert's note: *Masclon.*

[60]Joubert's note: Stomach colic.

9. Gout, decline, cold, catarrh, natural gout.

Gout is the disorder of the joints,[61] accompanied by inflammation, which the Greeks call *arthritis*, from the word *arthron*, which means articulation or joint, that is, the conjunction of at least two bones. The painful tumor or swelling is the result of the arrival of humors flowing into these joints, drop by drop, and hence the disorder is called *gout*.[62] There are some who call it *decline* at its inception, or *rheum*, or *catarrh*,[63] since the word *gout* is most disgusting, especially for young people. Sometimes it is called *natural gout*[64] so as to distinguish the ordinary kind, which is most often inherited, from the drops of the pox,[65] which each man acquires on his own, even though it can be transmitted to one's offspring.

10. Sciatica.

This is a corrupted form of the word *ischiatique*, which designates the gout of the hip, the hip being called *ischion* in Greek, at the point where it joins the thigh and affords movement to the upper part of it. Whence the gout in this joint is called *ischias* in Greek, but ordinary physicians call it *ischiatique*, and ignorant common folk call it *sciatique*.

11. Quinsy, the Adam's apple.

Quinsy is an inflammation of the throat at the larynx (commonly called the *Adam's apple*) choking and suffocating the patient. The Greeks call it *cynanche*, and *synanche*,[66] which signifies a cord or a throttling rope for strangling a dog or other animal. From this term the

---

[61]Joubert's note: Gout.

[62]The French term for "gout" (*goutte*) also means "drop."

[63]Joubert's note: Decline. Rheum. Catarrh.

[64]Joubert's note: Natural gout.

[65]The term *gouttes* refers to the fluid exuding from the sores of those suffering from syphilis. Rabelais refers to victims of the disease as *goutteux* in the prologue to *Gargantua*.

[66]Joubert's note: Cynanche.

corrupted form *squinance* was used for *synanche*.[67] As for the *Adam's apple*,[68] it is the top of the gullet and is composed of three pieces of cartilage or soft tissue, which are very prominent in a few individuals. It can be clearly felt in everyone, and because it is hard and round, people call it the piece of the apple that Adam did not want to swallow, repenting as soon as it was going down his throat and holding it there with his fingers. And so it stayed there and has ever since been the mark in that very spot of his action, even for his successors. But if that were true, women would not have one, and yet they all do, and in some it shows even more than in many men.

12. *Noli me tangere.*[69]

This is the name given to a chancre on the face because it must not be treated the least bit roughly or else it will get worse. The same is true of chancres on other parts of the body, but they are considered more dangerous on the face because they diminish its beauty and because of the imminent danger they present to the brain, which is so nearby, for they could thus result in death.

13. Nosebleed.

This is usually said of someone who lacks courage, as in the case of a person's undertaking or promising something that he cannot manage to make good. People say, "His nose is bleeding," or "He had a nosebleed." This is because bleeding, when it is copious, weakens the heart. For strength consists in blood and humors, which are both lost in such a case, and faced with this loss, the heart, made cold by it, becomes fearful and dares not act or move forward when the slightest danger is perceived.

---

[67]Joubert's note: Quinsy.

[68]Joubert's note: Adam's apple.

[69]Joubert explains this expression in the following section.

14. Migraine.

This is a pain in one side of the head and is a corrupted form of the Greek word *hemicranie*, which means half of the head. People began by using the corrupt form of the word, *micranie*, then *migranie*, and finally *migraine*, which means a pomegranate in Languedoc, a fruit thus named because of the large number of seeds, renowned for its refreshing and thirst-quenching quality. One of the kingdoms in Spain bears the name of the fruit, or else the fruit took its name from the kingdom.

15. Lunatic, and to be frantic.[70]

The Greeks called *seleniaques* (this is a word-for-word translation) those who, because of the moon, have lost their senses. Likewise, all disorders obviously linked to the orbit and the faces of the moon are called *seleniaques*, such as the falling sickness, called in Greek epilepsy, and a type of madness called melancholy. In this sense people commonly say that women are inconstant, since the moon governs the months and women have their purgations every month. Hence their purgations are called *months* and *menses*. Therefore, since they are controlled and driven by the moon, they are said to *take after it*, with the added phrase understood (so as to preserve their honor) to be the main thrust of their health, which is fecundity. People use the expression *to be a lunatic*[71] in another sense to mean being inconstant and changing like the moon, which changes its face every day. This is a quality commonly attributed to the female sex; still, it is a defamation of their honor, seeing that it proceeds from a great purity and simplicity of matter, which renders women light and changeable like the sky. In this respect I praise their condition, countering the opinion of common folk, in my *Popular Errors*.[72]

---

[70]Joubert's expression is *tenir de la Lune*, which Cotgrave translates as follows: "To be inconstant, variable, or changeable, as the Moone; also, to bee a little franticke."

[71]Joubert's note: *Tenir de la Lune*.

[72]Joubert's note: In chapter 6, Part Two [*PE* 109–11].

16. The falling sickness, earth sickness, Saint John's illness, cock sparrow's illness, high sickness.[73]

This disorder is called *epilepsie* in Greek, a word that means astonishment or suspension of all the senses. Hence it is that a man falls to the ground if he is not held up. For he loses in an instant his vision, his hearing, and his other senses as in a syncope, commonly called *swooning*, or in an apoplexy. But there is a big difference, in that with apoplexy and with a syncope there is neither movement nor sense perception, and in epilepsy the body moves in a most jerky way, seized with convulsions called a *spasm* in Greek.[74] It is given the term *falling sickness* because one falls, collapsing on the ground, just as a very old man, said to be falling when he is curved forward, bowing down to the earth, with (as people say commonly) one foot in the grave. For this same reason (in my opinion) people in Languedoc call this disorder *earth sickness*,[75] because it throws to the earth the people who are afflicted with it, however robust they might be, as if they had been given a blow to the head with a club. It is also called Saint John's illness because (perhaps) the head of Saint John the Baptist fell to the ground when he was decapitated, and it was later put on a platter to satisfy Herod.[76] In Gascony it is called the cock sparrow's illness because sparrows are very subject to it.[77] The average Frenchman calls it *high sickness*, either because of its great seriousness and violence, or because of the aforementioned reason, that it makes people fall from their high positions.[78]

---

[73]All these expressions are synonyms for epilepsy.

[74]Joubert's note: Falling sickness.

[75]Joubert's note: Earth Sickness [Joubert's term is *mau de terre*, literally, "earth sickness"].

[76]Joubert's note: Saint John's illness.

[77]Joubert's note: Cock sparrow's illness [Joubert's term is *mau de la passeras*].

[78]Joubert's note: High sickness.

17. *Mau-loubet.*[79]

This is one of the curse words of the people of Languedoc, as is the aforementioned *earth sickness*. I think it stands for the *loup*, which is an ulcered chancre on the thighs and on the legs (a disease without a real cure other than extirpation),[80] just as the one on the face is called a *noli me tangere*. In its diminutive form it is called *loubet*, which means "little wolf." For they say *loup, loubet,* for "wolf," "female wolf," and "wolf pup."

18. Plague-sore,[81] *la ghiandozza.*

This is a third curse word from the same country, designating the plague, namely, the tumor or pestilential bubo that (beyond any doubt) is vicious and fatal. Hence the Italians (as we have noted above)[82] say *la ghiandozza* as a curse word.[83] For the plague is, properly speaking, a bubo or a tumor and swelling in some gland (*ghiande* in Italian) among those in the neck, in the armpit, and in the groin.

19. Throttle.[84]

The *canne* is the gullet or the slit through which we breathe. People who are choked or strangled are deprived of their *canne* and are consequently *ecannez*, which the dialect of Languedoc (partial to the letter *s*) pronounces "escannats."

---

[79]For a discussion of this term, see *PE*, bk. 5, chap. 1, n. 2 (314).

[80]Cotgrave does not give a translation of this term but defines it as "... a malignant, and remedilesse Vlcer, or Cranker [sic], in the legs, which in th'end it wholly consumes."

[81]Cotgrave's translation of the term used by Joubert, *la male bosse*, is "a plague-sore, pestilent botch, contagious bile."

[82]In no. 6.

[83]Joubert's note: *Ghiandozza.*

[84]Joubert gives an explanation of the Languedoc form (*escannar* and *escannez*, from *canne*) of the French *escanné*, which Cotgrave translates as "stifled, throtled, strangled."

20. Be gone![85] To faint, spasm, fainting.

Avalir in the Languedoc dialect means "to be lost or dispersed," so as to be no longer visible, as if carried off by the devil or swallowed up by the earth. This word is often on the lips of our common folk in Montpellier, and it is also used jokingly and familiarly. It can be translated into French as "to faint,"[86] meaning to fade into the air and the wind, as when people say of something, "It faded away," when they do not know what happened to it. But *to faint* also means another thing altogether, which can be said in another way: to fall into a *swoon*.[87] And when all of a sudden all faculties fail us, we use the Greek term *syncopiser*. Spasm is another disorder,[88] of which epilepsy is a species, but this word is commonly misused to designate a fainting spell and a faint heart.

21. To dine, to drink, to take a repast, to have a snack, to have supper, to give the lie to.

To dine is literally "to break one's fast."[89] For one fasts until the first morsel one eats, and the syllable *de* is privative here, as in *dedire, demordre, defaire, dedier, denoüer, desalierer, desopiler, desenyurer, deployer, desennuyer, demembrer, demeubler, depriser, desobeyr, debonder, desengager, deshonnorer, dechausser, debander, detendre, decrouter, decrouller, deserrer, decoudre, decouurir,* and so forth. Thus "to give the lie to" means to remove the lie concerning some-

---

[85]One of Cotgrave's translations of the term used by Joubert, *aualisque*, is "auant, be gone; fie upon it: ¶ *Langued.*"

[86]Joubert's note: To faint [Joubert gives *euanoyr*].

[87]Joubert's note: Swoon [Joubert gives *pasmaison* (sic)].

[88]Joubert's note: Spasm.

[89]Joubert's note: To dine [Joubert uses *desieuner*, which means literally "to break one's fast," as in the English word *breakfast*; the *déjeuner* is the noon meal in France today, as it was in Joubert's time, but if we are to believe Joubert, it was the first meal of the day, which means that the French in the days of the Renaissance did not eat breakfast].

thing;[90] when somebody lies and you say that he lied, this is "to give
the lie to," which means "to take away or to deprive, to exempt and to
remove the lie." Thus it is with *desieuner*, privation of *ieusne*. Those
who use the phrase "*i'ay desieuné auiourd'huy deux fois, trois fois,
&c.*"[91] therefore misuse the term considerably. For one can only *desieuner* (which is to say, "break one's fast") once a day, and it is with
the first morsel one eats. For one is no longer fasting if one has taken
the smallest bite. Let the other meals be called whatever one wishes,
the first will always be "breakfast," whether it is taken at noon or in
the evening, in which case one will say, "I fasted right up until evening." And if one only has two meals, which one calls dinner and
supper, the dinner is actually a breakfast. If one has three, the first one
in the morning will be a breakfast and the second a dinner. But if the
first is taken rather late, it will be called dinner, the second a snack or
a repast, and the third, supper.[92] The word *supper* seems to be based
upon the word *soup*, which was eaten in the evening more than at any
other time. A *snack*[93] is so called because of its small size, especially
since it is like a tasting,[94] in which one tastes and samples some piece
of fruit, or one only drinks something with a small piece of bread.
Drinking is a term[95] used only in conjunction with the noon meal because the ancients, the first to eat this meal, did nothing more than
soak bread in pure wine and drink it, calling it *acratisma*.[96] Hence in
the Languedoc dialect the word *drink* is used only in reference to the
first meal, which the French call *desieuner*; and the word *desieuner* is
taken in a meaning contrary to that of "to fast and abstain." And thus
Italians say, "*Io son digiuno,*" when they mean "I am fasting."

---

[90]Joubert's note: To give the lie to [Joubert uses *dementir*, which Cotgrave translates as "to giue the Ly unto; also, to foyle; digresse, or derogate from; proue naught,
or false; doe contrarie to expectation"].

[91]Literally, "I have broken fast two times, three times, etc.," as in the English "to
have two or three breakfasts."

[92]Joubert's note: Supper.

[93]Joubert's note: Snack.

[94]Joubert uses the term *collation*.

[95]Joubert's note: To drink.

[96]*Acratisma* is a Greek word (*akratizomai*) meaning "to drink pure wine." The
term also meant "to breakfast" because this meal consisted of bread dipped in wine.

22. To sleep in.[97]

The morning is neither fat nor skinny, yet one often says "to sleep the fat morning" because sleeping in makes one become very fat. For it is the case that the first stage of digestion (through the action of the small intestine)[98] is slower at night while one sleeps than it is during the day while one is awake, and sleeping is more conducive to the second stage of digestion, which generates blood. Blood (since it is more plentiful and rich) produces fat. It is certain that sleeping late, as in the morning, puts on weight and makes one plump. People who study get up early and are usually deprived of this, for dawn is the friend of the Muses.

23. To treat a patient.

This is an expression and a manner of speaking used by common folk meaning "to advise, to see to, and to set up what is needed by a patient," and in fact to get one's hands involved if it is a question of surgery. One thus speaks of treating a horse, which does not mean to imagine them and have them in one's thoughts and cogitation,[99] but rather to curry them, to brush them, to wipe them down, to clean their hooves, feed them, water them, provide bedding, and so forth. It is therefore a caring for and a treatment that is in conjunction with what is needed by the patient, when he or she is treated by a physician or a surgeon, as if one were to say, "Think of the patient and see to what he or she needs."

---

[97]Joubert uses the expression still in use in modern French, *la grasse matinée*, which means literally "the fat morning"; this explains the opening sentence of his discussion.

[98]Joubert uses the term *ventricule*, which Cotgrave translates as "The uentricle; the place wherein the meat sent from the stomacke is disgested [sic]; some call so the stomacke it selfe; others expresse by it th'*Epigastre*."

[99]This confusion is because of the French verb *penser* ("to think") and its homophone *panser* ("to dress, to treat, to care for").

METAPHORICAL AND EXTRAVAGANT REMEDIES

1. To increase semen and fecundity.

People insist that eating fish engenders a lot of semen. It would have to be far more nourishing than meat, for semen is nothing more than the surplus of good food. It is true that eating fish increases the desire for coitus, since the semen that is produced from it is more milky or watery, and stinging, thus provoking the expulsive faculty. One can be mistaken in this, as if fish contributed to the abundance of semen, as in a person who never fished without having a huge catch. Perhaps the mistake comes also from the fact that fish are beyond comparison more fecund than any of the other animals; witness the infinite number of eggs they produce, whence someone was able to convince himself that eating fish creates in us the same ability or aptitude. For this very reason some people highly recommend eating carp (but especially the tongue as the most delicious part) in order to become more lusty in the venereal act and to have a lot of children, because the carp lays eggs five or six times a year and always in infinite numbers.

But one must understand the mistake in the projection: it does not follow that simply because some animal is fecund a man will become so as well for having eaten it; rather, to attain this end it is better to eat meats that are very nourishing in an effort to engender a lot of wholesome semen. This is perhaps why it is written that eating sparrows and cock sparrows makes a man more lusty in love, because the sparrow is very lascivious. But in that case (in my opinion) it would have to be young ones who have not yet made mad use of their bodies. Otherwise, inasmuch as cock sparrows live only a short time, one would have to admit that the man who eats sparrows would shorten his life, for the sparrow has a very short one indeed. And conversely, the man who eats ravens, crows, and deer would live forever. For it is said that a crow can live to be three hundred years old, and the raven nine times as long as a man. And there are deer that live for five or six hundred years. Using a similar logic, whoever wants to become very agile and quick should eat monkeys. In this same vein I remember the candid reply of a lady whose husband had been ordered by a doctor to drink goat milk for two or three months: "What! But, Doctor, they say that people who drink it for a long time become so excited that they do nothing but jump, dance, climb, and run about, to the point that they cannot be kept in one place. My husband is already jumpy enough, and I do not want him to be any more lusty than he is." It is also said that there was a woman in Paris who, because she had always been fed goat meat, was always ready to climb and jump about.

2. To deliver more easily and to avoid miscarriage.

Our midwives tie to one of the thighs of a woman in labor (depending on whether they think the child will be a boy or a girl), or on both so as not to make a mistake, a magnet so that she will have an easier delivery. And during the pregnancy, if a miscarriage is suspected, the magnet is tied to one of the arms or to both for the same reason. For a magnet (which is called a *calamita* in Italian and an *azimant* in Languedoc) attracts iron, and because of this the remedy is transferred to childbirth, as if the magnet were able to draw unto itself the child with even more strength. Granted, but a child is not made of iron, and a magnet does not attract flesh and bones. It is not possible to say that because it attracts iron that it will attract something else. For attraction is its natural property and not an animal force, as one would say of a man or of some animal, that is, if he is able to pull or carry a hundred pounds of iron he will easily carry thirty pounds of flesh. Still, the comparison is in no way fitting, for there is no way by any stretch of the imagination that the little magnet tied to the arm or thigh can attract a piece of iron as heavy as the child is. It can scarcely draw a large needle or move a metal punch. But there is something mysterious and secret in this manner of treating that the ancients prescribed (for this is not the invention of midwives) for some sound reason that is not allowed to be explained to common folk. I understand that several women also use magnets to provoke or to stop menstrual flow, for which application the same admonition likewise applies.

3. To break up stones in the body.

Because chickens digest stones and gravel, the opinion has developed that the tissue lining the inside of the gizzard or *perier*[100] (thus called because of the stones that are often found in it) is able to break

---

[100]The term *perier* is based on the word for stone (*pierre*), as Joubert explains, and is a synonym for the gizzard, according to Cotgrave: "The giserne of a Henne, &c."

up and dissolve stones in man. But what is not understood is that it is the fierce heat (along with the property of the very thick stomach characteristic of fowl) that allows fowl to digest tough things. This is shared by all birds. One must therefore not be astonished by the fact that ostriches digest iron.

Likewise, because lemon juice melts pearls, which are very hard, people thought it would break up the stones in the bladder and in the kidneys. And since the blood of a male goat cuts diamonds, which are stronger and harder than any other rock, it is inferred that it would break up all the better stones in the human body. But it must be determined whether it is not by some antipathy or strange property that the blood of a male goat breaks diamonds and no other type of stone. It is not to be scorned when it is properly prepared, for we use it to good effect in breaking up and dissolving calculi in man. This is done by feeding a three- or four-year-old male goat all the saxifragial (that is, stone-breaking) herbs one is able to make it eat, giving it good white wine, and forcing it to run fast every day. Its blood takes on, acquires, and retains the virtue of these herbs, just as does the vinous must that is also prepared for the same purpose. But there is more virtue in the male goat's blood, as we have often found through experience. As for the lemon juice, there is another reason for its ability to break up and dissolve stones in the human body, or at least to soften them, as vinegar makes the shell of an egg soft. But its added stinging quality is most harmful to the stomach and bowels if one takes a lot of it, as would indeed be necessary in order to dissolve a stone. Besides, the case is not similar, in that the pearl is submerged in the lemon juice, thus suffering its entire strength, whereas the lemon juice, taken orally, is greatly diluted and weakened by remaining in the stomach and several other organs through which it must pass, thus meeting up with more liquids and further dilution, weakening still more its strength.

4. Something bad for one's memory.

Eating rabbit brains is considered to be damaging for one's memory because this animal has such a short memory (residing in the brain) that, unable to recall a danger that just occurred, it never fails to return to the hole it just crawled out of a few seconds earlier. But one could consider all other brains just as dangerous since they engender pituitous blood, which is very deleterious to one's memory, as can be seen in the disorder called *lethargy*, a term meaning both forgetfulness and neglect.

SUPERSTITIOUS, VAIN, AND CEREMONIOUS REMEDIES

There are a thousand superstitious remedies having no founding in reason or in experience, although several people are mistaken in believing that they are well tested. The error comes from the coincidence of a recovery that occurs at the same time one of these remedies is being used, just as it happens when one recovers after using several different things that were administered, done, or said, and to which the entire recovery is attributed. I shall speak of a few such useless remedies and inept cures, which have been sent to me from several people in the greatest secrecy. It is absolutely true that in some instances there is some mystery involved, and that they bring about a recovery, not in and of themselves but by chance, as I shall be able to explain after presenting each one. Whatever the case may be, common folk are in error by virtue of the fact that they are ignorant of the true cause and attribute the whole event to what they are able to see, be it done, said, or applied.

1. To stop any type of bleeding.
   One must have a red-hot needle that was given by a groom on his wedding day. Squeeze very tightly the little finger of the one who is bleeding with the hand that corresponds to the part of the body that is bleeding. The bleeding will immediately stop, wherever it is occuring, even if it is from a wound.
   Likewise, the stone from the brain of a carp put in the fold of the little finger corresponding to the part that is bleeding stops the flow of blood, no matter how heavy it might be.
   Likewise, place a piece of straw in the shape of a cross on the back of the person bleeding, with his clothes on and without his being aware of it. Or have him bleed on pieces of straw in the shape of a cross.

2. For jaundice.

Find some plantain sprouting under a house. Have the person with jaundice piss on the plantain repeatedly until the plant dies. As it dies, the jaundice will go away.

3. For gout with cramps.

Wear all night long, against the ankles, as one would wear brace-lets, a flagon chain[101] made of freshly cast brass.[102]

4. To speed up teething in small children.

Take the quill of a feather and fill it with alum. Plug it tightly on both ends and have the child wear it hanging from a necklace.

5. To stop vomiting at sea.

Put salt on your head upon coming aboard.

6. To make a woman's milk dry up.

Have the woman jump three times, or three mornings in a row, on the sage in the garden of a priest.

7. For any type of fever.

Carry a live spider in a nutshell hanging from a necklace.

8. For a quartan fever.

Have a mendicant brother ask it of you for the love of God: you will lose it and he will catch it.

---

[101]Joubert's term is a *jazerant*, and the translation is Cotgrave's.

[102]Joubert's term is *letton vierge*; Cotgrave translates *leton* as "Latten (mettall)."

9. To make warts go away.

Touch the clothes of someone you know is cuckolded; whatever part of his clothes you touch without his knowing it will cause your warts to go away. People also say that if you are cutting up a hare, a rabbit, a partridge, some fowl, and so forth, and if you are having trouble finding the joints, think about some cuckold and you will find them.

Likewise, to get rid of warts, have a person younger than you count them; that person will catch them and will in turn be able to give them to someone who is younger still by doing the same thing.

Likewise, have anyone whatsoever touch them with pitch and that person will catch them.

Likewise, take a handful of salt and run and throw it in an oven, and the warts will disappear.

10. To cure the dropsy.

You have to piss on some horehound nine mornings in a row as soon as the sun touches it, and as the plant dies, the swelling in the stomach will subside.

11. For colic.

Wear a brass ring on the little finger. People say this remedy is also good for the falling sickness.

12. For suffocation of the womb.

The woman must wear on her finger a ring made of three metal wires twisted together: one of silver, one of brass, and one of iron.

13. Conjuring the womb.[103]

Withered womb, with your fifty-two roots,
Plus one nobody talks about,
Move away from the ribs;
That is not where you and yours belong.
Move away from the backbone;
You are not comfortable there.
Move away from the bottom of the belly,
Where you cannot stretch out.
Bump up against the belly button,
There where the Virgin [Mary] carried her [dear] son.
Crick, crack, womb, return where you belong.

    Our Father, Hail Mary. Must be recited
        three times.

FABULOUS STORIES

Common folk are mistaken in several sayings concerning animals, which they did not make up themselves but rather transmit from the ancients. The ancients either understood or explained them poorly or else (perhaps) made up such stories on purpose for some good reason, just as the wise and divine poets instructed bestial man in virtue

---

[103]Joubert first gives the following text in the Languedoc dialect, followed by his translation of it into French:

Mayre mayris, que as cinquanto dos rasits,
Et vno mays que l'on non dits:
Tiro te das coustas.
A qui non son pas tous estas.
Tiro te de la esquinas:
A qui non son pas tas esinas.
Tiro te del fon de ventre:
A qui non te podas estendre.
Mais bouto te à l'ambounil,
Là on la vierge [Mario] portet son [car] fil.
Cric croc, Mairo torno tel al loc.
      Pater noster. Aue Maria. Faut reiterer
        cela par trois fois.

through fables and pleasant stories. This has always been and will ever be permitted them, no less than it is for painters, as gentle Horace bears witness when he says:

Always equal power and temerity have had
Both the poet and the painter in what they wished.[104]

As for painters, consider how they represent an angel in the form of a youth, clothed in a white stole bound at the waist, bare-headed and with the wings of a bird, and the soul of man as a small child completely naked, the devil with horns and with a tail. And yet these are nothing but spirits without a body, resembling no visible creature. Thus hell, which is nothing but a state, is represented as a deep pit; death, which is nothing but the privation of life, as the bones of a dead person, holding a scythe. Thus love, which is nothing but an emotion and an effect, having no substance in and of itself, is painted and represented as a naked and blind child with wings and carrying a bow and a quiver filled with arrows. The four winds, which are nothing more than stirring and moving air, are painted as the heads of men with their cheeks greatly puffed out like those of a trumpeter. And when astrologers wished to use painters for the purpose of instructing the ignorant, they had the twelve figures of the zodiac (which are nothing but a few stars arranged in diverse configurations) represented, one in the shape of a ram, the other a bull, the third twin children, etc. Thus too the constellations in the heavens that are other than the signs of the zodiac: one is a bear, the other an eagle, the others a river, a harp, a dog, a dragon, etc. Then the planets, which are nothing but stars or asters: Saturn, Jupiter, Mars, Mercury, and Venus as persons with various countenances and clothes. The sun one way and the moon another. Painters have always maintained the representation of stars with five rays standing for their bright glowing, even though all of them do not shine in such a way, and it is well known that they are all round, without points or physical rays. As for the four elements, painters represent fire (which is invisible) as our own artificial fire, which is not all that inappropriate. Air cannot be painted any more than can the sky, both diaphanous and transparent bodies, yet they are represented with the color blue. Water is figured with waves and the earth as a globe, like a ball. As for the animals, painters make up some fabulous

---

[104]These lines are from Horace's *Ars poetica*: *"pictoribus atque poetis / quidlibet audendi semper fuit acqua potestas"* (ll. 9–10).

ones, such as the salamander, which is not at all as it is painted, nor is the dolphin as it is placed in mottoes and coats of arms. Not even the fleur-de-lis, which is quite common. And the heart, whether of a man or of some animal, does not look anything like painters make it. The pelican is painted with its sharp beak turned against its breast, which it spears so as to make it bleed in order to nourish its young until it dies from it; and yet we note that the pelican has a dull beak that is wide and flat, much more like apothecary spatulas, such that it could not wound its breast. Furthermore, the Greek word *pelican*, signifying a hatchet or an ax, clearly shows that its beak must be flat. Add to that the fact that it is said that the father pelican beats the little ones as if with lashes from a whip until they are near death, and that the mother wounds herself so as to bring them back to life with her blood. Now, lashes from a whip are delivered by means of something flat, and not with a pointed beak. The phoenix, which is represented burning itself up in a fire it made for itself, is even more fabulous.

But all of this is allowed in the case of painters and poets (as we have said) for some good purpose and hidden reason, which is not necessary to explain now, when I wish rather only to mention a few fabulous sayings that common folk hold for true and certain. In this they are quite excusable, for several great ancient philosophers and physicians have argued for such opinions.

1. About the viper.

It is a very ancient opinion that the female viper joins with the male by receiving the head of the male in its mouth for lack of genital parts elsewhere, and that the female, because of the pleasure she takes in it, closes her jaws so tightly that she cuts off the head of her husband, thereupon becoming pregnant. Then when the moment for delivery comes, the little ones, having no other exit and as if to avenge the death of their father, devour the belly and the flanks of their mother, causing her death. And this is why it is said of the posthumous child whose mother dies in giving birth, "He is like the viper, who never sees its mother or its father." And there is an emblem that the printer Jean de Tournes (among the best in France) has as a motto with the following inscription: *Quod tibi fieri non vis, alteri ne feceris.*[105] All of this is false and improperly stated because of a misunderstanding of what Aristotle said. What happens is that the viper conceives eggs that hatch in its belly and become little baby vipers. They come out already formed, having rid themselves of the membrane or case that had surrounded them in the womb. This is their afterbirth. But the last ones to come out, driven by impatience, eat through this membrane in order to come out more quickly, for the mother carries more than twenty of them and only has one of them a day. This makes the last ones impatient and forces them to eat their way through their tunic or membrane but not through the sides or the belly of their mother. There might have been a mistake over the origin and etymology of the word, as in the case of calling the viper *quasi vipariens*. But the word comes from *viuum pariens*. For no other snake but the viper brings its young into the world alive. The others lay eggs that, once outside the belly of the mother, hatch and make snakes.

2. About the beaver, also called the water-horse.[106]

It is commonly believed that this animal bites off its testicles when it thinks it is being tracked by hunters; it knows from instinct that it is hunted for its testicles. Hence people think that the name *castor* was given to it because it castrates itself and consequently becomes chaste. This is false, for as Dioscorides wrote long ago, it is unable to reach its testicles.[107] It is not a question of the two glands it has in the groin, like two apostemes full of fatty matter called *castorium*, for it does not bite these off either. And it is not called a *castor* after the verb *castrate* or the word *chastity*, but after the Greek word *gaster*, which means "belly," because it has a large belly, only the letter *g* was

---

[105]Jean de Tournes (1504–64) was one of the celebrated printers in Lyon during the Renaissance. He published editions of Rabelais, Louise Labé, Pernette Du Guillet, Pontus de Tyard, and Jacques Peletier du Mans. The inscription, literally translated, reads: "What you do not wish done to you, you shall not do unto others."

[106]Cotgrave's translation of the word used by Joubert (*castor*).

[107]Joubert's note: Book 3, chapter 23 [Dioscorides was a Greek botanist of the first century A.D.; he wrote a famous work, entitled *De materia medica*, in which five hundred plants are named and described; he is also thought to have authored *Alexipharmaca*, which treats the subject of poisons and their remedies].

changed to a *c*. See on this subject the last chapter of the second volume of Monsieur Rondelet's most learned treatise on fish.[108]

3. About the salamander.

There is also a grave error concerning the nature of this animal, said to live in fire and even to extinguish it. This notion was the basis for the emblem of the great French king François, first of this name, father of arts and sciences: *Nutrisco & extinguo*.[109] Dioscorides had clearly pointed out just the opposite,[110] and Galen as well, saying that the salamander lasts for a short while in a fire but burns up if it stays too long.[111] Yet people preferred to espouse the opinion of Aristotle, who said that the salamander does not burn up in a fire but runs over it and puts out both the flames and the coals.[112] Experience (which is mightier than all the authority of the wisest in the world) teaches us that none of this is to be believed. As for its face, the salamander that artists paint is imaginary and is made up by painters who pictured it thus in their minds and made it appear much larger than it is. It looks a lot like the little lizards that live in the walls and are called *laugroles* in Languedoc and *larmuses* in Dauphiné. The salamander is a little larger and is marked with several spots. Its body is full of a thick white juice like milk, which can be made to come out through its pores by squeezing it. This milk is so cold that the salamander is able to last a short while in a fire but not much longer without roasting, burning up, and dying, as we have witnessed several times. This is a long way from putting the fire out and still further from living in it, as the chameleon lives on nothing but air, if it is true what people say about it. I have yet to see any that live afterward in order to verify the claim.

---

[108]On Guillaume Rondelet, see *PE*, bk. 4, chap. 3, n. 3 (310).

[109]"I am nourished [by it] and I extinguish [it]."

[110]Joubert's note: Book 2, chapter 56.

[111]Joubert's note: Book 3, *On Temperament* [*De temperamentis*].

[112]Joubert's note: Book 5 of the *History of Animals*, chapter 19.

4. About the bear.

People say that a bear brings forth nothing more than a lump of flesh, without any animal form whatsoever, and that afterward it licks it so much that it forms its young and gives it its shape. This is a hyperbole for saying that the cub is very heavy at birth, completely covered with slime in such a quantity that it seems to be no more than a lump of flesh without any distinguishing parts. The mother quickly cleans it by licking off this liquid, causing the cub to appear afterward in the form of an animal. Hence anyone seeing a dog (or some other perfect animal) come out of the very sticky thick slime would not be able to recognize it at first sight. Once it is cleaned up, all its parts can be clearly recognized.

TWO OF MONSIEUR JOUBERT'S PARADOXES, TRANSLATED BY HIS SON ISAAC

TO MONSIEUR JOUBERT, COUNSELOR AND RESIDENT PHYSICIAN OF THE KING AND OF THE KING OF NAVARRE, CHANCELLOR OF THE UNIVERSITY OF MEDICINE OF MONTPELLIER

In Paris

It is very reasonable, Monsieur and most honored father, that I give you an accounting of my studies, both in order to comply with your wishes and to demonstrate through some good exercise (as I am always anxious to do) the progress I am making in my fledgling erudition since your departure. Monsieur Giraud, my good master and most methodical teacher, gave me as an exercise a few days ago the task of translating two of your *Paradoxes*.[1] Having approved my version (after making a few corrections on it), he accepted my idea of sending it to you to give you an idea of what I am able to do. Mademoiselle, and our most honored mother, continues along with us, all your children, to get along as well as possible in your absence, which, because we find it difficult to bear, diminished considerably our good cheer. But we hope to see you soon, now that you are toward the end of your term with the King, as you promise in all your letters.[2] May God grant us the grace of your return and keep you always in complete happiness. We all of us kiss your hands, begging very humbly your good graces. From your home, this first day of January (as a New Year's gift), 1579.

Your most humble, most affectionate,
and most obedient son, Isaac.

---

[1] On Joubert's *Paradoxes*, see *PE*, bk. 1, chap. 2, n. 12 (286), and bk. 5, chap. 1, n. 6 (315); see also *PE* (xiv, 105, 128, 134, 195, 271).

[2] Isaac is referring to Joubert's stay at court as *médecin ordinaire du roi*. He already enjoyed the title of first physician of the Queen of Navarre when Henry III called him to his court in 1579 in an attempt to bring to an end the sterility of his wife the queen, Louise de Lorraine. Joubert was not successful; historians lay the blame upon Henry III rather than upon the queen. See Amoreux (24–25).

1. Whether one can determine that certain poisons must not be given
on certain days and whether they will cause death within a certain
lapse of time.

To the most illustrious Doctor of Medicine,
Monsieur Pierre Perreau, Jr.[3]

You are able to explain this problem much more eloquently and
precisely than I, most learned Perreau. Yet, since you also wish to
hear my opinion on the matter of the limits and the potency of poisons
set to work on a specific day, I will tell you briefly my thoughts on the
subject. I have always thought absurd and ridiculous what is commonly
advanced: that poisons can be controlled by poisoners to work at a
certain time. For they are like drugs in that their administration is
certainly more practical, but even the potency of drugs (specified on
the notice limiting the quantity and the dosage for each person) can
only be learned through long and repeated experience and, once
known, still leaves one with an art that is far from certain but is, rather, conjectural.

I therefore see no justification whatsoever enabling poisoners to set
an exact time for the action of their poisons. For they have no opportunity to test them without danger or even without punishment, as one
does in experimenting with the action of health-related drugs. I am of
the opinion that they try their poisons on animals: dogs, pigs, and
birds, and that thereupon they set up their timetables, after observing
the various times it takes for death to occur, according to the nature of
the poisons. As if the natures, that of man (the most tempered of all
the animals) and those of the animals, were not all that different. Add
to that the fact that it is much easier to set a certain and precise time
for an animal than it is for people. For animals, deprived of reason,
have very little diversity within a given species, all eating the same
food and never taking up diverse studies (or trades). Thus it follows
that in the same circumstances animals experience almost the same

---

[3]Joubert's note: This is the last Paradox of the Second Decade [As is clear from
the above letter, Joubert's son, Isaac, translated this and the following paradox into
French from the Latin, the language in which Joubert wrote all his works, with the
exception of the *Popular Errors;* not much is known about Pierre Perreau, who
appears to have been a well-known physician in Joubert's time and is cited as the
author of *La Singuliere vertu de la fontaine en Bourbonnois* (Paris, 1600)].

feeling. But men, even though they belong to the same species, are nevertheless so different from one another that you will never find two alike (with the same face). And how many thousands of different complexions, conditions, and trades will you find? Indeed, in the sole species of man I think there are as many differences among each particular person as there are different species among all the remaining animals.[4] And so one must consider totally abusive and unfounded this claim made by poisoners, as can easily be seen from what I am about to say. Let us therefore begin our task.

Several people believe and maintain that Theophrastus (a most serious and highly considered philosopher)[5] is the source of this opinion because he speaks thus about aconite:[6] "People say it is prepared in such a way that it is able to cause death at a given moment, namely, in two months, three months, six months, a whole year, and sometimes in two years. And it is said that these latter die a more horrible death the longer they are able to resist. For the bodies of such people slowly fail, perishing in a long-lasting languor, and those who die from it suddenly have an easier death." But the authority of Theophrastus must in no way move us inasmuch as he is writing this as the opinion of others and not as his own, as the recited words very clearly indicate. And if anyone wants proof of this conviction, he will find two elements to it.

The first is the cleverness of men, who flatter themselves too much and make much of their vices. For will one not find many more willing to bear the remonstrance of their evils if they come from some external source than if they are said to come from the incorrect temperature of their bodies (or from their intemperance)? For even though no single vice can be said to be the cause of one's primary constitution, and cannot therefore be cited as the pertinent cause of one's imperfection, yet, because the vice is our own, we cover for it and

---

[4]The notion of the great diversity among men is expressed in *TL* in the preface to bk. 2 (65); it also appears in *PE* in bk. 3, chap. 2 (143–44).

[5]Theophrastus (ca. 372–287 B.C.) was a Greek peripatetic philosopher. A pupil of Aristotle, he became the head of the Lyceum in 323. His works include *Historia plantarum*, *De causis plantarum*, and *Caracteres*, a model for La Bruyère's work by the same name.

[6]Joubert discusses the aconites, along with other poisons, in *PE*, bk. 2, chap. 13 (125–29).

cherish it inordinately, to the extent that, if some misfortune arrives because of our imperfection, we fear that we will be taken to task for it. This is how it comes about that we much more willingly grant that the cause of the evil comes from outside than from inside. The examples are far more telling in those who are less educated, ignorant of the fine arts and of the sciences, won over by the simple force of their love of self. This is how old people are, and most idiots, who will accept nothing said about their misfortunes unless all is attributed to some saint, to some poison secretly administered, or to the witchlike appearance of some old lady,[7] whence the complaints Virgil speaks of, and in particular:

> I know not what evil stare
> Goes about bewitching my tender lambs.[8]

For unable to claim falsely with assurance that just now or a short while hence they were poisoned, one fabricates with more confidence that it was administered a long time ago.

The other reason for this conviction is the wild interpretation of astronomical theorems. For as is the case with astrologers, who infer (which is true) the diverse behavior of the passions or emotions from inferior heavenly bodies in diverse conjunctions, oppositions, and aspects as shifted from the superior ones, common folk have thereupon taken upon themselves the founding of the variety of effects on the slightest differences they observe in the heavenly bodies, such as when they infer that some plant is effective against fevers as long as it is picked before sunrise.[9] Now this error has gone too far. For not only from such differences (certainly very slight) have men commonly constructed the diversity of effects in kind, but they also expect the accidents of such effects to be diverse for the same reason, such as the time before the action of certain poisons. Theophrastus speaks of the

---

[7][Isaac's?] Joubert's note: The ignorance of causes invites all too often the unfounded suspicion of poisonings and witchcraft.

[8]The lines are from the *Eclogues* (3:103): "... *nescio quis teneros oculus mihi fascinat agnos.*"

[9][Isaac's?] Joubert's note: So it is also with herbs picked on the eve of Saint John's Day.

raving of such men when he writes: "Death comes in the same amount of time that the plant has been picked."

Let us therefore look for the true solution to this problem by using reason rather than the relating or witnessing of some person, which we will do very conveniently (if I am not mistaken) by beginning with the definition of the term *poison*, so that we might understand more easily what it is we are arguing about.

We properly call poison anything that, introduced into the body, so revolts the body's nature that it is unable to quell the poison but is, rather, changed by it in much the same way as food is normally changed by the body. All poisons share two distinct characteristics. For either they are enemies of human nature because of their manifest qualities, or they are hostile to it in their entire substance. Furthermore, some are able to kill quickly, others more slowly, according to their particular natures. Those which are carried immediately to the innermost parts of the heart kill suddenly, within a few days or hours. Such poisons are extremely hot and, for the most part, corrosive or putrefactive, called *septiques* by the Greeks, and possessing very subtle elements. For the cold and unrefined ones are slow acting and infiltrate little by little into the veins and arteries. There are some that infect and destroy our bodies with nothing more than their vapors or invisible exhalations, among which are numbered those occupying the highest rank of atrocity and malice: certain unnatural poisons which have such a subtle potency that, when rubbed or oiled into the stirrups, they penetrate the boots of the man on horseback until they reach the bottoms of the feet, whereupon they enter the body through the pores of the skin and corrupt all the organs of the body. Saddles and bridles are also infected with it, allowing it to make its way by means of natural body heat into the veins and arteries of the person on horseback through the pores of the hands and the thighs. Finally, clothes, beds, and covers are poisoned with it. In this type may be included those poisons that kill through the intermediary of the sense of sight, the sense of smell, or the sole sense of taste (without being swallowed), suddenly precipitating the victim into disaster without the slightest delay. All these poisons bring about instant fatality, allowing no time whatsoever to intervene for the miserable ones on the brink of death. I understand that such poisons are in frequent use among the Turks and other savages. From these are to be distinguished the less refined poisons, which are slower acting and take longer to have their effect.

But in the end they burn horribly, gnaw, eat away, and torment; over time they acquire greater strength and more maliciousness.

Now, not only are there different levels of efficaciousness among poisons of different types, but there is also a great variety in the amount of time they take to do harm, according to their compositions and according to the constitutions of those made to ingest them. Some feel the attack sooner or later than others when poisoned; some also survive. For it sometimes happens that the poisonous potency is mitigated and overcome by the complexion of the person given the poison, or that the person is of a strong enough constitution or made strong by the administration of an antidote, just as with those who are exposed to the same pestilential air: some do not catch the plague, and among those who do, some die sooner and others later, and some finally recover. If this is the case, it seems totally ridiculous when people say that it is possible to give someone poison that on a certain day at a certain time will cause death, and that this is a quality of the poison itself.

This error seems to engender another one that we overturned a long time ago: namely, that drugs steal our natural heat at the beginning of their decomposition, as Galen points out.[10] It would therefore follow that if they are administered too hastily they will produce their effect much later. But even if I were to grant them this point, it would still not corroborate what they are claiming here, except fraudulently. For suppose someone argues in the following way: "This drug has its effect later than that one; therefore it will have it at such and such a time." The argument is false and is called *elanche au consequent* by Aristotle,[11] neither more nor less than if one were to say: "The goat is an animal; therefore the goat is an ass." For *to take effect later* and *to take effect at such and such a time* are different types of what this action is at whatever the time.

Now, that such people take into account nothing more than the sole condition of the poisons is proof enough that you hear them take no account whatsoever of the bodies. They specify, rather, only the type of poison, to which they solely attribute the lapse of time for its effectiveness, and not the complexion of the man poisoned. But it has often

---

[10][Isaac's?] Joubert's note: Paradox 1, Decade 1.

[11]Joubert is referring to Aristotle's *De sophisticis elenchis* (167b).

been noted that among people given the same poison in the same amount at a banquet together, some died suddenly and others after a few days, and that on some it had scarcely any effect at all. We see the same thing happen every day with purgative remedies, which, given in the same amount at the same time and from the same preparation to different people, cause some to empty their bowels very quickly and others later, still others in great amounts, and others yet next to nothing; besides this, some void without any trouble, others with great difficulty, horrible cramps, and a recurring queasy stomach.

And what is the necessity of citing different men when in the same man the same medicine does not always produce the same effects? Since, then, according to the diverse and unique complexion and make-up of different bodies we see such things happen all too often, and since we cannot understand exactly the exact temper of each man, how will anyone be able to know how long someone's natural heat will resist a poison? Even if I were to admit that someone were such an expert poisoner, and that he measured with unfailing precision the potency of the poison, as exquisitely as one weighs musk on a scale, I would nonetheless never admit that one can determine with exactitude the nature of the person to be given the poison such that it will not fail to cause death at the very moment it was predicted. For the art of medicine itself is held to be [an art] founded upon conjecture when it is a question of prescribing for each patient the amount and the specific quality of its remedies, since one could in no way know, say, or write down the exact specificity.[12] As Galen says, in the third book of his *Method*, chapter 3, and a little later, in his *Art of Medicine*: "There is no single thing or remedy that cannot be named in its kind, but what is unable to be said or written, nor prescribed with certitude, is the quantity for each person." This he repeats often in the remarks that follow, pointing out that each man has his own particular cure, and that its natural property is unknowable and incomprehensible by means of exact science. Common physicians call this natural property *idiosyncrasy*, as Galen notes. And because all admit that it cannot be grasped, the true art of medicine is attributed to Aesculapius and Apollo.[13] For the principle, and the very foundation of the perfect, complete, and

---

[12][Isaac?] Joubert uses the expression *le justement propre*.

[13]On Aesculapius's role in ancient medicine, see *PE*, bk. 1, chap. 1, n. 4 (284).

infallible medicine (which Galen calls *the art of true medicine*), is the specific knowledge of various natures. This is why he adds: "If I knew how to recognize perfectly the nature of each thing in its specificity, I think I would be what it must have been, as I see it, to be Aesculapius. But since this can never be attained, I have vowed to conduct myself such that I will be as close to this state as can any man, and I exhort others to follow my example."

Thus, if medicine is conjectural and uncertain insofar as prescribing remedies for each patient, and if this cannot be made certain other than finally through long observation and experience, who will be able to convince us that poisons escape this limitation? For if, in the art of medicine, experimentation is dangerous, as Hippocrates most widely warns us,[14] it is easy to imagine how uncertain is the case for timed poisonings, for one is not at leisure to try out their potency, without danger and without being punished, as one may on various people with health-restoring drugs. And what their effects might be, as observed in animals, I have already spoken of above: it is inept to try to compare it to what happens in men, since the nature of man is very different from that of animals, if only on the basis of the proof that starlings live unharmed by hemlock and quail by hellebore, which are drugs and poisons for us. We are finally able to gather from these arguments that one must consider most erroneous and unfounded the art (if art it may be called) and the conjecture of poisoners, especially since a poison has its effect at times immediately and at other times much later, and this not so much because of its own properties but rather because of the nature and complexion of the body, the looseness or tightness of the passages, the strength or weakness of the natural heat, and the great or small amount of similar or different excrements. For the strength of the poison sometimes remains without effect or diminished, as in the case of those whose bodies have strong faculties and robust souls because of their very solid temper. This is why Galen believes that the structure and composition of the body is why hemlock kills men and nourishes starlings. In this he underscores the force of the refining and reducing virtues of heat, to which he also attributes the fact that cold poisons show themselves to have a more rapid and more powerful effect on hot natures. This might seem paradoxical to many,

---

[14][Isaac's?] Joubert's note: *Aphorisms*, 1, Book 1.

but since it was very clearly demonstrated by this author, I consciously omit the proof.

As for the nature of excrements, they weaken the action of poisons, which are quickly overcome by their repugnant qualities. For if there is an abundance of pituity in the intestines, the strength of a hot poison will be greatly diminished by it; and conversely, a hot humor will hasten the action of such a poison. Thus a copious amount of choleric humor will dull and overturn a narcotic that has been taken, while pituity intensifies it.

What these wicked poisoners are able to know is nothing beyond their knowledge of which poisons cause death solely because of the evident action of their qualities, and which ones cause harm with their entire substance. In this category are those that kill with a rotting or corrosive effect, and which also happen to gain strength over time, as Galen says, whereas the others become weaker with the passing of time. For all of these decompose over time, and more quickly the more humid and the hotter the climate is. And so time strengthens the action of those which have a rotting effect, because time favors rotting; and since they decompose continuously, they cause the body to decompose also. This is how it is that these poisons, principally of gross and earthy substances, cause death long after having been administered.

This is, as I see it, what poisoners might have learned through long observation, such that they know how to distinguish poisons that kill because of their notorious qualities from those that cause death with their entire substance.[15] Likewise, [they are able to say] that the latter, because of their very nature, have a very rapid effect on any person whatsoever, and that the former only unleash their strength over a longer period. Moreover, depending on the type, they kill quickly or slowly (without any regard for the victim's constitution), according to whether a larger or smaller quantity is administered. They are also able to moderate the poisons as they will and, weakening or strengthening them, make them cause death more quickly or more slowly, which is no great secret or miracle of nature. For we physicians also make use of such artifices every day in our purgative drugs, sharpening the weaker ones, giving them spurs, as it were, and, conversely,

---

[15][Isaac's?] Joubert's note: 1 [the Arabic numerals 1 through 4 enumerate the four points in the margin].

holding back the overhasty penetration of others by mixing them with those that are slower and less refined.

But we find absurd and completely ridiculous the idea that one can time the effect of a poison to take place on a certain day at a fixed time, especially since the nature of each person cannot be known in its entirety (as we have sufficiently demonstrated above), whence the highly uncertain term of each poison in causing death in man. For every natural action encounters diverse effects, depending upon the diverse dispositions both in that which acts and in that which endures. And this comes about not only by reason of the obvious qualities but also the hidden and specific ones, which is also the reason why that which harms one person considerably might do another a lot of good. Pietro d'Abano (the one called the Conciliator)[16] proposes, at the point in his work where he deals with this subject, that once the duration of a man's life is determined on the basis of the measured amount of his radical humor, it is possible to give him a poison that will consume him in ten years. From this he concludes that some people who are poisoned waste away continuously (they are commonly called *herbati & strigati*), and that in these cases it is sometimes possible to time the poisoning. But what he conjectures on the basis of astrology can scarcely be divined with any certainty. I grant that all those whom we see become little by little more ashen from being poisoned have a long-term illness but that they will die at a time that is unknown to us. Pliny does not give a more definite time for death resulting from the sea hare[17] (a poisonous fish) when he says: "People who eat it smell of fish, and this is the first sign they have been poisoned by it. Moreover,

---

[16]Pietro d'Abano, or d'Apono or d'Albano (1250–1316), was born in Abano near Padua. A physician whose interests extended to astrology, he was seen as a magician and accused of heresy. He was condemned to be burned alive but escaped by dying a natural death. The Inquisition sought to exhume and burn his corpse but failed to secure the body; he was later burned in effigy. Known as the Conciliator for his efforts to resolve differences between philosophers and physicians, his works include *Conciliator differentiarum philosophorum et praecipue medicorum* and *De venenis eorumque remediis* (published in the same volume, Venice, 1471), *Decisiones physionomicae* (Padua, 1474), *Expositio problematum Aristotelis* (Mantua, 1475), *Quaestiones de febribus* (Padua, 1482), and *Hippocratis de medicorum astrologia libellus* (Venice, 1485).

[17]The *lieure marin* is translated by Cotgrave as "the sea Hare; an ouglie, and venomous fish, whose left side nothing resembles the right."

people die from it in as many hours as the sea hare has lived." For who indeed will be able to guess the age of this sea hare so as to predict the time of death? And even if I were to tell how many days the sea hare had lived, I would still not grant that all men will die from it as many days afterward, since any given poison acts very differently according to the diversity of constitutions, as it has been more than amply proved. This is why it was never spoken more truly (which is what Pliny himself adds) when it is said that this poison acts in an unspecified time, as Licinie Macer[18] has said.

This, Perreau, dearest and most learned friend, is what seems to me to be the truth in this question. Forgive me if I was a little long in explaining it, and I want you to know that it was out of love for a few medical students who happened along when I was dealing with the topic. For they begged me to furnish them a copy of this lecture. Since I was not in good conscience able to refuse, I had to treat the question at length so as to accommodate their level of understanding. You, excelling in knowledge and understanding, would have easily understood in far fewer words my opinion on the matter, which is what you wished to have.

---

[18]Joubert has confused Lucius Clodius Macer, contemporary and opponent of the Roman emperor Nero, with Æmilius Macer, a contemporary of Vergil and Ovid who wrote about poisonous plants, or perhaps even with a later Macer who lived after Galen and to whom has been attributed a work on plants that came out in several Latin editions (Naples, 1477; Milano, 1482; Paris, 1506; Basel, 1527 and 1559; Freiburg, 1530; and Frankfurt, 1540) and later in Lucas Tremblay's French translation, *Fleurs du liure des vertus des herbes* (Rouen, 1588).

2. That there is a reason why a few people can live several days and even years without eating.

To the most renowned lawyer,
Monsieur Jean Papon,[1] counselor to the King,
judge, and lieutenant general
in the forest Bailiwicke[2]

The Christian religion teaches us that we must immediately believe the theological propositions recited to us, and that in things that cannot be proved, faith and firm acceptance is most pleasing to God, since He alone is able to break the laws of nature. But in those disciplines that deserve to be called mathematical and true sciences, inasmuch as they explain everything on the basis of causes, the idea of affirming something without demonstration and of ordering it as would a legislator is thought by us to be ridiculous. For nothing seems more absurd than hasty acceptance without counsel and without caution, especially among those who know that the human mind is most avid and most anxious in its search for truth.

Yet you see a lot of people who, if several others have said the same thing, will not contradict them and will think no further about whether it is more licit to tell the truth or, on the other hand, to lie because it is something everyone accepts. Oh how much better it would be to stop at this point and to doubt things the mind cannot comprehend. This is what I have the habit of doing, and because of it several people who are of a fearless consensus call me incredulous. For I have determined for some time now not to admit anything as true among those which can be proved by reason and argument, however great the authority might be proposing it. I admit outright that the cause of everything that experience teaches us has yet to be found and

---

[1]Jean Papon (1505–90) was a celebrated jurist of the sixteenth century. His published works include *In Borbonias consuetudines commentarius* (Lyon, 1550), *In sextum decalogi praeceptum* (Lyon, 1552), *Recueil d'arrets notables des cours souveraines de France* (Lyon, 1556), and *Le Notaire* (Paris, 1568). Joubert cites him on two occasions in *TL*, both times referring to him as "light of our time" (13, 69).

[2][Isaac's?] Joubert's note: This is the second Paradox of the first Decade [on Joubert's *Paradoxes*, see n. 1 of Isaac's letter to his father, Laurent Joubert, which introduces the preceding discourse on poisons, "Whether one can determine that certain poisons ..."].

known by us, just as I hold as most true several opinions that are paradoxical for the common man, inasmuch as they have not yet been argued before him. But since I do not want people to believe mine unargued, I likewise wish not to grant theirs until I have learned from their authors the basis for such effects or am able to understand them by reasoning through them myself. Would that all be free not to believe arguments without proof. For those who accept these admirable affirmations, moved by some unfounded opinion of a talker, seem most unadvised and (what is more) dull.[3]

Indeed, such is the one I was putting forth yesterday, most renowned President: that some people are able to live without eating, not only for several days, but for several months and even years. You prudently said that you would not accept such a notion before my proving it, especially since it seemed the most paradoxical of all those of mine you have heard. Yet it is most true, as are all the others, and after you have heard it, you will not contradict it. For you will not hesitate to espouse my opinion, since it is founded on very obvious reasons taken from natural things. I will not claim to have observed such a thing, but I will confirm that such a thing is possible.[4] If it were necessary to prove the phenomenon with witnesses, we would produce a few, unreproachable and of great authority.

Hippocrates sets the lethal fasting of a man at one week. But Pliny says it is not lethal at one week, since several people have lasted for more than eleven days. I understand that there is a sixty-year-old man in Avignon who eats very little and only at long intervals of five, six, ten, and more days. Albertus Magnus[5] writes something similar: that

---

[3]It is most interesting to read the first two paragraphs of this *Paradox* as precursors to the first two parts of Descartes's *Discours de la méthode*, published in 1637.

[4]This statement is as characteristic of Joubert's thought as are those which suggest he is of an empirical bent. In general, Joubert seems more theoretical in his Latin works, destined for his learned colleagues, and much less so in his *Erreurs populaires*.

[5]Albertus Magnus (ca. 1193–1280), born Albert of Bollstadt in Swabia. After studying in Padua, he joined the Dominican order before he was seventeen and began teaching in Cologne in 1228. He went to Paris in 1245 to study theology, at which time he began writing a vast series of works, the best known of which were on natural science, particularly *De vegetabilis* and *De animalibus*. He also wrote on metaphysics, ethics, logic, scriptures, and theology. In 1248, he returned to Cologne, where he was to instruct his most famous pupil, Thomas Aquinas. He was beatified by the Church in 1622 and canonized in 1931.

there was a woman who sometimes went twenty and often even thirty days without eating. He also says he saw a melancholic man who lived seven weeks without eating and only with drinking every other day. Athenaeus[6] recounts that the paternal aunt of Timon hid in the same manner as bears for two months each year, living without any food other than air, half-dead, such that one could scarcely recognize her. Serious people report having seen in Spain a girl who ate nothing, staying alive by drinking only water, and who was already twenty-two years old. Several people have seen in Languedoc a young girl who lasted for three years, and we know through the writings of some trustworthy and learned people that there is another one in Spires in Germany who lived just as long in perfect health with no food or drink other than air. Guillaume Rondelet[7] attests to having seen another girl who, similarly nourished, went to the age of ten before eating normally, and who then, when she grew up, married and had beautiful children. Giovanni Boccaccio writes about a German woman who lived thirty years without eating anything at all. Pietro d'Abano[8] (called the Conciliator) tells of a Norman woman who ate nothing for eighteen years, and of another who lasted thirty-six years without eating. It is held for certain that a priest in Rome lived forty years by only breathing air, the fact being well observed under the guard of Pope Leo (the Tenth) and by several princes, and faithfully witnessed by Hermalao Barbaro.[9]

But why not stop reciting these miracles, which might seem pure foolishness until such time as I have explained them through reason?

---

[6][Isaac's?] Joubert's note: Book 2 of the *Dipnosophiae* [Athenaeus was a Greek writer of the second century; the work cited in the marginal note is the *Deipnosophistai*, literally "connoisseurs in dining," and is a compendium of excerpts and anecdotes from ancient Greece].

[7]On Guillaume Rondelet, see *PE*, bk. 4, chap. 3, n. 3 (310).

[8]On Pietro d'Abano, see n. 16 of the preceding section, "Whether one can determine that certain poisons ..."

[9]Hermalao Barbaro (1454–93) was not a physician but a senator in Venice. He is nevertheless credited with contesting ancient remedies and left extensive works in spite of dying of the plague at the age of thirty-nine. His writings include *Castigationes Plinianae* (Rome, 1492), *In Dioscoridem corrolariorum libri 5* (Rome, n.d.), *Compendium scientiae naturalis ex Aristotele* (n.p., n.d., reprinted in Cologne, 1534, and in Venice, 1544).

Certainly the authority and the observation of others is of great weight, but it must not suffice when reason is not lacking for the confirmation of what one is maintaining. I am most happy that you do not wish to accept my proposition without reasonable proof; this allows me the opportunity to exercise my mind, to search out the explanation, just as I have for so long wanted to do.

I. It is a firm and ratified proposition that all living bodies, whether plants or animals, live by means of the heat that they have enclosed within themselves, by means of which they ingest food, digest it, take nourishment and sustain themselves from it, grow, and reproduce, with the difference that animals feel and move about. Furthermore, the more perfected they are in such activities, the more extensive is the strength and the nature of the heat. This is why Aristotle, who defined death as the extinction of a body's heat, left the reminder (as something that is widely known and repeated) that life is made up of heat alone, and that without heat neither animals nor plants can live. Imitating him, all the philosophers, without exception, define life in terms of heat and death in terms of extinction of heat. For however small the amount of heat a body might have, it nonetheless enjoys life because of it and produces its own activities, obscure though they might be.

This heat is nourished and maintained by means of a thick yet aerated humor, which, transversing the tissues of similar organs, is completely invisible. This is the primal (or principal) humor, common to all living things, from which the mind, bolstered by heat, takes foremost its substance and to such an extent that neither the mind nor heat can last for long without this humor. Hence the life and the longevity of animate beings lie in the consent and harmony of these two elements: heat and moisture. Heat is recognized as the operator of all actions; moisture is at its disposal, so that the heat will be more stable. And as long as this useful and delectable heat is able to sustain the vital heat, the animal or the plant will live. Thus it is that those who have a greater quantity of natural moisture or [those who have natural moisture] that is thicker and more resistant to dissipation will have a longer life. For its nature is to be heavy, oily, and sticky, so that the heat (which, enveloped by it, is taken and put to use in very small portions) might drink it up and absorb it later. Yet, before this happens, the animal gives its soul up to nature, because its own matter is withdrawn from it and the mind and the heat are languishing.

Now, since the bodies of living things are thus constantly spending and diminishing, if a substance similar to that which is being spent is not restored to it, they will certainly dry up and wither away. But there is not the wherewithal to replace the substantific moisture (as it is called) [that has been] consumed. I do not mean insofar as it continuously diminishes, but only a small amount of such a substance. For it has its origin in the semen and in the principles of our reproduction, and we do not see how any such substance could be added to our bodies, whence the inevitability of death, for there is no artifice for repairing what only heat can retain. The fleshy [moisture], spent during a weak spell, can be restored, but the primal moisture can never be restored. And as its very sustenance is consumed, so is the heat therewith; if it is that which consumes its sustenance (as it indeed is), it inevitably follows that heat itself is the cause of its death.

All that is left us to stop the vital force from going out (since we cannot stave off completely the cause of death) is at least to slow it down and keep it at bay, since its haste and its precipitation move it quickly, according to its nature, toward life's exit. This can be done through the intermediary of food, when, by adding some pleasant humor, the natural substantific moisture is maintained and thus better enabled to resist the voraciousness of its own heat. For it is thus preserved for a longer time when the natural heat is not free to exercise its force on the moisture, for its escape is somewhat hindered when it acts in the mass of the tissues and in the sustaining humors, and because of which it consumes during this time less radical humor. Yet, although there is always a small portion of it that is consumed, less is consumed when the other humor is present in sufficient quantity. And for this purpose nature has given from the beginning not only to animals but also to plants certain powers of seeking continuously after that which is lacking or missing in them, so that all will be preserved from death as long as possible. For all that is engendered and comes from nature has a deep desire to be around for a long time and to remain in the world. To this end animals have never learned from any other to eat, to drink, and to breathe but, from the beginning, have instincts that fulfill this instruction without any teacher.

From this it seems obvious to me that the use of food is necessary for all living things, if for no other purpose than for maintaining this internal humor (familiar and truly unique sustaining element of natural heat) so that it will not be too quickly spent. For as long as we are able to do this and to keep the natural moisture in a quantity sufficient for the maintenance of vital heat, so long will we remain alive.

II. From this we may deduce (for the second proposition we have to explain) that those who have less heat and are more languid do not need a lot of food because their heat does not seem to be very efficacious in consuming its moisture. It is just like a small fire, which, unable to support a lot of wood, nonetheless manages with a small amount; a large fire on the other hand goes out immediately for lack of fuel if you do not add to it a huge pile of wood. And this is why old people fast with ease, as Hippocrates says.[10] He goes on to say: "Next come those who have reached the end of their age bracket; far less, adolescents, and least of all, children, and among others those who have a quick mind and are very energetic. For those who are still growing have a lot of natural heat and thus need a lot of nourishment; otherwise their bodies waste away."[11] Old people have little natural heat, so they do not need a lot of food. In fact it would overwhelm them. "For just as with the flame of a lamp," says Galen, "although it uses oil for fuel, if too much is added to it all of a sudden, it will be more quickly extinguished by it than nourished."[12] Similarly, with old people and others who have a more serene natural heat, an abundance of food is harmful to them, stifling their natural heat and overwhelming it with its mass. Those who have a lot of natural heat (such as children and adolescents) enjoy an abundance of food because the matter of their bodies burns itself up fast, and their voracious heat causes the natural moisture to dissipate entirely if it is not reined in and held in check by the addition of a similar humor.

Thus the proportion and amount of food is calculated in terms of heat, without any consideration other than that of nature. For hunger, or the appetite that follows the natural necessity of nourishment, is its absolute rule, so much so that those who are subject to more frequent and more violent attacks of hunger are those who need copious and constant nourishment; those who are not hungry, or hardly ever and much less often, have no business eating food unless it be very little

---

[10][Isaac's?] Joubert's note: *Aphorisms*, 13, Book 1.

[11][Isaac's?] Joubert's note: *Aphorisms*, 14, Book 1.

[12]This is one of Hippocrates's aphorisms (I, 14).

and after long intervals. Workers, laborers, and others who work all day at hard tasks are forced to take in huge amounts of food and to have frequent meals because of the hunger that presses upon them, for the quality of the natural heat becomes more acrid and is used up by the exercise, such that those who give themselves wholly to physical labor are unable to fast without great harm to their health and their strength. Thus Galen points out that in *picrocholes*, that is in bilious people, abstinence from food is most detrimental; and in fasting for a long time they catch very fierce and very hot fevers, which can easily turn into hectic fevers, and in turn into complete dehydration.[13]

People of a sanguine complexion endure fasting more easily because they possess an abundance of substantific moisture and of nourishing matter also. In addition, their natural heat is more calm and less violent, as if checked by the moisture. They also take no pleasure in exercise but are always at rest and lazy; moreover, half-asleep like dormice,[14] they have scarcely any appetite and later become phlegmatic, most often beginning to eat without necessity, solely out of habit at the appointed hours. This type of complexion truly has a more attenuated and as though benumbed natural heat, which it would be better to excite and heighten through physical work, so that once the great quantity of superfluous humor is dissipated and the natural heat returned to a normal level, the appetite would return, which is nothing more than the natural desire for what each separate part is missing and needs, namely, the nourishing element that is to replace the substance that is constantly being driven off by natural heat.

When, therefore, there is no appetite, it is likely that the natural heat is acting upon some other humor, excremental and unnatural in nature. And since the consumption of such matter is in no way harmful, why should we be surprised if without any pain or discomfort the lack of appetite persists for as long as this accumulation of superfluous humor refuses to diminish, especially in view of the fact that the languishing natural heat of laziness is almost impossible to dissipate? This

---

[13][Isaac's?] Joubert's term is *marasme roti*. Cotgrave translates *marasme* as "a consumption in the highest degree; an extreame, or totall consumption; an exsiccation, or drying up of the whole bodie."

[14]The text reads *"endormis comme glirous,"* which is a printer's error for *glirons*; Cotgrave first translates the term literally ("a Dormouse"), then gives a clarification (*"Gras comme glirons.* We say, fat as pigs, or hogs, &c.").

is the second reason why old people can stand to fast more easily and without discomfort: namely, because aside from their small amount and feeble quality of natural heat, they consequently have a large accumulation of pituitous excrement, and because their bodies, being heavy, lazy,[15] and slow, are most inept at moving about and doing exercises. This is why they do not need much food, for their natural heat, on account of a lot of reasons, makes its way very slowly out of their bodies.

Now, what we have said to be the case for old people applies absolutely to similar complexions. For if someone is, either because of his natural complexion or because of the way he lives, more moist and more cold, he will have little appetite and will easily have his fill on a small amount of food, since he lacks the natural heat responsible for consuming large amounts of substance. This is why bloodless animals (called by the Greeks *anaimes*), finding the cold most unpleasant because of their small amount of natural heat, bury themselves during winter and live underground in warmer places without food. This we learn from experience, and it is perfectly consonant with reason. For if the need for food is linked to the replacement of that which is constantly being lost, so that the primal humor (the fuel of natural heat) might not be consumed too rapidly, those who lose next to nothing and who have practically no heat (at least for a time) have no need for food and derive no benefit from it.

Now, serpents and lizards, and other such animals, are cold by nature. The small amount of natural heat that they possess is lost extremely slowly, and even more so during winter, when it becomes more sluggish as a result of the vehemence of the cold. At this point there is scarcely any flow or dissipation, since the skin is thick and absolutely stopped up by virtue of the hibernal cold. And all the black excrement that there is, called up by their small languishing souls, gathers in the skin, which, finally becoming harder and rougher, loosens and separates from the underlying skin without harming their bodies. This is what is called the molting of the snake, which takes place in the middle or at the end of spring. Then when the sun returns to us and excites their natural heat, these creatures become more active and regain their original agility, having driven off the numbness, for it is heat that brings on and accomplishes movement. This is why Vitru-

---

[15]The text reads *"pigre."*

LAURENT JOUBERT219</>

vius used to say: "Serpents wriggle about horribly when the heat has purged the cold from their humors." During the short days of winter they do not move, benumbed by the cold that results from the change in the air.[16] That dormice and mountain rats (called the Alpine mouse)[17] not only abstain from eating all winter and do nothing but sleep, but also become all the fatter for it, is quite marvelous yet is confirmed by experience, whence that which Martial says of them in his *Distiques*:

> During the winter I sleep,
> And am fatter although
> I am nourished by nothing
> Other than sleeping very well.[18]

You will reply that small animals can go for a while without food, but not the larger ones. To which argument I reply by citing the crocodile (wild animal of huge proportions), the sole creature that is thought to grow throughout its lifetime, and which lives for a very long time. Now, Pliny writes that the crocodile spends four months of every winter in its cavern fasting. People also affirm that the bear can live all winter without eating. Just as old people, because of their coldness, do not have much appetite and do not need much food, thus it is too that all complexions that are more cold than hot can go longer without food. And what need of renewed nourishment have those whose natural or added heat is not dissipated? And what amount of fuel will a languishing heat consume? If it does consume some small amount, and if there is an abundance of substances slowing down consumption, the need will not be felt immediately but much later. Sometimes the mois-

---

[16][Isaac's?] Joubert's note: Book 6, *Concerning Architecture*, chapter 1 [Marcus Vitruvius Pollio was a Roman architect of the first century B.C.; the Latin title of this precious work furnishing much information about the period is *De architectura*].

[17]Cotgrave gives much detail in his entry on *marmotaine* [also spelled *marmotan* and *marmote*]: "Th'Alpine Mouse, or mountaine Rat; broad-backed, great-eyed, and short-eared; as big, but not so high, as a Conie; her haire is, as a Badgers, long, and of diuers colours; her voyce verie small, and shrill; her taile but short; her clawes so sharpe, as with them she quickly digs her a hole into the hardest earth."

[18]*"Tota mihi dormitur hiems et pinguior illo tempore sum quo me nil nisi somnus alit"* (*Glires*, XIII, lix).

ture from nutriments and other times the moisture from excrement will slow down the dissipation of our natural humor. When our natural heat acts upon and dissipates these two types of moisture, less damage is done to our natural humor.

III. From this the third proposition can be drawn, which will serve as proof for the proposed conclusion: namely, that a small amount of natural heat in and of itself does not make fasting any easier, but that it is the large amounts of superfluous humors accompanying it that preserve our natural heat. For the various nutriments that are cast about here and there in the body, nourishing its members and complementing our natural humor, sometimes ensure a copious accumulation in the body of excremental humors, which have a calming effect on the vehemence and persistance of the natural heat, thus stopping it from assailing a more refined substance by offering itself in its stead. When the small intestine is full of pituitousness (unless it happens to be sour), we have no appetite and are disgusted by food; and (in my opinion) we do not have much need for food until this material has been digested or sent elsewhere.

It is quite possible that, while the stomach refuses to accept food (because it has no need for any fresh nutriments), the other members of the body also endure a natural hunger, but which is not felt, and thus languish and waste away if nourishment is not given to them. For this reason it is often better to supply the stomach with food before it finishes completely its previous contents. Yet, it would be better still to purge artificially beforehand (if this is possible), so that the new supply of food will not be tainted. If the entire body were filled throughout with the same humor as that of the stomach, each member would not have to seek out its portion and would not need food as long as such a humor was sufficient to maintain its natural heat. But the stomach is all too often overstuffed because it receives everything first and because its cavity is larger. It happens far less often that all these types of excrements wander throughout the body. This does happen, however, with old people and with others who are cold by nature, because their feeble amount of natural heat is unable to digest the food sent to each member but, rather, leaves all about a considerable amount of undigested matter. These humors are pituitous and mild, perfect for the nourishment of natural heat if they are further refined. For physicians maintain that pituitousness is brought to perfection by the action of natural heat in the veins, where it is slowly refined and converted into wholesome blood. For (as they say) phlegm is nothing more than unrefined blood and will serve to nourish the organs of the body after being carefully enriched. It is therefore imperative to allow our natural heat to perform such praiseworthy work and not to let it be disturbed by the constant arrival of swallowed food.

This is the function of fasting, most healthy for those who have accumulated throughout the body an abundance of humors that are pituitous, mild, or insipid. This is why Hippocrates strongly advises fasting for those who have moist constitutions, because natural heat takes delight in using up humors, even if they are still rather unrefined, scarcely more than food recently ingested. For food is far less similar to the form blood possesses and far less similar to the nature of the various organs than is pituitousness, and our natural heat will sooner be able to prepare the humor already at hand than it will to prepare food. And if it does not act in this way, every time new food is furnished it will inexorably turn bad, and the whole of it will become excrement. When this excrement is retained in the body, it spawns all sorts of disorders related to this type of humor: edemas,[19] vitiligos,[20] *alphes*,[21] scirrhi,[22] *loupes*,[23] knots, and [[other]][24] countless afflictions in the phlegmatic category, which can be avoided by the person who will allow his natural heat to elaborate and to refine to perfection this cold humor by not taking in any food or, at the very least, by taking it in much later and in small amounts.

---

[19]Cotgrave's definition of *oedeme*: "A painelesse, waterish, and flegmaticke swelling, which pressed downe with the finger, retaynes the impression thereof."

[20]*A Physical Dictionary* (1657, cited in the *Oxford English Dictionary*) defines *vitiligo* in a way that clearly separates it from its modern medical usage: "A foulness of the skin with spots of divers colours. Morphew."

[21]Cotgrave's definition of *alphe*: "A morphue, or stayning of the skin."

[22]Cotgrave's definition of *scirre*: "A hard and almost insencible swelling, or kernell, bred between the flesh & skin, by cold, or of thick and clammie flegme."

[23]Cotgrave's definition of *loupe*: "A flegmaticke lumpe, wenne, bunch, or swelling of flesh under the throat, bellie, &c; also, a little one on the wrist, foot, or other ioynt, gotten by a blow whereby a sinew being wrested rises, and growes hard...."

[24]An editorial note at the very end of this discourse explains the use of these double brackets. See p. 230.

For if we admit that it is our natural heat that must be the sole agent in this activity, [we know that] it is distracted from it by the ingestion of new food, which is useless and even harmful. But when our natural heat has used up what it had found at hand for the maintenance of the organs it must nourish, soon afterward each of them begins to develop a fierce appetite and to indicate its lack, by means of mutual communication, to the small intestine. Yet, as we were saying just above, sometimes the stomach desires nothing (because it is full of humors) even though the other organs are fasting; and, conversely, other times the stomach can be empty and famished while the other organs are completely satisfied. And so, constrained by severe hunger to take nourishment, we try other means in order to purge the other organs of their humors, so that our natural heat will not be overwhelmed by their excessive quantity. But if this repletion is common throughout the entire body to the point that the small intestine as well as all the other organs feel as though they are full of pituitous humor, and if there is no appetite, the temperate natural heat has enough to do in taking care of the task at hand and there is no need for food. For the natural heat has much to do and little strength, and so it does not consume a noteworthy amount of the natural moisture of the organs while it is enjoying another moisture that it finds more to its liking: that of a mild pituitousness. This does a great deal of good for those who fast for three or four days and longer. For what is the point of bringing in food when the entire body is spilling over with cold humors and is having a hard time dissipating them, simply because the appetite springs from the fact that the previous meal has been swallowed some time ago?

Stop and think! If someone has a strong dislike for food and becomes nauseous from merely looking at some, is this not a definite indication that he does not have [[much]] need of food, for which nature itself has instilled the desire without ever having to learn it from anyone? And who can tell us at what time we should eat and in what quantity or of what quality? In these matters we follow our own natural inclination and desire, free from the dictates of reason. Thus a person who abhors food completely does not have [[great]] need of it, inasmuch as it is a natural appetite and not a voluntary one nor one that obeys reason.

It is thus more than sufficiently confirmed now through our arguments what experience bears out: that several people have lived several days without eating and without any damage to their strength or their health. Not only that, it is believed that they have thus prevented diseases that were threatening them, or that they escaped from some they actually had. For disorders will threaten those who are overwhelmed with humors and replete with them throughout their bodies if too much food is taken in, because it will all unavoidably turn bad. This is why Hippocrates says that the more one nourishes those who are unpurged, the worse off they become.[25] From such a disease, made worse by ill juice in the body,[26] the German girl escaped who fasted for three years. For they say she was sweet and resigned, taciturn, lazy and sleepy, covered with blisters and scabs because of the abundance of a thick and sticky pituitous humor. After having sustained with her own forces such a long period of fasting, and after the humors were finally consumed and the substance of her disorder was removed, she regained her health and started eating again. This should not seem at all absurd, since the mind easily comprehends that not only can this happen but that it is accomplished for the better health of the person in question. Perhaps it is difficult to admit that the action of our natural heat can take two or more years to consume humors once they have been assembled. You will certainly grant that the longest period of fasting is limited to a week or two, as Hippocrates and Pliny have said. But I will make it so that the length of time will not be an obstacle for your coming over completely to my side and sharing my opinion. I, who am certainly the last person to be accused of credulity, am not convinced of such things without the support of reason. And I ask that you consider the source of my conclusion, that this argument can be made, after you finish reading the few words that have yet to be said.

IIII. When the pituitous humor that saturates the body and pleasurably drenches its organs is in copious supply, it constitutes a sort of nourishment that lasts a long time; when it is in short supply, as soon as it is consumed the appetite returns. Now, if this humor is not only abundant but unrefined and sticky as well, who will still doubt that life cannot be prolonged for a long time without adding any other nourish-

---

[25][Isaac's?] Joubert's note: *Aphorisms*, 19, Book 2.

[26]"Ill juice in the body" along with "euill digestion" is Cotgrave's translation of the term Joubert uses, *cacochymie*.

ment? Let us moreover grant that we have a person with a frail, languishing natural heat, either by nature or by accident: it will not be able to dissipate very many humors, which will consequently hold strong for a very long time. In an old man, a girl, or a priest, the natural heat is less strong and more calm because of the age, the sex, and the peacefulness. And the abundance of sticky humors in these people can be so great that the natural heat will be no less pleasantly entertained by their presence than by the daily arrival of some fresh food. This will continue as long as the natural heat is furnished with an abundance of humors; and it is furnished for a long time, since, because of their density, viscosity, and coldness, very small amounts of them are consumed by the natural heat, which is neither vehement nor acrid. And although it might have on a few occasions been violent and acrid, at least for now it is quelled. And so we have found that the salamander (an animal incorrectly thought not to be consumed by fire, as Dioscorides had said)[27] put into a fire is able to resist being burned for a long time and is able to put out a small fire because its body is completely full of a thick and viscous humor, more like milk than blood. A similar matter (in my opinion) fills the bodies of those who abstain from food for several years. And I suspect the same to be true of the nature of the chameleon, if what Pliny writes about it is true: that it spends its life with its mouth open, never eating or drinking and living on no food other than air.[28] For what he himself says concerning the *astomes* [[that is, people without a mouth]], who live on the sole exhalations and odors they take in through their noses, occurs somewhat differently, if you accept the very clever reasoning of Marsilio Ficino, which runs as follows: "People say that in certain hot climates that are full of powerful odors, several people who have slight constitutions and weak stomachs live almost entirely on odors. It is (perhaps) because the nature of the place reduces to mere odors almost all the juices of the plants, grains, and soft fruits, and this same nature dissolves into spirits the humors of the human body. If such is the case, what is to hinder their being nourished solely by vapors, since all

---

[27][Isaac's?] Joubert's note: Book 2, chapter 6.

[28][Isaac's?] Joubert's note: Book 8, chapter 33.

things alike are nourished by like things."[29] But those who were observed living without food in Europe were full of a cold and viscous juice. We can add to the aforementioned conditions the closing of the pores in the skin, which Alexander Beniven[30] recognized as having a considerable role in this matter, when, speaking of a man from Venice who fasted for forty days straight, he noted not only that the man had cold limbs, filled with crude and unrefined phlegm, but also that the pores of his skin were plugged.

Now, if one will allow me to transfer what happens in plants to what happens in animals, I have several experiments to cite. For onions, garlic, and wheat, several months after they are removed from the earth (which was furnishing them with food), not only live but also germinate, because they have a thick and copious humor, which, highly resistant to wilting and to drying, maintains the natural heat even without the support of newly received humor. Thus sengreen,[31] a plant called *sempervive*, aloe [[called *perroquet*]], and the plant commonly called *faba inversa* (this is thought to be *telephion*, called by the Romans *illecebra* and in shops *crassule maieur*, once pulled up by the roots and hung upside-down [outside]), live for a very long time because they have an abundant supply of viscous juice in their very thick leaves. And what need do they have of frequent or continuous nourishment, since they have such a gluelike sap that it can hardly be consumed by severe heat waves?

And, so that nobody will make fun of this argument (in which plants and animals are compared in their ability to go without food unperturbed), I insist that everyone realize that it is much more diffi-

---

[29][Isaac's?] Joubert's note: Book 2, *On the Triple Life*, chapter 18 [Marsilio Ficino (1435–99) was an Italian humanist whose translations and commentaries of Plato were an important impetus to neo-Platonism during the Renaissance; *De triplici vita* was one of these texts].

[30]Joubert must be referring to Antonio Benivieni (1443–1502), a Florentine physician and surgeon enjoying numerous clinical successes. He was often associated with Poliziano, Marsilio Ficino, and Alexandro Benedetti, whence Joubert's possible confusion. This group sought to break with the Arab influence, and Benivieni might be credited with providing the foundations for anatomical pathology. His works include *Abditis nonnullis ac mirandis morborum et sanationum causis* (Florence, 1506) and *De regimine sanitatis ad Laurentium Medicem* (n.d.).

[31][Isaac's?] Joubert's term is *ioubarbe*, which Cotgrave translates as "Houseleeke, Sengreene, Aygreene, Bullocks eye, Jupiters beard."

cult for a plant to go for a time living without sustenance than it is for animals. For why is it that plants must always be attached to their roots if not so as to continuously draw in sap, which is constantly necessary for their existence? Nature gave movement to animals because it was necessary for them to look for food only occasionally. And this is why you see that animals that have been deprived of food still live for several days at least, whereas almost all plants wither as soon as their nourishment ceases, and especially the family of grasses. Nevertheless, those which have a lot of humor and thick and dense tissues have a longer life and last longer after being uprooted. For they retain a portion of the gluelike humor in which the soul is preserved, and it is enough to make it last for several days. Hence the branches from many trees die only several days after being cut. Hence the limbs cut from an insect continue to move because the tenacious humor is slow to dissipate and slows down [the departure of] its soul, as though surrounding it and hampering it so that it will not escape so soon. This is also why the beautiful bloodless ladies (as we have shown above) are able to live for a long time without the benefit of nourishment.

V. I think that nothing further hinders me from concluding as true (as most sufficiently proved) that such a great abundance of coarse and viscous humors sometimes gathers in a cold body that the natural heat will do nothing over a period of several years other than consume them. During such time the body has no need of new nourishment, the sign of which is a total absence of appetite. Experience first taught us this fact; reason proves the very same thing through the comparison of several things that are similar. Please examine this more carefully, most renowned Papon, and you will no longer be able to contradict it but, rather, will subscribe to our opinion and marvel (as is fitting for every man of intelligence) at how from the simplest and most commonly accepted principles I have won you over to the opinion you had judged to be most untenable. It is the strength of the demonstrations with which geometricians (with much more certitude than the others) infer their conclusions, based on suppositions known and admitted by common folk. For they first speak of nothing more than lines, points, surfaces, squares, angles, circles, and other such things; then suddenly they deduce so much from one after the other that in the end, using no craftiness or sophistic cleverness but simply unerring consistency, they lead their disciples by the hand in the measurement of the greatness of the skies, the distance of the planets, the behavior of eclipses, and other very hidden things.

Similarly, he who has expertise in physics and in natural phenomena, knowing how to find through a sure method the principles and causes of everything, can easily affirm propositions that are paradoxical (yet perfectly true) and prove them by appealing to what the senses and experience confirm. This will suffice for you, who are well versed in every discipline and not remiss in confirming my argument, which, at the beginning, you thought not to be even the slightest bit likely. With anyone else I would debate for much longer if these demonstrations had no effect on him; but you yield already (I know full well) and add your allegiance.

After having finished this, I happened upon a passage of the Arab Avincenna[32] that confirms our opinion on the phlegm. He thinks that when it is more abundant it is possible that we could live longer without eating because it takes the place of food. And he does not deny that this cannot be the case in healthy men. I am most pleased that such a great author approves my opinion, which I thought not to have been treated by anyone.

What follows is translated from the second part
of the opuscula of Monsieur Joubert,
page 136, where it is noted,
to be added to this Paradox

Now, I easily foresee that two sorts of people might react to this, either because of the subject of the argument or because of its proofs. The former are ignorant of natural philosophy and of medicine, venerable people for their simplicity and piety, like common folk and all those who do not apply themselves to studying the cause of each thing. The others are diabolical, taxing with impudent calumny that which they know is well stated. I will give no time to such as these because they do not await the explanation [[of my statement]] and because they

---

[32]On Avincenna, see *PE*, bk. 1, chap. 2, n. 6 (285).

distort and infect with their poison all that comes into their impure thinking.[33]

As far as the other group of people is concerned, it seems fitting to me to satisfy them gently and sincerely. I see that one could make the following objection to my argument.[34] The fasts of forty entire days, which Jesus Christ, Elias, and Moses underwent (as is witnessed in the Holy Scriptures, dictated by the Holy Spirit), would no longer be considered as miracles if for some natural reason fasting for a period of several months and years can be endured. It would certainly be true if one did not recognize that these cases of fasting were given in flagrant contradiction with the laws of nature to men who were in perfect health and through a certain privilege, as we piously believe. For a temporary exemption from infirmity was divinely granted them, such that their condition was for a time other than that of humankind. But those we have learned of from profane accounts to have lived several years without eating (if they are true) must all have been unhealthy and full of a cold humor on which the body was able to feed for a long time, as I have demonstrated at length in the above argument. And so we learn from what happens daily that several sick people have no appetite because their small intestines are full of bad humors, and they eat less food in a week than they would eat every day when they are healthy. But that a man with a heart in perfect condition is able to go only one [[or two]] days without food and not be hungry exceeds the limits of nature and is a divine miracle. How much more admirable it is that such a man is able to fast a full forty days, such that he does not feel any hunger, does not have to combat the desire to eat, and does not seek out food or drink any more than does one of the angels? We believe that Jesus Christ had an extremely pure and temperate body, even though he was subject to disease, according to the condition of human nature. We likewise recognize that Moses and Elias, when they abstained for forty days from eating and drinking, were perfectly healthy and for that period (through a certain privilege) were exempt from the ordinary lot of man. Hence it follows that one may

---

[33]One might compare the tone of this passage with Rabelais's disgust with the evil reader in the prologue to the *Tiers Livre*.

[34][Isaac's?] Joubert's note: Objection.

rightly consider these cases illustrious miracles, through which the authority of these prophets and of Jesus Christ was established.

Now, it is nothing new for similar things to occur through the order of things that God, most good and most great, has prescribed for nature, and by an obvious miracle against the laws of this same nature. For such fevers, and many other diseases that the saints cured, physicians also can heal. But the means they use make for a great difference. For the saints through their mere words or touch undid (by means of the grace of God) the causes of such effects, within the confines imposed by nature. Physicians do nothing more than impose upon the natural causes other similarly natural causes, through which, if the virtue of the remedies given by the Creator is more potent, and if He does not wish them to be powerless in that instance, the cause provoking the disorder is erased. Jesus Christ heals completely inveterate menstrual blood through the sole touch of the hem of his robe. We through our medicinal arts, of which He himself (as a good father having pity on the human condition) is the author and true founder, remedy similar disorders by using certain drugs.

Thus it is most certain that an excess of phlegmatic humor can induce fasting [[naturally]], as was the case in the aforementioned cases of men in excellent health, by the sole will of the most high God. But aside from these there is an infinite number of miracles that surpass our understanding and that neither human arts nor nature itself can begin to imitate in the slightest. Examples of such an instance are the healing of blindness from birth, driving out demons from the human body, raising dead bodies that are already half decomposed, and other such feats that confirm the authority of God Almighty. I think it is clear from this that things said to come about through a certain law of nature (albeit rarely) do not put into doubt true miracles or diminish their veracity, and that a person who searches diligently into the causes of such events does not contradict the Christian faith. Rather, does one not better question the truth of false miracles by taking away forthwith the occasion for impostures, so that people with little expertise will not be easily abused by them? For if someone from among those who live without eating because of their cold temperature and excess of phlegm wished to pass himself off as a prophet inspired by God, how many thousands of men would not be precipitated into error and ruin? Certainly most impious is he, and ignorant of true (that is, divine) philosophy, who, reflecting upon these things and carefully weighing them, would pronounce impious and irreligious those who try to distinguish, through unadorned arguments, between the works and (as some of our people call them) miracles of nature and divine miracles. Such a desire is what all good and pious people will confess openly to be most fitting for a good, religious, and notably charitable man.

What is surrounded in the text by these marks [[]] is by the author, after having recognized and approved the version of his son.

END

APPENDICES

APPENDIX A

A COMMON QUESTION

WHAT LANGUAGE WOULD A CHILD SPEAK IF IT HAD NEVER HEARD SPEECH?[1]

That a Person Deaf from Birth Is Necessarily Mute:
(As Is One Who Is Raised among Deaf-mutes)
and That, Conversely, a Person Mute from Birth
Is Not Necessarily Deaf;
and Why It Is That Man Is So Slow to Learn to Speak

It is popularly believed and held as true[2] that man would speak the language of Adam if he were not taught another language from child-

---

[1] A note at the end of this brief treatise clarifies what is meant by "children who had never heard speech": "... if they were brought up among deaf-mutes."

[2] Joubert's note: The popular opinion.

hood, as in the case of being brought up by deaf-mutes or in some desert entirely uninhabited by men, where he would never have heard speech. Herodotus in his second book recounts that Psammetichus, king of the Egyptians, tried once to prove as much in an attempt to determine which was the oldest and most natural of all the languages spoken in the world.[3] He had two children brought up by women who were mute in the middle of a forest where they would be able to hear no human voices. After two years they were brought before the king. They pronounced the word *bec*, which in Phrygian means "bread." From this it was gathered that Phrygian was the first language of man.

But (as Saint Augustine says in his ninth book on Genesis)[4] these children could have learned and retained this word from the sheep among which they had been raised. For, as he demonstrates in his work on the quantity of the soul, all speech comes from hearing and through imitation. Still, in his book *The City of God*,[5] he thinks and believes that, before the confusion of tongues, which came about with the raising of the Tower of Babel, the Hebrew language was natural to everyone,[6] as if speech were an action proceeding from natural instinct, or from a simple movement proper to the soul, and as if it has of itself and within itself certain natural inclinations that it manifests and puts into practice without having learned them, such as knowing how to suckle, scream, cry, laugh, move the feet and hands and, when enough strength is gained, to walk. A young goat, a lamb, a young horse, and other such animals, as soon as they are born, seek out by themselves the udder, knowing naturally that therein is their nourishment. After they are grown, they choose from among a thousand different plants found in the pastures of their regions, those which please them and satisfy their particular complexion. They bay and neigh right from birth, which corresponds to the crying of children,

---

[3]Joubert's note: The experiment of a king of Egypt to determine which language is the most ancient [for an analysis of this and other stories from Herodotus, see O. Kimball Armayor, "Hecataeus' Humor and Irony in Herodotus' Narrative of Egypt," *Ancient World* 16.1–2 (1987): 11–18].

[4]Joubert's note: The opinion of S[aint] Augustine [Saint Augustine speaks of the origin of language in *The City of God* (XVI, 11); the work referred to here is his commentary on Genesis, the first parts of which were published in A.D. 414].

[5]Joubert's note: Book 16, chapter 11.

[6]Joubert's note: Refutation of the second point of Saint Augustine.

and all without ever having learned how, either through example or imitation.

Man has such ability to represent in common with other animals, simply from his nature and without having to learn them. But speech,[7] which is a meaningful vocalizing, expressing the conceptions of the rational soul, proceeds entirely from learning or instruction and is grasped through the sense of hearing, such that it is impossible for a person deaf from birth and remaining so ever to learn to speak, even if his tongue and the other organs destined to this purpose be in such perfect order and condition as to leave nothing to be desired.

And just what will someone who has never heard anything say? Language is [from] instruction no less than is music. Both are learned through hearing; and so it is that the child, wherever he may be nurtured and brought up, learns and retains the common speech (which is called the vernacular or the native), whether it be Hebrew, Greek, Latin, or some barbarous language. One is not more difficult than the other, for having had none by nature, he is indifferent to all, just as white will receive all colors, and water will make all flavors fade away.

Adam did not speak naturally any more than we do.[8] But God breathed into him a soul able to speak the language He wished him to speak, as He did with Eve. Their first children learned to speak from them, as ours do from us. Now, from these first parents already corrupted by their transgression we have and keep all our inclinations and natural conditions, and especially that greatest imperfection of being more inclined to evil than to good, [a consequence of the] truly original sin. But as for speech, we have but the aptitude and ability, as is the case in learning anything else. And this is what is truly innate within our souls, themselves bound in bodies of such and such temper, temperature, and complexion, besides being what man must have for his own development. For the person who is stupid and witless from birth is like a child in its first years, incapable of reason because of the body's lack of development, likewise those who through the misfortune of some disease or violent passion (such as love or anger) become mad, besotted, maniacal, and senseless. And in all these cases the soul

---

[7]Joubert's note: That speech is gained through learning or through instruction.

[8]Joubert's note: That Adam did not speak spontaneously or naturally.

remains the same and loses nothing of itself; it is nevertheless unable to exercise its reason because the body is not under its command.

Aristotle has very well shown that the soul is ignorant of everything[9] and is like a fresh tablet, smooth and polished, on which nothing has yet been painted or inscribed, when it is sent from heaven and infused into the soul, according to our belief. It is all simplicity, sincerity, purity, facility and ease, inclination and aptitude for every art and science, for all knowledge of things human and divine (which is the true definition of philosophy), with the exception of those powers and faculties required by a living soul, as in that of animals, which our souls exercise over our bodies from the very start even before the child is born, without learning or instruction, as has been demonstrated above. For to live simply (which is defined in animals and limited to the two principal actions of feeling and moving) the soul has no need of instruction. Learning is only required for the arts and sciences because the soul has none in itself, even though the divine Plato says the opposite,[10] claiming that the rational soul has knowledge of all things when it is joined to the body, but having been plunged into and, as it were, submerged in the humidity of the body, it forgets everything, as does one who becomes oblivious (in Greek the term is *lethargic*) as a result of the phlegmatic humor that drowns his brain. But later, as the body loses this excessive humidity and slowly dries out, the soul remembers small bits and pieces and understands everything that is shown it or pointed out to it, as if it were recognizing and remembering instead of learning anew.

This is the opinion of our dear Plato, which supports those who claim that we all have some natural language coming to us from our first parents, Adam and Eve, and that we would speak it over time if the other language that we hear ordinarily and familiarly were not preventing it. But the truth is that our soul in no way knows, or holds in itself, any language,[11] nor is it inclined or given to any particular one but, rather, is drawn equally and indifferently to all languages,

---

[9]Joubert's note: Opinion of Aristotle, that the soul has nothing of its own as far as learning is concerned [Aristotle's famous *tabula rasa* doctrine was also the subject of Joubert's letter to Marguerite de France, translated in *PE* (26–31)].

[10]Joubert's note: Opinion of Plato contrary to Aristotle's.

[11]Joubert's note: That our soul knows no natural language.

such that one does not hinder any other, as might be the case (perchance) with a natural language, if there were any such thing. At the very least one would detect in it some trace, as in those who cannot rid themselves of their accents or pronunciation habits in certain words and expressions of their native language.

The rational soul, having therefore no language of its own, is highly apt and disposed to comprehend and to express, by means of its properly functioning instruments, any and all languages, as is written of the king Mithridates, who had such a good memory that he spoke perfectly well twenty-two different languages. We have from nature but voice alone,[12] common to all animals who breathe, and different in each according to the species. For each animal has its own voice, which expresses only roughly its feelings or emotions; this voice cannot be marked or represented (says Ammonius in commenting upon Aristotle) by means of letters or syllables any more than one could the sounds of the sea or the wind.[13] Man also, in his first months, when he lives as simply as an animal, has only voice before learning to speak and, while deprived of it, is said to be mute, even though he has not lost his voice.

This is why Aristotle says in his *Problems*[14] that only man can be mute. Now speech is nothing more than fashioning and articulating one's natural voice by adding consonants to the vowels, combining them and interlacing them so as to express meaningful words that reveal and (in a manner of speaking) give birth to the conceptions of man, which are infinitely more varied and in greater number than those of other animals lacking reason and speech. And yet it was necessary for man to learn to modulate his voice in order to respond to what was held by the great capacity of his understanding. The child gathers and assembles various conceptions in its mind, along with the words it hears accompanying certain actions, all having meaning. This the child understands little by little, retaining it by frequent repetition. Later, when its tongue is more in control, the child tries to reproduce what it had retained, stammering. Finally, it speaks after a long apprentice-

---

[12]Joubert's note: That voice alone is from nature and speech is not.

[13]Ammonius (Ammonios) Saccas was a philosopher from Alexandria (third century A.D.) who founded the school of neo-Platonism.

[14]Joubert's note: *Problems*, Book 11, 57.

ship, no less than does a parrot, after having for a long time listened. For, otherwise, neither one nor the other would have any more than its gibberish (which is its natural voice) expressing nothing more than certain feelings or emotions, as we have said above.

Let us now see what Aristotle says about this[15] in his *History of Animals*.[16] "Animals that speak have of necessity voice; but all those that have voice do not [necessarily] speak. For those which are deaf by nature are also mute. Hence they are indeed capable of vocalizing but not of speaking." And in his book on sensation and its organs,[17] where he draws the comparison between people blind and deaf from birth, he calls them deaf-mutes, as if the two conditions were necessarily connected. This is why Alexander of Aphrodisias[18] in his *Problems*, having asked why people deaf from birth are also mute, responds genuinely that they cannot utter what they have never heard.

In order better to confirm this notion we must add what Aristotle said in this same book[19] concerning the voice and the song of birds, which is in part simply natural and in part stems from some learning among themselves.[20] For I do not wish to adduce at this point that which man teaches a bird: to reproduce a language other than its own, but the teaching that mother and father birds give to their offspring. From this it can be easily understood that if birds have a natural song (which is the voice common to the entire species) and still another, learned or instilled while living in their particular surroundings and which it would not have if it had been taken from the nest and kept apart, then it is likewise with a child who has been kept away from all people who speak and who by their conversation teach it to speak: it will only have its natural voice, as when it was born. "The voice that is made manifest," says Aristotle, "(which is, as it were, the speech of

---

[15]Joubert's note: Difference between voice and speech.

[16]Joubert's note: Book 4, chapter 9.

[17]Joubert's note: Chapter 1 [Joubert is referring to the *De anima*].

[18]Joubert's note: Book 1, problem 133 [Alexander of Aphrodisias, another in a long series of Aristotelian philosophers, began lecturing in Athens around A.D. 198; he was the author of several commentaries, among which are his *Problems*, often cited in Renaissance texts].

[19]*Historia animalium*.

[20]Joubert's note: That the singing of birds comes in part from learning.

animals) differs among animals, both from creature to creature and from place to place. For example, partridges from different regions sing different songs, for some prattle and others screech. And there are small birds that do not sing as do their parents if, taken from the nest, they have not had the parental instruction; they imitate and take on the manner and the singing of the other birds. In fact, nightingales have been seen on occasion teaching their refrain to their little ones, giving them some songs to imitate. For speech does not spring from nature, as does voice, but it can be acquired by study and instruction. This is also why men speak different languages, even though all have a similar voice, etc."

It is, it seems to me, sufficiently proved that speech is a thing learned through hearing, and from this it inevitably follows that people born deaf, and those who have never heard speech, are consequently mute,[21] unless over time, finding their ears unstopped, they acquire hearing, as we have sometimes observed and even treated, in the case of children who had not spoken before seven or eight years of age.

Now I wish, in passing, to touch upon a point that is apropos: whether there is a difference between the speech that a child has learned and that of a parrot, a starling, a magpie, a lark, a linnet, a thrush, a crow, or a jay, similarly learned. It is certain that, inasmuch as their souls are different, so too are their languages, in that the child understands what it says and wishes to say in this way or in a better way if he were able, in order to express and make understood his conceptions. The bird, on the other hand, has no idea of the meaning of what it is pronouncing. This is so much the case that if the bird asks or answers in an apropos fashion it is by chance and quite out of the ordinary, unless prompted or made to say something expressly. Still, the bird will always add some word out of place, which sufficiently argues for its not understanding, whence the common expression for a person who talks and does not heed what is said: "He talks like a parrot." In the same way, one can learn in German, Polish, Basque, Breton, or other unfamiliar language some stupidity or cursing that one will unknowingly use as a greeting and that people will laugh about. Indeed, several people pray to God in Latin without any knowledge of what they are asking of Him.

---

[21]Joubert's note: Conclusion, how people deaf from birth are also mute.

There still remains,[22] since the person deaf from birth is consequently mute, the similar question of whether a person mute from birth (because of some defect in the tongue or other organs necessary for speech) is consequently deaf. Lactantius Firmianus in his book on the work of God[23] believes this to be so, but because he is an unrefined atomist (as can easily be seen from his argument), [his belief] must not be taken into account. Alexander of Aphrodisias, in the place cited above, seems to be of the opposite opinion (but without good foundation) when he posits that there is a pair[24] of nerves coming out of the brain, with one group going to the mouth and the other to the ears, and that because of this the affections of the tongue and the ears are easily communicated to each other. And inasmuch as one of these nerve groups can be injured and damaged and not the other, it thus comes about that a person can become deaf because of some sickness without becoming mute, and conversely.

But his hypothesis is groundless, as is the argument of certain modern physicians, following Pietro d'Abano, surnamed the Conciliator,[25] claiming that the sixth pair of nerves from the brain, which controls the tongue, is firmly connected to the fifth pair, which provides for hearing. For, just as I refuse to allow that the inability to speak is a consequence of deafness because of a lack of communication or bond between the tongue and the ears but rather because of a lack of instruction, I also refuse to grant that hearing is affected by the malfunction and defectiveness of the organs of speech. Nor is the condition similar, since these organs contribute neither to the soundness nor to the composition of the ears, and even less to any learning

---

[22]Joubert's note: II. Whether the person mute from birth is, as a consequence, deaf.

[23]Joubert's note: Chapter 11 [Joubert is referring to Lactantius's *De opeficio dei*; this third-century A.D. philosopher was a convert to Christianity].

[24]The text is defective. The base edition gives *"vn paer de nerfs,"* but on the same page *"le sixsieme pareil des nerfs,"* which is the standard term for the branching of nerves from the spinal cord.

[25]Pietro d'Abano was a thirteenth-century Italian physician and philosopher who promulgated Arabic medicine and the doctrine of Averroës. Denounced by the Inquisition as a heretic, he was pardoned in Paris, but his works were not published until the fifteenth century; his *De venenis eorumque remediis liber* was published in Mantua, circa 1472, and went through four editions.

gained through hearing, which in order to function has no need of the slightest instruction, not any more than vision or any of the other senses require anything other than that they be open and free of obstacle and that their objects be at a relatively close distance. We thus both see and hear naturally, without having to learn or to be taught.

Since, therefore, the sense of hearing (in its simple act of hearing) takes or borrows nothing from the organs of speech, nor even from the faculty of speech itself, a person who because of a defect in the tongue is mute from birth will not be any more deaf than a fancy talker whose tongue has been yanked out. Indeed, one sees every day that those whose tongues have been cut out still hear just as well. It could be countered here[26] that it is another thing altogether to have one's tongue mutilated after birth than to suffer from some congenital defect, since we also see that those who have become deaf following some illness do not lose the faculty of speech, even though people deaf from birth are necessarily mute. But no further proof of our first proposition (that muteness is a consequence of natural deafness) is required[27] than the fact that people who become deaf through some accident are from that point on unable to learn new languages, unless it be by means of writing, for the learning of which hearing was, again, at one time necessary.[28] For since it is the case that the written letter is the vicar of speech, it is impossible for a person to know how to write or to understand writing (even though one may copy it, as in painting, through imitation) without ever having been able to hear. If, therefore, it is true that the organs of speech neither commune nor are joined with the ears in any particular way, and that speech has no effect upon hearing, as, on the contrary, hearing not only affects speech but is its very condition, then it clearly follows that a person who is mute by nature will because of it hear any less well (it being granted that the organs of hearing are in no way defective), whereas the person deaf from birth will be necessarily mute even though the tongue and the other organs of speech suffer from no defects whatsoever. Note that throughout I say "from birth" and "by nature" indifferently so as to

---

[26]Joubert's note: Reply.

[27]Joubert's note: Rejoinder.

[28]Joubert's note: That one can learn neither to read nor to write intelligibly without first being able to hear.

designate the deaf or the mute person from the very beginning. And I say "mute from birth" and not "one who does not speak" (for we would thus all be mute) but "one who is unable to speak."

Let us come to the third point.[29] Why is it that man, having a mind so subtle and quick that he understands everything in such a short time, is nonetheless so slow to learn how to speak and articulate his voice? Animals, immediately or shortly after birth, have the total and perfect use of their voices, as much as they will ever have. Aristotle in his *Problems*[30] gives the answer that man's voice has great variety; the other animals form few if any letters (two or three at most) and no consonants, which, joined to vowels, allow for speech. Now, speech (he says) is not simply a matter of voice but is brought about and perfected by meaning, through modulation and control of the voice, and the modulation of the voice [produces] the letters. This is why children, before they know how or are even able to pronounce letters express their emotions (no differently than animals) with their natural and wholly untaught voices, common to all children from whatever their countries. But speech differs from town to town, and even within the same town, because of the artificially articulated voice, through the great diversity of letters coupled and interlaced in infinite combinations, from which proceed the words designating an infinite number of things. Therefore, since there are so many varieties of speech, and since with five or six letters fifty completely different words can be made, it is fairly easy to understand why the child takes so long to develop its voice, as compared to animals, which have such a simple voice and (as Alexander of Aphrodisias says)[31] more natural than animal. For that which is extremely diverse and must be differentiated in many ways cannot be handled in a small amount of time, both because of the soul, which deals with the learning of speech, and the tongue, [which deals with] the articulating of it. The tongue also takes some time to become agile and trained, as does the hand in the case of [playing] a musical instrument. Thus in the beginning, from the state of being mute one progresses to being a stutterer, unable to sound out all the letters or to pronounce words properly because of the lethargy of

---

[29]Joubert's note: III. Why it is that man is so late [in learning] to speak.

[30]Joubert's note: Book II, problems 58 and 60.

[31]Joubert's note: Book II, problem 143.

the tongue and its clumsiness in a new trade. There is another uncertainty in this matter, which is less easy to explain. Aristotle treats it in his *Problems*.[32] How is it that some children begin to speak before the age at which one normally forms words and, after having pronounced a few words perfectly, fall back into their first stage and remain there until the normal time for beginning to speak? Several people think this is a prodigious feat, especially when it is said that a few infants have spoken from the time they were born. This is truly most exceptional and difficult to believe, yet it can come about with a natural explanation. It is that the child, at the same instant it hears, understands and is able to repeat. But most often and ordinarily, hearing precedes understanding, and understanding precedes speaking, by a considerable amount of time, especially since the organs of speech do not yet have the means to express what the mind has conceived. On the other hand, some talk before they are able to understand (just as we have said concerning the parrot and other talking birds), mouthing words they have heard up to the time required for being able to do both, that is, to understand and to speak. Those, then, upon whom the objects of the sense of hearing make an impression on the soul before the speech apparatus is perfected pronounce several things after having heard them said, especially after sleeping, when the humors, having become more abundant, are able to make an effort and force the tongue to articulate distinctly. But inasmuch as this activity is not maintained, it does not last; this is why the child reverts to his former muteness.

In the same way we too are sometimes disposed that, without thinking about it, there come out of our mouths phrases and sentences so appropriate that we would be hard put to come up with better ones; conversely, other times it is impossible for us to express what we know perfectly well. Likewise, it can happen that a child will say something, only to have its tongue return to its original state and become mute again until the latest moment for its normal development.

Still another case[33] is that of children who become mute because of deafness after having already begun to babble or even to speak intelligibly. We know through sound sources that this is what happened

---

[32]Joubert's note: Book II, problem 27.

[33]Joubert's note: Concerning those who stop speaking because of deafness.

to all the male children of Monsieur Antoine Butin (the well-known apothecary of Toulouse who has the sign with the three kings) but not the female children. They all spoke up until about the age of four, when they become so deaf they could no longer hear the slightest noise, and little by little they stopped speaking. This is mainly because, no longer able to hear, they quickly lost the small amount of language they had learned in their younger years, for children are very forgetful because of their great amount of moisture, and especially those of Monsieur Butin, who were very rheumy. Therefore, no longer having the means of learning to speak through hearing, they become mute, as does the man who learns a few words in German, Basque, or Breton and, for lack of continuing to practice them, forgets the little he knows, or the one who fails to keep up his grammar, or some other exercises or the playing of musical instruments, and quickly forgets all.

This fact still confirms our first proposition, in support of which we have argued as above. For if after having been able to speak one can become mute because of deafness incurred through some accident, who will then doubt that a person deaf from birth will inevitably be mute? I will add another well-known condition that has some bearing on this argument:[34] those who through some wound or other illness of the brain lose their memories completely, even of how to speak. They learn little by little to speak again, as do children, having at their disposal the sense of hearing and the organs of speech in proper working order. Witnesses who are dependable and trustworthy claim they have seen people wounded in various parts of the head, even in the eyes (concerning this, Monsieur Rondelet[35] relates a story from his practice in the appendix of chapter 21), who have actually forgotten their own names and who had to learn everything all over again, as though they were children. They all return, then, to the pristine state of a child at birth, except for their native language, which a few of

---

[34]Joubert's note: Concerning those who forget everything, right down to their own names.

[35]Guillaume Rondelet (1500–1584) preceded Joubert as regent and chancellor at the Faculté de Médecine at the University of Montpellier. Known as the father of ichthyology, he was the author of the first major treatise on fish, *De piscibis marinis,* and the *Universalis aquaetilium,* both of which were translated into French a few years after their publication in Latin (1554).

them still possess. But the acquaintance with foreign languages, with acquired knowledge in the arts and sciences, with everything they have seen and known previously, all is erased from their souls by the inundation and flooding of the illness.

Having finished this argument, I was informed that Monsieur Pero Mexía had touched upon this question in his *Diverses leçons*.[36] He arrives at two conclusions: that children who have not learned any language would speak in Hebrew, or that they would make up on their own a new language, giving things strange names. Since we see that children by nature apply names to what they desire, it would seem that nature teaches them to make up an entirely new language before they learn the language of their fathers. That is an interesting opinion, and worthy of a simple gentleman, but not one that will be accepted by a demanding philosopher, who weighs everything on a more refined scale than do others, and who judges (as they say) with the rigor of the law.[37] The reasoning we have furnished above argues and concludes of necessity that a child born deaf, or who otherwise has never heard, will also be mute, and that he will in nowise be able to invent a language, nor even know that things have names. This the child learns from others when they point them out to it, calling them by their names. From this it afterward recognizes these things when they are named, as when things are pointed out to the child and named, one after another, such as switches, a knife, bread, an egg, shoes, etc., and it understands what each is, with its name, through frequent repetition. Otherwise, it would never occur to the child to name anything, for it would not even know (as it is said) that it is a question of giving things names if it had not learned it from someone.

As for the strange and bizarre words children use, most of them are learned from women who chatter with them, imitating other children, who pronounce very indistinctly those other words they seem to be making up and applying to various things. These words are but corrupted forms of true words, which they twist and deform in diverse

---

[36]Joubert's note: Book I, chapter 33. Opinion of Monsieur Pierre Messie [Pero Mexía, a Spanish compiler, served as historiographer to Charles V; his *Silva de varia lecion* (Seville, 1542; 1548) enjoyed great success and was translated into most of the languages of Europe—French translations appeared as early as 1526 in Rouen and Lyon].

[37]Joubert's note: Refutation of said opinion.

ways or else take one and use it for another; or they are words that they are familiar with, but, [having] badly stored [them] in their memories, they take the head of one word, the tail of another, and, adding to them the belly of a third, make up a chimera of a word. In doing this they make us laugh, as does a German, an Italian, or a Spaniard who, pretending to talk French (of which he knows only half, or a third or a fourth), pronounces untoward and foolish words. Will one say that he is inventing them in order to found a new language? Not in the least, in my opinion; rather, he is fooling and abusing himself in thinking he is speaking properly by only using a few words he once learned and perhaps took in a sense other than that which they have in normal usage. So too the child, while it is learning to talk, confuses, corrupts, twists, deforms, and counterfeits words, through ignorance or through inability, in a strange way, just as one who is learning music makes irregular chords, or an apprentice painter or writer produces strokes that have never been learned anywhere, or a novice logician advances crooked syllogisms such as have never been seen in Aristotle. This is how it is in every discipline: those who fail to represent clearly what they wish to imitate or fashion seem to want to found a new art after their own fantasy.

But could one not defend in some way the opinion of Monsieur Pero Mexía? Yes, if one presupposes that several children are together, and not taken separately.[38] For a child who is alone has nothing to ask about, to discuss, or to communicate. It consequently has no need to speak nor to find words to express itself. But children who are in one another's company will most likely, in order to communicate (as man's nature would have it, being that of a social animal), apply names to the things they see and talk about together. For we possess naturally in our souls the faculty or ability to speak and to express through certain instruments of the body all our conceptions, just as we have the ability to walk, run, grasp, pull, lift, and perform other actions with our hands and feet. It is but a matter of the will's inviting and moving us to do so as soon as our hands and feet are strong enough. And these faculties or abilities are relegated to and brought into action by our control, without any teacher other than nature.

---

[38]Joubert's note: How it could come about that children make up a language.

It is therefore quite possible that the faculty of speech goes into action on its own when necessity requires it.[39] Such is the case when, in an effort to communicate, people, who must say something and express their thoughts through words invent and agree upon words together, accepting and retaining terms they find to be satisfying. But a person born deaf, and one who has never heard anything named, will not even know that it is a question of speaking or of making oneself understood by using words. Such a person will therefore only move the lips and make a few gestures with the hands, the head, and other parts of the body, just as he sees others do. Such people will thus always remain mute, as if they had always been alone, for they are unable to communicate words to others, which are received [only] from others. And so their souls will indeed have the power to speak, but only in vain and without effect, in that it is not solicited by any act of the will (since for an unknown thing one cannot have any desire) or by any necessity. For people born deaf, who neither know nor feel the need to speak, will never try to do so, nor will those who have always been alone. But when two, three, or four are together and want to associate with each other, then in order to communicate and live in fellowship, as the human condition dictates, it is highly likely that, even if they had never spoken to each other, their souls on their own would draw up and fashion for the occasion a language that would be entirely different from all others that, because of a similar occasion and need, would likewise be invented elsewhere by other people of another society. For if the soul is not impeded or frustrated by corpo- real instruments required for the execution of its faculties and powers, it takes them up on its own and puts them clearly into action when the occasion and the necessity moves it to do so.

Therefore, children who are not born deaf and who have at their command the organs of speech, if they have never heard speech and if they find themselves together, will ordinarily be able to make up some

---

[39]Joubert's note: See what is noted concerning the son of Croesus in the preface of the second book of Laughter [Joubert is referring to the following passage in *TL*: "Herodotus writes, and several others after him, that Croesus's son, mute because of a natural impediment, upon seeing his father in danger of death, suddenly began to speak and cried out, 'Do not kill the king'; and for the rest of his life he spoke most distinctly. This is because with the very great fear, accompanied by a very great desire to speak, he was able to produce such a great effect" (68)].

language among themselves, over which they will easily agree and have secret intelligence, no less than mutes make up signs through which they make themselves clearly understood, for each sign stands in the place of one or several words. Moreover, most of them make entire sentences, as do the hieroglyphic notes of the Egyptians. But children born and conversing among people who speak do not experience any need to make up a language by applying names to what they see and discuss, because they learn and help themselves to the words they hear spoken normally. And it would be the case with any language other than their native language, were they to be transported elsewhere, such as a child carried from France to Germany before learning or barely beginning to speak, for it will quickly forget what it had learned in French and start learning the German language.

I therefore do not contradict Monsieur Pero Mexía, except when he says that the gibberish of children and their bizarre words are of their own invention (they are, rather, the result of corrupted words they have [already] learned) and when he insists that a child can on its own make up a language. From this it would also follow that a child born deaf could likewise speak, which is patently false, as we have sufficiently proved with our entire argument.

End of the argument on the question in which it is asked which language children would speak if they had been brought up by mutes, by M[onsieur] LAUR[ENT] JOUBERT, Counselor and the King's Ordinary Physician, First Doctor Regent, Chancellor and Judge of the University of Medicine of Montpellier.

APPENDIX B

ON THE BEVERAGE OF MONSEIGNEUR
THE MARÉCHAL D'ANVILLE[1]

The beverage that Monseigneur uses,[2] in the place of the customary wine greatly diluted with water, is a light decoction of sharp-pointed dock[3] into which, upon cooling, cinnamon is infused, whereupon
with powdered sugar it is decanted and clarified through a long filter of
the kind used for making hippocras. Such a drink can be called a thin-
syrup *bouchet*[4] in apothecary's terms, and *propoma* in Greek.

The proportions[5] of the four simple ingredients of this composition
are: eight pints of water (which are about equal to eight medicinal
pounds),[6] one and one-half ounces of diced dock in summer or two in
winter. The sugar and the cinnamon are according to Monseigneur's
taste, namely, four to five ounces of sugar and two to three drachmas
of cinnamon.

Now, the virtues[7] of this drink are easy to understand, given the
nature of the ingredients. I leave aside the water,[8] the common and
natural drink of all animals, which cools and moistens the body most

---

[1]The modern spelling is Damville. This is the name assumed by Henri Ier de
Montmorency, the younger brother of François de Montmorency.

[2]Joubert's note: What the beverage is.

[3]Joubert gives the spelling *parille*; Cotgrave shows only *parelle* and defines the
term as "the hearbe Dockes, or the Sharp-pointed Docke; also, Patience, Monkes
Rhubarbe...."

[4]Cotgrave defines *bouchet* as "a kind of broth for a sick bodie; also, the sweet
drinke, Hydromel; or a drinke made of water sweetned with sugar and cinnamon; or
as: *Eau de bouchet*. A certain compound water, which with that of Corianders, makes
a kind of Hipocras."

[5]Joubert's note: The composition of said beverage.

[6]We recall that the *liure medicinale* was reckoned as follows, according to Cotgrave: "The Physitians pound; contains also 12 ounces; but they be diuided into 96
drammes, they into 288 scruples, those into 576 Oboles, they into 1728 Siliques, and
they into 6912 graines."

[7]Joubert's note: What virtues this beverage has.

[8]Joubert's note: Concerning water.

fittingly to ward off thirst coming from contrary causes. This is why water is a proper thing with which to dilute wine and to use as a base for all artificial beverages. Its goodness and perfection consist in having none of the known qualities of color, odor, or taste, such that water that is sweet, unsavory, or dull is rightly condemned by all.[9] And if occasionally one speaks of good water as being sweet, it means that it is drinkable and pleasant tasting, not actually sweet, as milk is, or honey. For it must have its comeliness and its fullness; otherwise, the stomach will find it unpleasant, becoming sickened and upset by it. This is why I am unable to see how one could maintain that the frequent use of sweetened or honeyed water is good for one with a weak or upset stomach, or one subject to indigestion, since it furnishes matter to be spit up often while eating, because the stomach is continually made queasy by the fluid flowing down from the back of the nose.[10] There would at the very least have to be something astringent in this water, as is rosewater in Alexanders julep,[11] for which sugar is only present to make it palatable over the astringency of the rosewater, which fortifies the stomach and stops the runny nose.[12] Still, I would not want this julep to become a daily drink taken with meals.

But a beverage in which sweetness is the main component, dominating the other qualities without being curbed in any way, is certainly gravely harmful. It is especially so for those with weak stomachs and delicate appetites, who spit up easily, complain about nasal discharges, and are quick to vomit their food, as is the case with Monseigneur. And it is especially so if taken at the very moment they wish to enjoy the pleasure and benefit nature has incorporated into the moderate use of the most tasty and the most healthy fruits during their season, creat-

---

[9]Joubert's note: That sweet water is bad.

[10]Joubert uses the term *cerveau* ("brain") because it was believed such discharge came from the brain.

[11]*Alexanders* was another term for horse-parsley (*Smyrnium olusatrum*). Henry Lyte speaks of it as follows: "In Frenche *Grand Ache* or *Alexandre* ... in English, *Alexanders*" (Dodoens' *Niewe herball or historie of plantes*, trans. 1578 [cited in *Oxford English Dictionary*]).

[12]Joubert's note: That astringency must be accompanied by sweetness.

ed to refresh and moisten our bodies in the face of the fierce heat and dryness of summer.[13]

As for the two other ingredients, which are drugs, namely, the sharp-pointed dock and the cinnamon, they are not able to counteract sufficiently the sweetness of the sugared water.[14] For because the extraction of the dock is so light and the infusion of the cinnamon into the extract is done when cold, their qualities are not drawn out enough to overpower in any significant way the sweetness of the sugar. And it is indeed better, or at least not as bad, to proceed in this manner so as not to cause as much harm. For if these two drugs were to infuse the water with any more of their virtues, as would be the case if one were to boil the one mildly and use hot infusion with the other, this water would cause more damage upon encountering the food, especially in those who were cold stricken and in all who were subject to indigestion. For cinnamon provokes discharge, as does wine, because of its potency and its penetrating virtues, by means of which it thins humors and renders them more fluid. This is why hippocras (as it is called) makes a lot of people hoarse even if it is diluted, as I have often seen and noted in several cases. And so those with whom wine does not set well, such as people with gout, congestion, or colds, must also abstain from cinnamon in any form or amount whatsoever; and *bouchet* will not be any good for them either in however small an amount.

An alternative would be to do the very opposite in the preparation of this beverage, that is, not to use at all the cinnamon infusion (which contains only the most subtle and therefore the most harmful part) but rather the grounds of the cinnamon and put them into hot water, from which one would make a strong extraction, so as to remove from it the astringent, dry, and earthy qualities. Or else, if the cinnamon has not been weakened by a preliminary infusion, boil it so violently that its potency will be dispelled and lost. For it is specifically rough matter that fortifies the stomach and stops discharges, just as does coarse,

---

[13]Joubert's note: The eating of fruits does not interact well with having sweet beverages.

[14]Joubert's note: Concerning sharp-pointed dock and cinnamon.

unrefined wine, called *stomachal*,[15] and not the subtle and heady kind, which is strictly forbidden for the cold stricken.

As for sharp-pointed dock,[16] it is somewhat astringent but the subtle virtues of its leaves are separated from its astringent qualities by gentle cooking and are clearly dominant, for the greatest astringency remains in the grounds. Thus the aforementioned extract thins the humors much more, just as does cinnamon, rendering them more able to flow. For it must be understood that sharp-pointed dock, along with every other sudorific agent, only provokes sweating by dissolving coarse humors, which are thick and clotted, thereafter voiding them through the pores of the skin. It is not a fierce heat of the kind brought about by guiacum, Indian root,[17] or dock and other similar agents that provoke sweating, but a thinning of the humors with a certain dissolving action brought about by a light astringency. Otherwise, it would have to be the case that wine, which is even hotter than the aforementioned drugs and is extremely subtle, would bring about more extensive sweating than an equal quantity of guiacum extract. Those who love wine would be more than happy to undergo this treatment often!

If, therefore, sharp-pointed dock has as its principal virtue, at least on the surface, that of breaking down and thinning humors, and said virtue is driven off in boiling, the water that remains will provoke discharge more than it will curb it. It would be necessary to treat it in the same way we do cinnamon, so as to draw from it its astringent quality. The other great disadvantage with such drugs is that they can only tend to force undigested food out of the stomach. Hence the cold is not countered, and a thousand other ills will result from it.

Concluding, then, our remarks on the nature of this beverage,[18] which is an effect of the mixture, of the water temperature, of the

---

[15]Cotgrave defines the term as "stomacall, cordiall; of or in the stomache; hurting, or helping the stomache. *Mot stomachal*. Earnest, comming from the heart; also, uttered in choller." The word might have been translated as *cordial* were it not for this term's pleasant connotations in English.

[16]Joubert's note: Concerning sharp-pointed dock.

[17]Joubert's term, *chyne ou apios*, is translated by Cotgrave, who spells it *chine*, as "a red, and spungious Indian root, good against the Gout." The *Oxford English Dictionary* identifies Indian root as "(a) *Indian physic*; (b) the American spikenard, *Aralia racemosa*."

[18]Joubert's note: The virtue of this beverage.

sugar, of the sharp-pointed dock, and of the cinnamon, I maintain that it has a thinning virtue without being a violent astringent and is of a temperate heat with more of a slight moistening tendency than of a drying one. Hence the stomach is not only relaxed and mollified by it, but its flowing action is stimulated by it. For if the concentration of the dock and the cinnamon were increased, the flowing action would be so excessive that it would result in provoking a sweat, since sweat is also caused by flowing humors, but through the skin.

The undigested food is in part moved out of the stomach by this beverage, forced by its thinning action, which the relaxed stomach is unable to resist. Plain water would be much better in my judgment,[19] for it does not weaken the stomach with a cloying sweetness, gives off no vapors, does not excite the humors or thin them in any way but, rather, encumbers them, and, by supressing the vapors that rise toward the brain, curbs discharges. Stop and think! Is it not reasonable that when one is in good health, one should abstain from medicinal beverages, which ought to be reserved for serious use? For otherwise their strength and efficaciousness will abandon us when we need them, since things we are familiar with and accustomed to have no effect on the body.[20] This is why Celsus warns us most wisely not to take or make improper use of drugs when we are in good health.

One can always refute this by saying that Monseigneur is nevertheless in very good health and, since he has been using this beverage, feels even better. I deny that it is because of this drink; it is rather because of the preceding diet and the other good remedies that his stomach has improved. And I ask you: must something that has worked well in the past necessarily be continued? If this were the case, one would be justified in continuing to use opiates, lozenges, powders, pills, clysters, inhalants, medicinal broths, and other drugs once one has recovered, never ceasing to take medicine, never being exempt from apothecary fees, and never returning to one's former state of health.

---

[19]Joubert's note: That plain water would be better.

[20]Joubert's note: That medicinal beverages are not indicated when one is in good health.

I would very much like to know what is so bad about wine that cannot be easily corrected,[21] and why it is we have to have recourse to so many different drinks and be making an artificial one, rejecting the natural one, especially when the person in question has from childhood been brought up on wine. I maintain that there is nothing troublesome with wine other than its strength and vaporous quality, which might provoke a cold. But if it is well diluted and mixed with water ("baptized" as people say commonly), its strength is reduced and its vapor quelled, especially if wine thus watered down stands for an hour or two. For it is so vanquished and flattened by its contrary that it no longer has any vigor, remaining like a body without a soul. Yet it is in just this state that, because of its delightful substance,[22] it pleasantly calms the stomach and the liver, makes the heart of man rejoice, as the wise man says, raises the spirits, and contributes to our natural heat, weak as the wine may be, causing a healthier digestion throughout the organism. If one has the time to dilute it a long time beforehand, one has only to put a little bread in it, and it will absorb and retain most of the strength and vapor of the wine, the only troublesome qualities for cold-stricken people; conversely, the body or substance of wine diluted and weakened in this way is infinitely profitable for them and necessary for the maintenance of the health of their stomachs and the curing of the indigestion they are subject to more than all others, which is the cause of such disorders as windy colic, kidney stones, gout, and countless other illnesses.

Saint Paul, who knew many of God's secrets[23] and was aware of the secrets of nature and of our medicinal art, itself instituted by God (as Ecclesiasticus bears witness), strongly advised Timothy to drink a little wine to correct the weakness and queasiness of his stomach. For Paul knew how many illnesses come from indigestion and how much the use of wine is indicated to strengthen the stomach.[24] Jesus Christ, instituting his Holy Supper, chose to use wine as the most proper and fitting liquid for maintaining the health of our souls. And one of the greatest strikes of retribution to the entire Muhammadan sect is their

---

[21] Joubert's note: Concerning wine.

[22] Joubert's note: Effects of corrected wine.

[23] Joubert's note: Saint Paul's advice concerning wine.

[24] Joubert's note: On the dignity of wine.

abstention from wine, which cuts them off from the possibility of communicating with and being a part of the blood of our Lord Jesus Christ, as we are able to. These are sacred and most mysterious things, surpassing the natural order yet basing themselves on the natural, ordained by God for the service of man. It pleases God to honor thus his principal creatures. As if to demonstrate the excellence of wine, and the need we have for it, He compares it to his precious blood.

Let us come back to our physicians and doctors. All the great philosophers agree that wine is a necessity, provided it has been moderately diluted, once one has passed adolescence and the fervor of tender youth. For old [wine that is] even only very slightly diluted is like milk for infants. In fact it has an infinite number of uses for people of every complexion,[25] for it tempers the sharpness or acrimony of choleric humor and gives it easy expurgation through sweat and urine. It breaks up and dissolves phlegm, finally converting it into good blood, and softens melancholic humor, which engenders sadness and spitefulness, especially in people who have heavy responsibilities. I wish also to recall another very pleasant aspect, involving the use of ripe summer fruits and referred to at the beginning of this discourse. For it is certain that people who drink wine or plain water (such was the late Monsieur Rondelet,[26] a noteworthy *philopore*, that is, a lover of ripe summer fruit, which he ate in excessive and almost unbelievable amounts) are able to eat much more freely and healthily such fruit than are drinkers of *bouchet* and other sweet drinks.[27] For those fruits called perishable[28] in Latin have a laxative effect on the stomach, which must be tightened and closed with a little wine or cool water in order to counter their effect. Aristotle in his *Problems* calls for undiluted wine or for pure water. Our common folk have more willingly retained the former than the latter and as a rule have a swallow of wine after soft summer fruit. But this is not the maxim of the philosopher, who understands by this that the whole meal is limited to fruit, taking for granted that fruit was served at the beginning of the meal. For if greatly diluted wine, or water, is drunk afterward, then the

---

[25]Joubert's note: Wine is appropriate for all complexions.

[26]On Rondelet, see *PE* (xiv, 310) and n. 35 of appendix A herein.

[27]Joubert's note: That by drinking wine one is able to have more fruit.

[28]Joubert's note: *Fugaces* (fleeing) because they cannot be kept.

swallow of pure wine will not be able to maintain its strength in the stomach nor have its usual effect.

Still more mistaken are those who drink *bouchet* or some other sweetened beverage in allowing themselves to eat melon freely, so long as they have a swallow of pure wine immediately afterward. In this one at least recognizes that when the stomach is full of such sweetened or insipid water it is not ready to accommodate melon, and that wine is required when one wishes to eat this kind of fruit. But since wine does not remain pure in the stomach and is mixed and diluted with the sugared water that they drink throughout the rest of the meal, would it not be better to dilute this swallow of wine with plain water, which would not weaken the stomach? Those who request or order sharp wine (as the Italians say)[29] to drink with melon are much better informed, condemning evidently all sweet beverages, even though they might be more pleasant to drink. But one must be able to accept the corrective agent when one wishes to enjoy eating any food that is quick to spoil;[30] this is just what one does when one puts lots of salt on melons and figs, so as to counter their cloying sweetness and fortify the stomach with a slight astringency, with a healthy moderation.

This is what I have to say on the subject of the beverage Monseigneur has taken to using for the past several years now. It cannot be recommended for settling the stomach or dissolving the remnants of indigestion, and still less for curbing common nasal or intestinal discharge. On the contrary, it does just the opposite. And even if it were the best and the healthiest remedy in the world, it should still be reserved for times of need, as any other medical remedy should be; one should not be allowed to become accustomed to it when one is in good health. Coarse, dark red wine that is well diluted and left to stand for an hour or two before drinking has no troublesome vapors and is every bit as good as people claim medicinal *bouchet* to be. Besides all this it

---

[29]Joubert uses the expression *vin garbe* and supplies the following marginal note: "That is to say, brisk (*brusc*), having no sweetness." Cotgrave's translation of *brusc* (also spelled *brusque*) is useful here: "Briske, liuely, quicke; also, rash, hairebraind, headie; also, wild, fierce, rude, barbarous, unciuile, harsh.... *Vin brusque*. Wine of a quicke, sharpe, or smart tast."

[30]Joubert's note: Conclusion [the marginal note is set upside down in the Micard edition].

brings countless benefits to our bodies, even to those raised on wine from infancy.

Dated in Beaucaire this tenth of August, 1573. JOUBERT

APPENDIX C

THE HEALTH OF THE PRINCE,[1]
CONTAINING TWO PARTS

In the first the prince is advised to be timely and orderly in his every-day activities.
In the second he is advised as to what is to be expected of his physicians when he is in good health, and of what their duties consist.[2]

CHAPTER ONE

EXHORTATION TO THE PRINCE
TO BE MINDFUL OF HIS HEALTH AND REGULATED IN HIS
ACTIONS BECAUSE OF THE DUTY OF HIS CHARGE,
HIS REPUTATION, AND THE GRANDEUR OF HIS HOUSE.

Man, whose principal condition draws him to be a sociable and a political animal, is born not only for himself but also for his kin and for his country. The prince even more so, in that he is the principal commander of many men and has a definite strong obligation to those over whom God has put him in charge and who are to be ruled and governed in obedience to him, as their earthly lieutenant. So that he

---

[1]This tract appeared in the 1579 Millanges edition of *Les Erreurs populaires*, but for reasons of space and because the subject is more closely related to matters treated in the second part of the work, it was not translated in *Popular Errors*, although the chapter headings were given in appendix F (*PE* 281). The title page reads as follows: *"La Santé du Prince par M. Laur. Iovbert Conseiher et Medecin ordinaire dv Roy, et du Roy de Nauarre [,] Chancelier de l'uniuersité an Medicine de Montpellier. A Bourdeavx. Par S. Millanges, Imprimeur ordinaire du Roy. 1579."*

[2]This statement of structure corresponds, as can be seen in the chapter headings, to a division of the six chapters into two groups of three; chapters 1 through 3 are devoted to the first and chapters 4 through 6 to the second.

will be fit for the task, God gives the prince, along with the authority and the power, a heroic majesty, a perfect understanding, an admirable prudence, and the wherewithal to manage the greatest affairs of the world. For it is God's wish that the great multitude of men depend entirely upon the prince, whom He sets over them as the head.[3]

Now it is from the head that all movements of the other parts of the body receive their directions; hence if the head is in pain the entire body suffers from it. It is therefore of crucial importance for a kingdom, or for any other monarchy, and of obvious concern to all of its members if the head is not always most healthy and well disposed to attend to all the functions required of its preeminence. For otherwise, if he is ill, then we all of us are most unwell, troubled in our senses, dazed, confused, weak in our movements, flagging and unresolved in our efforts, marred in all our actions; we are, in short, all of us lost, beaten down, without our bearings, fainthearted, drained, and completely impotent. This is why one has every reason to pray to God ceaselessly that He will maintain our principal member, given to us by Him, in sound health of mind and of body, upon which the public health and safety depend entirely.

Because of this very interdependency the prince also owes it to himself, for three reasons, to be mindful of his own health no less than of the public health. First, he must serve as a true model for his subjects and deputies and must be of a great perfection, more divine than human in sobriety, countenance, and rectitude (which is the principal political condition) and in every form of modesty. For all will conform to the manners of the prince. And it will be much easier for him to govern and manage his people if, by imitating him, these people are well-disposed and well-mannered and follow the same rules, as opposed to being given over to every kind of disorder and dissolution.

Secondly, a prince who enjoys good health is more useful and helpful to his subjects, in that he can easily attend to and keep up regularly with the affairs of state and public matters, not finding himself time and again hampered by various illnesses, to the point that he must interrupt his praiseworthy actions, namely, the exercise of justice and arms, to which he is called in order to allow his people to live in peace, tranquility, and assurance. Now, if the prince is ill-disposed in

---

[3]Joubert uses the term *chief*, whose etymological meaning of *head* was still very resonant in the term and serves as the basis for the anatomical metaphor he develops.

his person, it follows that he must either put off such affairs until a later time or must entrust them to another; both avenues are most unacceptable and prejudicial to his subjects. For they would always rather, if at all possible, see the face of their prince and receive directly from him justice and military orders, or at least be assured that all laws and orders proceed from his free and healthy will, from his sound knowledge, true understanding, and straightforward intention.

Thirdly, a prince who takes care of his health lives longer, a most desirable thing in the eyes of his subjects. For the switching of a superior, under whom one has been nourished, to whom one has become accustomed and for whom one has developed affection and loyalty, is most unpleasant and most troublesome for subjects, especially since this change sometimes shakes, startles, and throws into disarray or bewilderment the condition of the nation or kingdom. We presuppose that the prince is an affable, legitimate ruler with the support of his people, subjects who would be very concerned if the good prince were not to live very long and rule over them for at least as long as a well man who took care of his health might be expected to live. It is therefore in the reciprocal interest of all for the prince, in his duty to his people and in his search for their loyalty, to be very mindful of his health and not to be merely sober or continent, controlling his appetites and banishing all voluptuousness unseemly for his grandeur and his sublime station, but also to measure most modestly all his actions, affections, behavior, dealings, designs, and undertakings with the strictest codes and rules he can possibly manage to apply, as much as the unexpected, uncertain, extraordinary, and emergency circumstances will allow. For a great nation is subject to many accidents. Beyond such occurrences, it is simply a matter of the prince's normally submitting himself to such ordered and regulated conduct as he would expect others to observe in his laws and ordinances in order to ensure that his subjects live holy, healthy, and peaceful lives in the fear of God, in clean habits, and in the enjoyment of their possessions.

And is it not logical that he begin with his own person, upon which all else depends, and which belongs less to him than to his subjects? For God, to Whom we all belong, has given to us the life of the prince, whence the logic of the prince's being the first to obey this law of being vigilant about preserving his person from every evil, harm, and trouble. And since everyone willingly complies with the wishes and practices of the prince, is it not the prince's duty to discipline himself to the point of being a model and an example of all good, useful, and necessary behavior characteristic of human life, such that one may live a holy, healthy, and peaceful life in all piety, honesty, and modesty, as befits a Christian man, a rational, social, and political animal? It is said that the prince is the living law, and that his life therefore preaches, invites, exhorts, and persuades each person to live an orderly life, away from confusion, disorder, and excess and governed by order and harmony. He should be the common clockwork indicating to each of us the proper behavior and manners in all our actions. Does one not, from the appearance of a principled man, sense the presence of the inner principles, just as from the outside of a watch one can tell whether the internal movement is working properly? It must not be doubted that from the external actions of a man the tenor of his prudence can be determined, as well as his capacity to control others and to govern them, if he is able to control and to govern himself properly. For most men's words speak louder than their actions, but it is a great confirmation of doctrine, law, and order when the life of the one giving orders also follows them.

It is therefore in the people's best interest if the prince is careful both for his health (which is for the good of the nation) and his reputation and in the example he sets for good conduct, most necessary for his high station, so that his subjects, more highly edified, better educated, and better fed, will more readily obey his commandments. It goes without saying that a prince who has such an orderly conduct will beyond any doubt have a household with the same conduct. For whoever is so properly behaved himself will not be very patient in allowing any disorder, confusion, abuse, or misbehavior in others. Such vices corrupt the general healthiness of the nation and cause its goods to be squandered. It also goes without saying that such conduct on the domestic front will also be observed in all the cities, communities, and provinces, which all ordinarily imitate the behavior of their princes. For each is convinced that such a household is a mirror of the highest perfection, since it is the policy observed in that of the prince, in which only the most perfect people in the world reside, graced with every sort of wisdom and experience, corresponding to the grandeur of the master.

Now it is of no mean importance that a princely household be well disciplined (causing each of its domestic servants to be much better off and much healthier, both in body and in mind) and that it be filled with the best people that can be found. For how can the prince govern and rule over his provinces, his country, or his kingdom if he is unable to govern and rule over his own household? And as for his domestic servants, who must be (as I have said) excellent, is it not fitting that he take his officers, his magistrates, his financiers, and others who must command in place of the prince as his lieutenants from diverse members of his obedient subjects? Having been trained in his own school, familiar with the practices of his household (which ought to be the model of every republic), they are the most appropriate people to be charged by the prince, especially since they are the best informed about his intentions.

CHAPTER TWO

THAT THE PRINCE OWES IT TO HIMSELF TO SET UP A SOUND REGIMEN MODELED AFTER NATURE IN ORDER TO KEEP IN GOOD HEALTH.

Man is called the little world, in Greek a *microcosm*, because he represents in miniature everything that is in the world and in nature. Now nature is the order that God has put in the things of this world so as to maintain it and keep it going until Judgment Day, at which time He will remove man from the world, for whom it all was made, the heavens, the earth, and the other elements, along with everything in them.

And this order is regulated by time, which is a definite number or count and interval of all mutations, alterations, reciprocations, generations, and disintegrations of all that is in the world. And within time we observe distinctly the years, clearly ordered and divided into seasons and quarters, months and days, hours and minutes. Springtime is of another condition than is autumn, and summer differs from winter. Day differs from night, morning from evening, noon from midnight. The sea also has its ebb and flow, so obvious and so regular that the beauty of this order cannot be ignored. The sun, advancing each day by a degree, makes the days lengthen and shorten so evenly that the difference is always in the same amount. The moon, always to the same degree and in regular intervals, changes its face, and in its inconstancy there is nonetheless a fixed regularity.

Such is the manner in which everything is maintained and preserved, the smaller bodies governed by the larger, well-ordered, and
well-ruled heavenly bodies, which make everything return and revive
in their exact seasons, now this particular species, now that one, some
in spring, some in summer, some in autumn, some in winter, whether
they be plants or animals. From all this is taken the time to plant and
to harvest, to plow and to cultivate, to sow, water, graft, prune, plant,
seed, weed, and perform other acts of husbandry, all governed by the
phases of the moon and by months or other divisions of time. This is
so much the case that whoever might wish to do otherwise and go
against nature would be sorely mistaken and come to nought or would
have his labor prove to have fruits of short duration, for things that are
forced with violence cannot be maintained.

The same is true in the little world, which is man. Everything must
come in its own time, season, hour, and moment, just as in the large
world (which it figures), without confusing things and without forcing
nature: sleeping at night, designed for man's rest; awake by day,
meant for accomplishing work; eating and drinking at the proper times,
and eating first and drinking afterward; exercising the body and the
mind during the proper hours; voiding excrement and superfluous
matter, which can be reduced to reasonable amounts if all the rest is
well managed. For nature loves and revels in fixed order as long as it
is not upset. And it is to nature that must be entrusted the governing
and the maintenance of the body, through a diligent search and strict
observance of its appetites and movements, all of which the trained
physician can understand very quickly.

Animals (if I may speak of them in this manner)[4] live better and
more wisely than men, and especially those that live in the wild. For
those we have domesticated are forced to do many things outside their
natures. This is also why savage beasts living in the wild are ill far
less often and live much longer; they let themselves be governed by
nature, the servant or lieutenant of the Creator. That is, they live
according to the order established in the weak and mortal things of the
world, so that they will last until their assigned term expires, preserving their species until the end of the world. Animals observe fixed
hours for sleeping and for being awake, for drinking and for eating,

---

[4]Joubert is acknowledging the infelicity of the French term for animals (*beste*),
which can also mean "stupid."

for playing and for walking about, for running and for resting; they observe fixed seasons for their mating and coupling, for purging themselves and using herbs, for migrating and returning home, for hiding and coming out of hiding. All their actions are regulated and controlled in much the same way as is the conduct of the heavenly bodies and of nature, which guides animals wisely and is wisely obeyed by them.

Would man, for whom all creation was made and who is in the image of God, being able to comprehend all human and divine knowledge, having perfect familiarity with the order and the movements of nature, forget to such an extent his duty (he who is like a small God presiding over this world) that he would be without any order and discipline in his daily activities of rising and going to bed, eating and drinking, working and resting, enjoying his wife etc., scorning his natural instincts, unable to hold a tight rein on his wild desires or to keep in check his unruly appetites, which are more prodded and encouraged than they are spontaneous or internal, this same man (I say) who claims to dominate the entire world and subjugate everything at his feet? To this, precisely, he is called, but how will he accomplish the greater things if he cannot manage the smaller? How could he possibly govern the cosmos if he cannot properly run his own life?

When the order God has instilled in the things of this world comes to an end, when all that is perishes, how can one expect that man, this microcosm, more frail than anything else, will last for any length of time if it is not regulated and disciplined? I say "last for any length of time," for it is crucial to think ahead and to see farther than the end of one's nose, as people say commonly. One must not live on a day-to-day basis, saying to oneself, "I'm doing fine living a disordered life, without any rules." To which I would quickly reply that a sound edifice with a strong, well-built foundation can stand many blows and onslaughts, such as not being properly covered, abandoned to the rain, not being kept clean and dry, not being lived in and kept in repair, but that in the end it will not last as long as it would if it had been well maintained and will often fall to pieces for lack of only a little support. The slightest disorders corrupt the soundness of the body little by little, just as the slow dripping of water hollows out and eats through hard and thick stone, so that in the end its constitution, unable to withstand the shock of a serious disorder (namely, some illness or disease) succumbs and is brought low. Its strength is sapped and barely holds, held upright only by wooden pilings. And it seems to be as strong as it was in its fuller form, for it is said that a straight timber can carry a great burden. But the fire of a fever will consume this wood (which is its only strength) and will bring the edifice to ruin in an instant, for it has lost its foundation or the network and integrity of its masonry.

This is why we often see several people who, seeming strong enough after doing something to excess, are knocked down and undone in only a few days by the first illness that assaults them, for they have no resistance because of their failure to maintain their health and because of their abuse of their strength and youth, having scorned all order and discipline. And, conversely, we see many sickly and unhealthy people live long lives, escape and come through the most violent and dangerous diseases simply because they live orderly and well-disciplined lives, taking good care of themselves; they thus avoid the clutches of many diseases and, when they are assailed by them or in their grip, they have the wherewithal to fight them off. What then would it be if good, sound health were safeguarded and maintained as well?

One could reply at this point that the prince, given the great charge and duty of preserving a great kingdom constantly menaced with ruin if he is not watchful, cannot have his schedule restrained in any way nor his activities held in check by some order. For matters that are important and of extreme consequence pay no heed to orders given by physicians. And if it were for that reason alone (someone might say), such rules are pernicious and noisome because they render a man so soft and weak he would not be able to endure the upset of a serious matter. For if he were to stay up all night or have one of his meals an hour earlier or later than usual, he would not feel well because of it. And so it is better to be loose and not observe any rules, schedules, or system.

I have already answered the first part of this objection when I said in my preceding exhortation "with the strictest codes and rules he can possibly manage to apply, as much as . . . circumstances will allow."[5] For necessity is not subject to the law. And as for the other part of this objection, I wholly deny that a person accustomed to an orderly routine would be weaker and less able to put up with a disorderly situation. For, on the contrary, he would be able to stand it much more easily, as one who is strong and robust, healthy and sound, not sapped

---

[5]Joubert is referring to chap. 1, par. 5, of this tract.

or undermined. It is true that his schedule must include, above all, hard work and exercise, so as to strengthen his members and not be weak in any way.

The first item is that he must eat moderately, preferring wholesome foods to lighter and more toothsome ones, so that he will have firmer flesh, stiffer nerves, and an entire body that is stronger. It is also required and most necessary that his schedule be not so tight and hurried nor that he be so constrained by it that if the prince were not feeling well he could not be dispensed from observing it. For it is expedient to become accustomed out of necessity to breaking with routine in a few places. This is why I find so very relevant to the subject I am treating the advice Celsus gives to a person who is healthy and of sound constitution, not under a physician's care and feeling very good: "The healthy man, while he is feeling well, belongs to himself and does not have to follow any rule or diet nor consult a physician.[6] He must have a varied manner of living, now in the country, now in the city, but more often in the country, sailing, hunting, resting at times but exercising more often. For idleness and laziness make the body blockish; work toughens it. The former ushers in old age, the latter prolongs youth. It is also good to bathe occasionally, sometimes using cold water, at times anointing or perfuming oneself, at times doing without, fearing no kind of food people normally eat. Sometimes enjoy a feast, sometimes withdraw from it, eating now beyond all bounds, now soberly. Have two meals a day more often than just one, and always eat a lot as long as you are able to digest, etc. As for carnal copulation, it must not be overly desired nor overly feared either. When it is infrequent it stirs up the body; when frequent, it relaxes it, etc. This must be observed by those whose health is sound; and watch out that the remedies for the sick are not taken by the healthy."[7]

There you have in a few words the manner of living of a healthy man, and especially of one whose profession is arms, who must be indifferent to all things, fearing neither wind nor rain, bright sun nor nightfall, heat nor cold, sleeping on hard ground, suffering hunger,

---

[6]As was the case when Joubert cited this passage in the *Popular Errors*, he omits Celsus's "rubber and anointer" (*iatroalipta*). See *PE*, bk. 1, chap. 18 (85, 292).

[7]For the reference, as well as for the passages Joubert omitted from this quotation, see *PE* (292).

thirst, nor any discomfort when it is necessary to bear these things. But aside from the necessity hindering us from doing so, it is better to live according to some routine and to have a schedule, observing order and measure in all of one's activities as much as possible. This is the first and most important point in the discipline required of a prince in order to keep him in good health, which I now wish to explain and discuss in detail.

CHAPTER THREE

WHAT REGIMEN A PRINCE CAN OBSERVE
IN HIS DAILY ACTIVITIES.

Just as there are four main seasons in the year, spring, summer, autumn, and winter, so too are there four main parts corresponding to them in a normal day: morning, noon, afternoon, and night.[8] And in one's daily activities there are four principal moments particularly observed in the life of a prince: rising, the noon meal, the evening meal, and going to bed. These can be evenly proportioned so that from rising to the noonday meal there are four hours; from the noon meal to the evening meal, eight; from the evening meal to his going to bed, four; and from going to bed until rising, eight.

For example, he might rise at six in the morning, have his first meal at ten, his evening meal at six in the evening, and then go to bed at ten; or, rise at seven, have his first meal at eleven, his evening meal at seven, and go to bed at eleven. For the schedule must be changed as the seasons change, getting up earlier on days with more daylight and when the weather is hotter, such as for the four months that have no *r*, May, June, July, and August, during which one can rise at five, eat one's first meal at nine, have the evening meal at five, and go to bed at nine. In the months of September and October, March and April, which correspond to one another, one might rise at six, have one's first meal at ten, the evening meal at six, and go to bed at ten. For the other four months, during which the days have less daylight and are

---

[8]Joubert's terms are *"le matin* [morning], *le midi* [noon], *le soir* [evening], *& la minuit* [midnight]. *"*

colder, one might rise at seven, have one's first meal at eleven, one's evening meal at seven, and go to bed at eleven.

There would thus always be the specific intervals of four and eight hours in the calculation: those times at which one rises, sits down to table, and goes to bed. And in so doing, the prince will not always be following exactly the same schedule (and indeed one should not) but, according to the seasons, making considerable changes every four months. For nature's order and movement must be observed as precisely as possible; one must not stubbornly maintain a single schedule but, rather, one must move back or ahead as does the sun, our great guide in nature.

We have established the limits of the four daily activities of human life, in which reside the most remarkable: those of nourishment and conservation of health. And they must be understood to have a certain amount of latitude and not to be fixed. For it is enough if the approximate time is observed. Furthermore, one should assign a certain amount of time for each activity, namely, an hour for the first meal and almost the same for the evening meal; for one should always eat less at the second meal than at the first if one wishes to live a healthy life.

As for the prince's rising, we assign one hour also; he has much important business to consider. This goes from the time he awakens until he is dressed and ready, for he can discuss matters while still in bed and give ear to the most urgent affairs for the first half-hour and the rest while putting on his shirt, his doublet and breeches, and right up to his housecoat. No sooner is he out of bed than he gives thanks and prays to God, leading the prayer himself in a loud voice, as chief of the group, so as to give the best example of piety to his court, and consequently to all his subjects, and even to all men on earth, who have their eyes attentively fixed on the actions of the prince.

Then, before he begins to cope with matters, it is a good idea for him to go to the privy even if he does not feel the urge, for by forming and retaining this good habit, nature will little by little lend itself to observing such a time (which is most fitting) if the rest of this schedule is respected. After this he will comb his hair by himself as a means of loosening and exercising his arms. He will clean his ears, wash his hands and eyes, and (if he wishes) his entire face. One must not forget to wash the mouth in order to ensure keeping one's teeth and gums and a fresh breath, all of which are most important for good health. For the air one breathes in through the mouth is infected if it encounters foul teeth and gums and, being thus corrupted, taxes the lungs and the heart with its foul nature, to the point that for this sole reason several people end up becoming poisoned. This washing of the mouth should be done with dark red, coarse wine that has been well diluted. The same should be done (I say it here in the event I forget to mention it later) after each meal.

Here then is our prince ready after about one hour. He may then, for about two hours, be about his daily business or in a council meeting, unless he should want to go to Mass on that particular morning, in which case he will have to put off some of his business until after his meal. For it is imperative to exercise every morning for one hour before breakfast. The best exercise is tennis,[9] because it exercises equally (or very nearly so) every part of the body. If the weather is not fair enough to allow going outside, one can fence, vault, dance, or wrestle, so that the body will have sufficient exertion. When the prince comes to the table, he must leave behind all serious and grave matters, all that is plaguing his mind, so as to be able to converse pleasantly, whether it be about hunting or other relaxing subjects, or to hear discussion and debate over various topics in theology, philosophy, and natural sciences, such as the nature of foods, unusual and miraculous cures, the mechanical arts, war, diverse inventions, and sometimes to hear music, now vocal, now instrumental.

And so that there might be a pleasant orderliness, and also so that the gentlemen and other lettered people who might wish to speak will be able to come prepared so as to give even more enjoyment to the prince, it will be good to limit the subject matter thus: on Sunday, sacred to God, nothing but theology and the virtues will be discussed; Monday, dedicated to the moon, will be for astrology and the arts of divination. Tuesday, which is named after Mars (the god of war),[10] will be for the military arts. Wednesday, the day of Mercury,[11] to whom all the commodious arts are attributed, will be for the discussion

---

[9]Joubert uses the term *jeu de la paume*; according to Cotgrave, the English term was already "tennis."

[10]In French, *mardi* (Tuesday) is based on two Latin etyma: *Mars + dies* (day).

[11]The French *mercredi* comes from *Mercurius* (Mercury).

of the so-called mechanical arts. On Thursday,[12] which is attributed to Jupiter, author and protector of life, everything concerning medicine will be the topic, including surgery and the apothecary arts. On Friday,[13] which belongs to the goddess of love, decent and conjugal love will be the subject, along with marriage, household management, government, and all that concerns jurisprudence. Saturday will be for poetry and will be a catchall for all other subjects, in an attempt to drive out the grave severity of the great father Saturn.

The entire procedure will be academic in form, and all matters that might prove controversial will be resolved by the prince, according to his sound and quick judgment. These matters will come to a halt as soon as the tablecloth is withdrawn, only to be taken up again at the evening meal. After giving thanks to God (it is supposed that a benediction was also pronounced upon arriving at the table, with the prince seated or standing), the prince will walk about and give ear for approximately one hour to those who need to communicate with him or to report to him, and then he will go about his business or into a council meeting for two or three hours, according to the work that must be done.

The remaining time before the evening meal will be spent in amusement, conversation, reading, writing, or walking about until about an hour before eating. At this time he will engage in some strenuous exercise such as horseback riding, running at the ring,[14] or playing tennis. Two or three times a week he can spend the greater part of the day (after breakfast) in the pleasure of the hunt, during which he will not fail to discuss, while coming and going, to consider, and to give thought to several important matters. During the evening meal all will transpire as during the morning one, and in just the same way the prince will, in the hour following, grant audience and then will go about the business at hand, if necessary, for no more than an hour.

---

[12]In French, *jeudi* (Jovis).

[13]In French, *vendredi* (Venus).

[14]Cotgrave gives more detail concerning this activity: "... also, the Ring, whereat gallants run with launces; (whence, *Courir la bague*; to run at the Ring;) also, the reward bestowed on, or prize gained by, him that does the best in a publicke Game, or Exercise; as tilting, wrestling, running, leaping, &c; (and hence;) *Il a gaigné la bague*. He hath woon the spurres, or carried away the Prize; the victorie, or day, is absolutely his."

After that he will relax by playing or conversing for an hour, leaving aside from that point on all matters of importance (so long as they are not pressing and can be delayed or put off) until the next day, so as to be able to sleep soundly and peacefully, as is necessary, in order to be better disposed to take up once again these serious considerations when his mind is refreshed. We allocate one hour for getting ready for bed just as we do for getting ready in the morning. He first will say his prayers in an audible voice, as in the morning, and, once he is in bed, will have read to him some good book, of history or ethics, for about half an hour, until he is able to fall asleep.

This is how the twenty-four hours of each entire day, divided up and filled with the ordered and disciplined activities of the prince, will transpire and be profitably put to use. From this schedule two great benefits will be derived: the first is that he will feel much better because of it, both in mind and in body, and will resist more and more any disorder or interruptions in it. For he will have to interrupt it occasionally, out of necessity, and sometimes even on his own (as we said above) so as not to follow ceaselessly the same routine. The other benefit will be the profit for the prince's household. For there will be better order, discipline, and management throughout, from which will flow countless advantages, as can be easily understood. It is certainly a great boon and gain both for the master and for the servants when everything is done according to a timetable, when everything is well organized, structured, and controlled.

On this very subject I once saw a venerable and prudent man who, upon arriving in a place to conduct some business and in an attempt to gain knowledge in a legitimate way concerning the politics of the city and whether or not it was well governed, asked only if the town clock was running properly. This would be an indication that, if people were careless in organizing their activities according to a timetable, this could scarcely be a well-ordered city. The same can be said of a house in which a clock serves no purpose. For one does not know how to run one's life in such a place nor how one ought to conduct and govern one's personal affairs, any more than a ship can without a rudder. Thus all its members will be troubled and confused in their actions, having greater difficulty and making much less progress than if there were time limits on everything that had to be done.

We have finished half of our undertaking,[15] which was to persuade the docile and gentle prince to regulate his activities and relegate them to specific times in order to preserve his health, his reputation, and the well-being of his household. This third point, his household, although incidental, must not be underestimated, in that it is most useful to him in maintaining his grandeur and will provide a sound argument in favor of his prudence. Let us now come to the second point and make known to the prince what he should expect and obtain from the service of physicians in preserving his health, and what their proper role is.

CHAPTER FOUR

ON THE CHARGE THE PHYSICIAN HAS
WITH RESPECT TO A PRINCE, AND HOW IMPORTANT
THE PREVENTION OF ILLNESS IS.

The charge of a physician is greater than all those of the other advisors of the prince, except for that of the theologian, who bears responsibility for the prince's soul. For the others have only to answer for the state of his affairs, of his provinces, his domain, his finances, his household, and his furniture. The physician is responsible for his health and his life, if his master does him the honor of trusting him and depending entirely upon him. I am speaking of all the physicians that the prince has in his service, if he has several serving three-month terms. For each is responsible, during the time he is serving or has served, for any breach in the prince's health, either through negligence, carelessness, or oversight, in that he has failed in his duty of supervising and healing the minor conditions (which end up causing serious illnesses) by means of light and mild remedies, such as the ones we shall be recommending shortly.

But let the prince be aware that he should not have physicians around only to be called to his side when he is ill, just so help will always be ready. For it is incomparably better and much more desirable to be kept in good health and to render it so sound, strong, and sure that no illness happening along can shake it, overturn it, or destroy it, unless there be by chance some external event, which is not in

---

[15]Joubert refers to the twofold division of this tract.

our purview to control or foresee, such as a fall or a wound, which a physician can well treat but not prevent. The other illnesses, which have their origins within the body, can and must be hindered by the physician from forming, growing, and becoming strong. This can be accomplished if he diligently watches over all actions of the prince, who expects such service from the physician.

And this is the principal, the most valuable, and the most desirable part of our art, which is called prophylactic or preventive. It can be compared to the prudence, industry, and skills of a ruler over a kingdom whose state is subject to change, tumult, sedition, and ruin, but who still maintains his province in such restraint, justice, order, and discipline that no movement, trouble, war, or damage ever comes about, while other provinces are put to the torch, ravaged, pillaged, and destroyed. Is not the ruler who has preserved his domain more to be praised than one who, through negligence, carelessness, or oversight and (perhaps) his own ignorance, had left it open to similar excess and ruin? This is so even if he is later able to control them, manage them, and return things to their previous state. For during this time the people would have suffered the mobs, the torment, the extreme sufferings, and the evils spawned by the rebellion and rage of civil strife, which should more rightly be called uncivil. And whatever pacification might follow, the province still suffers from the loss of strength, weakened both in its people and in its resources, both fixed and movable, to the point that several years will go by before the country will be healed and restored to its former state, with its houses rebuilt, its cities restored, and its fields replanted, not to mention the irreparable damage: people who have died either from wounds or unaccustomed distress, fear, sadness, or suffering. It could be argued that others will be born to take their places, or will come from elsewhere to people the region. This is true, but the province would be much stronger if both these and the others could be there together. The same is true also of the money, merchandise, and furniture that were carried off: it is possible to replace it as well, but the country would be much better off if none of it had been lost, for now there would be twice as much.

And so it is truly a praiseworthy practice and service and is far more worthwhile (to those who are able to grasp it) to block the arrival of illnesses caused by the sedition, rebellion, and revolt of perverse, corrupt, and rotten humors, which provoke combustion (called fever), destruction, and ruin in the body, rather than to combat and vanquish them after they have become entrenched. For during such time the patient has already suffered because of it, undergone much pain, unpleasantness, and worry, spent sleepless nights, and come close to death, in much anguish and terror. And (what is a rather important point) there remains in all of it an irreparable loss, which will be responsible for his never being ever again quite as rich in physical strength (and consequently will not live as long) as he would have been if he had not been thus afflicted. For natural moisture (which is the principal substance supporting our strength and the length of our lives) is diminished and irreparably weakened far more in an illness that lasts for fifteen days than it is through normal dissipation in fifteen months. And when it is said that one's strength is restored after an illness to what it was before, I reply that the body would be all the more strong if the two strengths were combined. I am not speaking of the strength in the arms and legs, of the head and shoulders (as common folk understand it when they say somebody is strong and tough), but rather of the natural resistance one has, residing internally in those parts controlling nourishment, namely, the stomach, the liver, and the heart. In that type of strength children and those who are still growing are more endowed than they will ever be. For this type of strength is always constantly diminishing right up until one dies, but only little by little when one lives a disciplined and sensible life; conversely, if there is an illness (which is a serious disorder) one's strength is taxed and spent most prodigally.

Thus, let him who would wish to live a long and happy life in this world exercise care in choosing a prudent, knowledgeable, careful, diligent physician who is dedicated to his responsibility, which is, first and foremost, always to preserve the health of the person in his charge and, secondly, to prevent illnesses by stopping their early stages from developing and becoming a threat. In these two efforts resides the whole of a proper physician's duty, be it toward a very good and intimate friend, a person who has retained him at great price, or a great prince in the service of whom he has been honorably called. In both the first and second case much loyalty is required, but the service owed a prince is of an even higher order, as is the concern, care, and vigilance; for the health of the prince is the health of the nation and is of infinitely greater importance and consequence than is that of a private individual.

This is why I wish to point out specifically to physicians who have the honor of being called or taken into a prince's service how they can fulfill their duties worthily and faithfully, deserve the good graces of their master, and expect honor (the principal wages of virtue) and appreciation for their services, aside from the other compensation and rewards that will not fail to be forthcoming from a good ruler. And this follows the beautiful admonition in Ecclesiasticus of Jesus of Sirach, who most rightly says: "Honor thy physician with the honor he deserves for the need thou hast of him: for the most High has created him. For all healing is from God: and he shall receive honor and wages and shall receive presents from kings. The skill of the physician shall lift up his head: and in the sight of princes he shall be praised."[16]

CHAPTER FIVE

ON THE VIGILANT CARE
THE PHYSICIAN OWES THE PRINCE,
AND ON THE GOOD THAT COMES FROM IT.

We are each and every single one of us expected to know ourselves, according to the inscription on the Delphian temple of Apollo: *gnothi seauton*, that is, "Know thyself." And Celsus wisely points out that one should first and foremost be aware of one's own body, that is, know one's own particular nature and complexion, know that which is good and that which is harmful among all the things one eats, studies, does, and makes use of, so as to retain and continue that which is useful and good for one's health and to despise and reject that which is found to be harmful and could in the end provoke illness.[17] Each individual is expected to do this, but few people listen to reason, won over by their desires and unruly appetites, forcing nature and ignoring its

---

[16]Joubert cites somewhat loosely the biblical text from Ecclesiasticus (38:1–3).

[17]Joubert's note: Book I, chapter 3 [containing Celsus's injunction, *Ante omnia autem norit quisque naturam sui corporis* (sec. 13); also appearing marginally next to Joubert's rendition are the corresponding Latin terms: *Assumenda, Educenda, Facienda, Admouenda*; "... *de toutes les choses qu'on prand, qu'on fait, & qu'on s'applique* ..."].

dictates, movements, and tendencies. This is why it is that most men who are not of good birth live miserably, more often ill than in good health, gout-stricken, full of gallstones and kidney stones, colicky, suffering from stomach disorders, pursy, feverish, benumbed, phthisic, subject to migraines, rheumy, dizzy, epileptic, scurfy, bald, ulcerous, deaf, one-eyed or blind, noseless, toothless, racked with pain, crippled, paralyzed, deformed in some member, full of lice, mangy, linty, pox-ridden, measly, leprous, etc. All of these could have been healthy and strong without the slightest touch of disease if they had taken the trouble to know themselves and to govern themselves according to nature under the guidance of reason. For those animals that are guided by nature live incomparably more healthy lives than does man, who nevertheless enjoys over the animals the advantage of having reason, which allows him to know himself.

Now, since no one is dispensed and exempt from this duty to oneself, the prince, who must be more careful about his health than all others, both for himself and for the public, has numerous physicians, like guards and sentinels, who watch vigilantly over all his activities, observing most diligently what is good and bad for him, but only after having meticulously calculated and considered his complexion, condition, and endurance. In this they must be keenly attentive, so as to fulfill the first part of their charge and duty. For the prince, called upon by God to tend to the sovereign affairs of this world, is not as able to see to his personal health as easily as a private individual. This is why the physician is more important to the prince than any other person, and why he is highly recommended in Ecclesiasticus.

It is therefore necessary that the physicians, in whose care the prince puts himself, study very closely his nature, complexion, and all that springs from them; it is necessary that they know how to read the signs of his body as though it were a book, the internal organs being no more hidden from them than is his face. It is crucial that they understand most precisely the quality and quantity of his humors and the profile of his behavior, which follows the temper of the body or, put in other terms, the temperament and complexion. This can be done very quickly (if they are able people) by studying his constitution, his corpulence, his posture, his height, the proportion of his limbs, his physiognomy, his appearance, his skin, his hair, his countenance, his remarks, movements, agility, and behavior, what he likes to do, how he occupies himself, and what he hates and disdains; next, what he drinks and eats, his appetite, the order he observes in eating his food, the times and the number of his meals, the hour at which he goes to bed and gets up, how well and how much he usually sleeps, whether he likes to have lots of covers, whether he is more sensitive to heat than to cold, or conversely.

They must also examine very carefully all that comes out of his body, his urinary, fecal, nasal, aural, and oral excrements. For from what we void we are alerted as to what becomes of the food we eat every day; and as to how well those parts assigned with digesting and breaking down our food are functioning so that good blood can be produced from it; and as to how well also those parts assigned with removing superfluities are functioning, and whether these superfluities are being properly voided or whether a part of them has been blocked and stopped. For it is necessary that the various excrements correspond to the quantity of food and drink taken in; otherwise, there is a mass of superfluities that builds up somewhere in the body and which can end up causing a serious disorder. It is also necessary to examine the person very closely, smelling the bed linen and nightshirts, for the nature of the sweat and black stains that soil clothing helps us to understand more thoroughly the body's complexion and the quality of its humors. It is said in this respect of Alexander the Great (a most kind, magnanimous, and heroic prince) that he had such a perfectly tempered body and such perfect blood that the linen and other clothes he used had a sweet odor given off by his person.

It is also important that the physician examine from close proximity, touching his master's skin often so as to note the quality of his natural heat and the rate of his pulse. For how will the physician be able to tell precisely whether the pulse is stronger, more violent or more weak, faster or slower, sluggish or quick, powerful or faint, even or uneven, if he is not well aware and informed as to what his normal, everyday pulse is? The same is true of the prince's natural heat. Who can tell if it is stronger, sharper, or more vehement than it ought to be, or less so, if one does not know its usual state? Furthermore, it is not enough to feel and evaluate the pulse and the temperature when the patient is resting in bed if one wishes to have a perfect understanding of them; they must sometimes be taken before and after sleeping, after meals, and when he has finished exercising or doing some other strenuous activity. For all this changes one's pulse and temperature, and it is especially important that the physician take note of how and in what way they change, quickly or not so quickly, as well as the types of changes, because if he is not well versed in this and very sharp, he could often be mistaken over the birth and origin of diseases that he will fail to catch in time, misjudging the pulse and temperature that have gone awry, ignorant of their nature and condition when the prince is healthy, and from what point they are greatly or slightly differing and changing.

This is of enormous importance if one wishes to counter illnesses and combat them at their inception, stopping them from getting out of hand, as physicians who are always close to their master can and must do, if their counsel is heeded. The soldier on sentinel duty does not wait until the enemy has climbed the walls, for he will be afraid that if he is attacked by him he will not be able to dispose of him as he would wish; and so he would rather fight him while he is still climbing up the ladder than when he is over the wall. So too the wise and prudent physician must never allow disease to set foot in the body over which he is put in charge. He must sense its arrival so as to cut it off and immediately to set up every sort of obstacle to its approach. For at the very beginning more can be done with a finger, a stick, or a stone than can be accomplished afterward with a battle-ax, a pike, or a harquebus. The same is true in the matter of healing: one can do more starting early with an ounce of medicine than one can do later with four or five pounds. Moreover, a nascent and developing illness can be driven off and defeated (note, if you will, what a beautiful practice this is) without remedies or drugs (most unpleasant for anyone), if the physician has sure knowledge of the inner workings of the body because of the aforementioned observations and if he is fully aware of the illness that is threatening. And the same is true of a cook, a gardener, or a cellar master, who is able to change subtly the quality and quantity of the production and gently nudge the enterprise in a certain direction, so as to hinder the development of any number of foul conditions, as long as close attention is paid at the opportune moment. Otherwise, one must have recourse to the drugs of the apothecary or to the instruments of the surgeon. Is there anything in the world that is more pleasant than to be able to do without drugs and to recover through some other means?

This is the great advantage the prince has when he has his physicians constantly at his side, provided these physicians (who we presume are among the most skilled) are careful, diligent, clever, prudent, and loyal in the service of their master. They must be well informed of his condition, complexion, and state of health through frequent observation of his daily activities, his life-style, his excrement, his pulse, and of the other things mentioned above. For those who do not have the means of having physicians at hand in this way cannot be as effectively cared for when they become ill, mainly because ordinary physicians do not have such particular and close knowledge of their normal condition. And so they are obliged to observe the standard rules of the art of medicine, which teach how to heal a patient generally, but not in each specific case, as with Henri, François, Catherine, or Marguerite,[18] whose specific treatment is left to the prudence of the physician as he tries to accommodate the general principles to the case at hand.[19] And in such an instance it is, beyond comparison, done more fittingly and more precisely because of the specific knowledge possessed. Our Celsus has rightly said in connection to this that if a physician is ignorant of a patient's nature and condition he must rely solely upon common and general practices. The physician who is able to know the specifics will be in a better position to apply the general principles. It follows from this, he goes on to say, that (since knowledge behaves likewise) the physician who is a friend and familiar with the case is better for the patient than an unknown physician.

We have sufficiently pointed out to the physicians of the prince what care, diligence, and vigilance they must exhibit in his service. Now let us in turn inform the prince that he must expect nothing less from them and should wish that his court physicians faithfully practice what we have indicated. So as to convince the prince of the importance of this, I will limit myself to demonstrating the point through some simple examples taken from my own recent treatments, so as to encourage the prince to keep a close watch on himself and to encourage others to study him very closely, in order that they might have a precise knowledge of his nature and complexion and thus be able to preserve him in good health and defend him against illness.

---

[18]Joubert has chosen as examples of specific cases the Christian names of the members of the royal family he was called to serve as court physician. For details on these individuals, see *PE* (283), n. 1 of the dedicatory letter to Marguerite de France.

[19]Joubert's note: In the preface of the First Book.

CHAPTER SIX

CONFIRMATION OF THE PRECEDING
THROUGH WELL-KNOWN EXAMPLES.

The human body can be compared to the works of a clock, which are easily upset. And it is not too difficult to maintain them if one is willing to be attentive to them. Now, a person who knows intimately the inner workings of a clock—how the drum is made and works, with its mainspring, how much its chain pulls, how its spindle is turned, how the large gear, the pawl, and the ratchet work, along with the dial gear, the balance wheel, the pivots, the sprockets, the pegs, and the whole mechanism—will know how to put it all together properly even if everything were dismantled. Otherwise, he would only know how to wind it, pull on its chains, and move its hands ahead or back a few minutes, which is a rather crude knowledge and wholly insufficient for the proper maintenance of the entire clock, including its movement. So too will the physician be of poor assistance who does not have extensive familiarity with the patient, especially in comparison with another who knows thoroughly the patient's nature and complexion. This can be made even clearer through an example taken from the military arena (for we too are at war in dealing with diseases): the difference there is between the physician who does not have specific, intimate, and perfect knowledge of a patient and one who knows the patient only superficially or through the report of another, merely as a man of such and such age, weight, hair color, and skin, having such and such eating and personal habits, from which the physician understands generally and roughly the patient's complexion, be it sanguine, phlegmatic, choleric, or melancholic.

Could not this physician, who has no more of an exact knowledge of his patient yet is otherwise skilled and competent, be properly compared to a wise and valiant captain in charge of defending a city with which he was unfamiliar but to which he was suddenly called to defend since it was about to be sieged or was already under siege? He has only a rough knowledge of the situation, the buildings, the munitions, and the strengths of the city and knows no more from the report given to him than he can glean from observation. Will he not have greater difficulty and will he not be less effective than another captain who is from the very city or who has at least visited it often? He would have a good knowledge of its setting, of the points from which it could be controlled, of the depth of its moats, the height and thickness of its walls; he would be well informed about its flanks, places of refuge, ravelins, bulwarks, casemates, spurs, scarps, counterscarps, parapets, outer walls, etc., and about the ways of digging in, erecting barricades and gabions. He would know well the weakest points and the strongest, likewise be duly aware of the quantity and quality of supplies within, either in public storage or in private houses, of the powder, sulfur, and saltpeter, lead, tin, copper, and other metals. And for the fabrication of firebombs he would know where there was pitch and resin, wax and grease; he would know the exact number and type of arms and of people at his disposal, right down to their complexion and local customs, whom he might trust or mistrust, and finally what support he could depend upon and what its sources would be, along with all the other specifics that simply cannot be transmitted or explained.

This is the way it is with the physician who undertakes the maintenance and defense of the human body against the diseases that assail it frequently. This same comparison also serves in the case of a physician about to lay siege to and drive out an illness that has taken hold of a body and is occupying it, either secretly, as if through some act of treason, or through some upset and disorder. For the physician having perfect knowledge both of the outside and the inside, as well as of the strength of the disease holding up in the body, what it can take over and convert to its advantage, what it can use for its reinforcement and maintenance, will when called upon for help be able to make it victorious over the disease, with the help of God's grace, so long as the body is able to offer some resistance and opposition to the enemy it has within itself. Just as a brave captain coming to lay siege to a city so as to drive out those inside—if he has perfect knowledge of the place, of the forces, means, and expectations of the enemy inside, if he is well informed and takes all into account—will secure the place with far less expense, loss, and damages than another who had never seen it or known of it until the time he had to secure it. And so he only knows it from afar, unable to approach it in any practical way, and can in no way obtain precise knowledge of what is inside. Hence such a person upon laying siege will go about it in a very rough and general way, according to common principles and methods he might have of a place having a similar situation, similarly surrounded with a ditch, similarly walled with similar defenses, similarly supplied, which can be mined or sapped, attacked between the bulwarks or in a pincer, or in some other way. As for the rest, he learns in the field from what he is told, very often of dubious worth, coming from people who are unable to judge what is most important, or of most consequence, or of most use. Such a captain is much less able than he would be if he had had the means of knowing in detail everything concerning the site, inside and outside. So too is the physician who only knows superficially or has never even seen the person brought to him for help unable to treat as precisely, deftly, and resolutely as another physician who has greater familiarity with the individual and who is no less skilled.

And so let the physicians of princes be exhorted and advised (I pray them fraternally to take in a positive way this warning I am giving, for the honor of our profession and for the purpose of noting that through the prince we make all men beholden to us) to be attentive in their duty, in a charge that is as onerous as it is honorable. Let them serve carefully, not only out of a sense of duty to these people who represent God on earth, nor for the profit, fees, pensions, gifts, and other advantages they hope to gain, as do vile mercenaries, but out of love, affection, devotion, and zeal in the service of princes, to which a generous heart must be brought, and not a selfish or avaricious one. Whosoever is driven by such sentiment will, I hope, do his duty completely and happily and will have all to his honor and all to the great contentment of the prince, whom he cherishes and faithfully serves.

END

APPENDIX D

ON NIGHTFALL,
WHAT IT IS,
AND WHETHER IT FALLS ON US

From the popular expression, and from the ordinary manner of speaking, it is my understanding that people think that nightfall is a certain rheumatic quality in the evening and night air that falls from the sky. But in fact nightfall is nothing more than the air of the evening, falling upon us no more than that of the day and surrounding us all the time. And as for its quality, it is more or less cold according to the season. For it has no bad or evil quality. And where would such a quality come from? The stars or the moon, which are coming out to guard and watch over the countryside? It is certain that the striking of moonbeams and moonlight on our heads excites flow and makes things considerably more sluggish. This is why the moon is said to cause colds in David's *Psalms*.[1] The stars are not suspected of this, although every other planet causes colds at night and excites rheum in those who are susceptible and disposed to it, but not for any reason other than that of the chill of the night. For just as the heat of the sun melts and makes the thick and coarse humors of the brain agile, and in so doing causes discharge and catarrh, so too does the chill of nightfall and of night itself provoke colds by squeezing out this moisture by pressure on the brain, much as if a sponge loaded with some liquid were being squeezed.

And so nightfall is nothing more than the air of the evening, chilled because of the absence of the sun shortly after its setting and most harmful to people subject to catching cold, such as those who have loose cranial seams, thin skin, and highly dilated pores. For the penetrating cold easily presses upon the brain and squeezes out the moisture and even engenders more, thus cooling the brain, making it ill-disposed and thick with vapors. This is why nightfall is more dangerous to those who are overheated, such as in summer, for there are more vapors on the brain then, and the chill penetrates into it more easily. If in the course of the day one has become accustomed to the cold, nightfall does not do as much harm, for it encounters pores that are more

---

[1] Joubert's note: Psalm 121 [Psalm 120 of the Vulgate, *Levavi oculos*].

closed and no massive evaporation takes place. For the same reason in regions that are warm and anywhere the air is thin, nightfall will cause more colds, for it will penetrate more easily. Even in a city there will be places where nightfall will have more of a capacity to cause colds, according to how hot or cold the air is there, and to what degree it is thinner or heavier than usual. On this matter Monseigneur the Conte de Joyeuse[2] has assured me he has often felt this difference in certain streets of Avignon; but it is everywhere the same, if one but takes note of it.

Now in order to avoid any harm coming from nightfall, which is as we have described it, the principal remedy is to have one's head covered, so that it will not feel the coolness of the air, and even to have a hat that has a large brim so as to protect the face, for the air we breathe out, caught by the brim, warms the air that comes in contact with our eyes and the rest of the face, areas through which we can easily catch cold. And so it would be better still to close the coat tight against the face, and women should not forget their masks or scarves.

And this is what confirms once again my arguments that there is no evil quality in nightfall air, and that it does not fall on us. But to make them stronger, I will add that the air of a very cool cellar will be as harmful and to the same extent for people susceptible to colds as will nightfall if they stay in it for any length of time after the setting of the sun whose warmth it has accumulated. For if one stays in a cellar all day long, because one becomes accustomed to such cool air, it will not be as harmful in the evening, as can be easily understood from what we have said above. And from this it can also be understood that nightfall is not only air that is uncovered and (as people say) in the open, but it is the same everywhere except that it is more active and more penetrating in the open than under some cover, since under the cover of a house, a roof, or a porch, the enclosed air is less cold than elsewhere.

Furthermore, I maintain that nightfall is not something that falls on us from the sky, except metaphorically speaking or in some other form of poetic speech, such as when the poet, speaking of night coming upon us, says that the shadows are falling from the high mounts. And yet night is nothing more than the obscurity or darkness of the air as a result of the absence of the sun. And so one may finally resolve by

---

[2]On Anne de Joyeuse, see *PE*, bk. 3, chap. 7, n. 5 (308).

discursive reasoning all of the questions raised concerning nightfall. For instance, "Why is it worse in the city than in the countryside?" Because in the countryside people become more accustomed to the air in the course of each day, and there is no sudden change. "Why is it worse when night first comes, rather than later?" Because at nightfall, since it is a first encounter, the air catches the body more open. Once accustomed to it after two or three hours, even if one is under a roof, it no longer seems so different, for the pores have slowly closed. "Why is it more harmful to those who have closely cut or shaved heads?" Because the seams of their skulls, through which the night air, as we have said, can penetrate, are less tight. Some people have seams such that they can go out at nightfall without hats, or only with light hats; but they are very much at risk because of their ears, through which the air can easily penetrate into their brains, and so it would be better for them to cover their ears than to wear big hats. "Why is nightfall worse when the air is thin than when the air is heavy?" Because such air is often quick to become heated and cooled, as Hippocrates says of clear water. And for this very reason, after a very warm day nightfall will be much more harmful. And those who live in warm houses or in cold houses where the air is enclosed have much more to fear in going out at nightfall.

But is it true that nightfall makes a man's hair become gray or white? Yes, for those who are sensitive to it and who are more subject to it, as is commonly said. For such people are rheumy and pituitous, a condition causing the hair to whiten in old people, and before their time in those whose brains are more moist.

END

INDEX
OF NAMES, PLACES, WORKS, AND SUBJECTS, INCLUDING ALL ANATOMICAL, MEDICINAL, AND PATHOLOGICAL TERMS

Abano, Pietro d', 209, 213, 238
Abditis nonnullis ac mirandis morborum et sanationum causis, 225
abdomen (lower),
  governed by sixth couple, 107
abortion, xv
  caused by bloodletting, 84
  danger of to women, 152
  popular expressions for, 170, 175
aconite, 202
  and venom, 149
acratisma, 186
Adam, 233
  language of, 231
Adam's apple, 170, 180
Aesculapius, 206, 207
afflictions (phlegmatic), 221
Africa, 27
aging, countered by laughter, 142
agones, 173
Agrippa, Cornelius, 125
ague, 35
air, xii
  cooling with water, 55
  importance of fresh, 55
aislerons grands, 14
Albertus Magnus, 212
alcohol, 41
ale, 27
Alexander the Great, 96
Alexander of Aphrodisias, 236, 238, 240
Alexanders julep (horse-parsley),
  rosewater in, 248
Alexandria, 235
Alian, Monsieur, 16
almond extract, 100
aloe *(perroquet),* 41, 225
Alphabet anatomique, 4
alphes, 221
alum, 192
America, 27
ammary, neck of, 14
Ammonius (Ammonios) Saccas, 235
amnesia, 242
anaimes, 218
anchovies, 110

ancients, 179
  love for blood of hares of, 75
  prescribed use of magnets, 189
  teachings of on bloodletting, 82
angel, 195
anger, 34
  and fat people, 138
animals,
  as physicians, 149
  bloodless, 218
  health of sea vs. land, 149
  live more wisely than men, 260
  putrefaction of, 145
  venomous, 131
  voices of, 240
anthos, 176
antidote, 131, 205
antipathy, 190
anus, 108
Anville, Maréchal d' (*see* Damville and Montmorency), 247
aperients, 64
Aphorisms (Hippocrates), 60, 65, 81, 88, 89
Apollo, 206
  Delphian temple of, 272
apoplexy, 26, 178, 183
apostemes, 34, 156
apothecary, 125, 168, 241, 247, 275
apothecary,
  delivers medicine, 100
  fees of, 251
  pleasant items from, 61
  understands poorly physicians' prescriptions, 101
  use of goat blood by, 74
apozem *(apozeme),* 64
appetite, xii, 216, 222, 223
  and swimming, 142
  heightened at sea, 160
  loss of, 135
appetites,
  controlling of, 66
  sensual and animal, 28
apple, 94
apple water, 27
Aristotle, 40, 197-98, 205, 244
  defining death, 214
  Historia animalium, 236

Nicomachean Ethics, 38
on the soul, 234
Problems, 235, 240, 253
armpit, 184
arrierefosse (reffiron), 14
Ars poetica, 195
Art of Medicine (Galen's), 206
arteries, 49, 74, 204
arthritis, 180
arthron, 180
ashes,
  as remedy, 132
  watered, 41
Asia, 27
astomes, 224
astriction, (stomach), 108
astringency, 248
astrologers, 195, 203
astrology, 209
Athenaeus, 213
Athens, 236
Aubenas, 28
Augustine, Saint, 232
Augustus, time of, 85
authority,
  medical and theological, xv
  vs. experience, 198, 211
authorization to print, 3
authors, Greek and Arab, 177
avalir, 185
Avenzoar, 83
Avignon, 15, 212, 281
Avincenna, 227
azimant, 189
Babel, Tower of, 232
Babylon, 56
back pain, 158
backache, 28
bacon, 149
balm, 41
balousse, 72
baptismal font,
  superstitions about pregnant
    women and, 162
Barbaro, Hermalao, 213
barbers, 133
  and bloodletting, 86, 88
  and wound dressing, 127
barley broth, 93
barley soup, for the sick, 61
barley water, 31
bashfulness, 143
Basque (language), 237
bastards,
  intelligence, strength of, 148
bathing, 263
baths,
  and rubdowns, 49

and the pox, 163
bats,
  blindness and urine of, 150
beans, 111
  and fear, 152
bears, xv, 171, 199
Beaucaire, 255
Beauchastel, Christophe (Chri-
    stophle), xiii, 16, 115, 169
Beaufort, Monsieur de, 16
beaver (water-horse), xv, 171, 197
bed (patient's), 55-56
bedcovers, excessive, xv
bedrooms,
  cooling with water, 71
  fresh air in, 72
bedwetting, and wine, 136
beer, 27
belly, and dancing, 144
Benedetti, Alessandro, 225
Beniven (Benivieni), Antonio, 225
Bertrauen, Louis, 8
beverages, xii
  avoid during fever, 57
  made from grain of fruit, 27
  used in place of wine, 247
Bèze, Théodore de, 38
Bibbiena (Bernardo Dovizi), Car-
    dinal, 113
bile,
  in stomach, 140
  yellow, 46
birds, 141, 145, 201
  song of, 236
  talking, 241
biscuit bread, 61
bite, venomosity of, 149
bladder,
  organs next to, 46
  orifice of, 14
  stones in, 190
bleeding,
  internal, 40
  stopping, 171, 191
blind (people), 236
blisters, 223
blood, 37, 77, 181, 221
  amount of drawn in phlebotomy,
    83
  and intelligence, 152
  and semen, 111
  clots, 40
  generated from digestion, 187
  male goat, 190
  menstrual, 78
  naturally preserved by nature, 78
  nefarious effects of menstrual, 78
  of bull poisonous, 149

of hares, 75
of lambs and kids, 74
of pigs, 75
ox, sheep, goat, 74
passing in urine, 135
pituitous, 190
polluted by bad humors, 77
produces fat, 187
quickly corrupted by air, 75
sausages, 74
thin, 154
vomiting of, 40
wine produces, 144
bloodletting (phlebotomy), xii, xv,
    121, 138,
    and barbers, 86
    and season of year, 88
    at the buttock, 159
    causes abortions, 84
    Celsus on, 85
    cools the body, 47
    extreme, 91
    fear of, 78
    indiscriminate use of, 86
    natural, 79
    necessity of, 77
    of pregnant women, children,
        elderly, 82
    physicians blamed for prescrib-
        ing, 80
    proper weather for, 154
    virtue of first use of, 80
blood sausage, 137
    as traditional gift, 75
    origin of, 74
    symbolism of as gift, 75
Boccaccio, Giovanni, 213
bolus (see gobbet), 95
bones, 141
    broken, 137
Boniface VIII, 12
Book of Curing through Phlebotomy
    [De cognoscendis curandisque
    animi morbis], 83
borage soup, 99
Bordeaux, 15, 137
bouchet, 31, 247, 249, 253, 254
boughs, 55
bowel movement,
    bloody, 121
    what constitutes good, 109
bowels, 178, 190
    blood sausage made with, 75
    fetid matter in, 63
    loose, xv, 107
    medium laxity in, 108
    move after meals, 150
    panada and loose, 142

rinsing of, 97
tight, 109
brain, 234, 251
    chilled when extremities are cold,
        107
    coarse humors of, 280
    cooling, 73
    danger to from chancres, 181
    inflammation of, 178
    penetrated by drug vapors, 95
    size of man's vs. animals', 152
bran, and bowel movement, 136
brass, 192
brass ring, cure for colic, 193
bread, 111, 130, 232
    and hemorrhoids and constipa-
        tion, 136
    crust of soaked in water, 68
    in wine, 252
    moldy, 132
    soaked in wine, 186
    toasted, 100
    wheat and rye, 136
breath,
    foul-smelling, 130
    shortness of, 68
breathing, difficulty in, 39
breezes, nefariousness of, 145
Brete, Monsieur de, 16
Breton (language), 237
Breuiarium practicae, 12
Breyer, Lucas (book merchant),
    xii, 4
bronchial tubes, 39
broom flowers, 41
broths (and soups), 29, 108
    as lavative, 98
    as remedy, 108
    black hen, 161
    for the sick, 61
    given at midnight, 62
    medicinal, 251
    proper times and quantities of, xv
    taken before dinner, 97
bubo, 184
bull blood, poisonous, 149
bullion, 29
burns, 152
Butin, Antoine, 241
butter,
    as remedy, 108
    vs. oil, 161
buttocks, whipping as treatment,
    108
Cabrol, Barthélemy, xiii-xiv, 64,
    115, 131, 153, 169
    first royal surgeon, 4
    letter to Antoine de Clermont, 6

letter to Neufville, 4
cagasangue, 178
cake, bad for stomach, 154
calamita, 189
Calandra, 113
calculi, 179, 190
calves, meat of as food, 128
canal, great, 14
canne, 184
cannibalism, and leprosy, 145
Canons, 99
cantharides, 111
Capel, Guillaume, 17
capons, 74, 111, 143
  and gout, 129
Capots, 136
Caracteres, 202
carbuncles, 127
care,
  excessive, xv
  for the ill, xv
carp,
  stone from brain of, 191
  tongue of, 188
cartilage, 181
cassia, 91, 96
Castigationes Plinianae, 213
castor, 197
castorium, 197
castration,
  and gout, 129
  yields better meat in animals, 150
catarrh, 170, 180, 280
  caused by dew, 154
Catherine de Medici, 113
Catholicon, 134
causes, true, 191
Celsus, 87, 123, 251, 263
  on copulation, 92
  on phlebotomy, 85
  on the body, 272
  on use of drugs, 251
cerveau, 248
cervix, 14
Cévennes, 137
chaff, used in mattresses, 56
chameleon, 198
chancre, 178
  on the face, 181
  on thighs and legs, 184
character, men and horses sharing
    same, 147
charcoal, blessed, 41
Charles IX, 13
cheese, 71, 152
  and aging, 160
  ripening of, 129
  vs. broth, 154

cherries, 70
chestnuts,
  and lice, 152
  and lust, 112
chickens, 74, 189
child,
  breathes in the womb, 151
  in the womb, 130
children,
  and fright during sleeping, 144
  and loose bowels, 109
  and tight clothing, 139
  at birth, 141
  bare-headed, 138
  bizarre words used by, 243
  cries of inside womb, 157
  diet and activity of, 142
  diet of very young, 158
  eating bread without meat, 133
  health of those born in seventh
    month, 156
  memory capacity of vs. old
    people's, 149
  must not hold their urine, 47
  phlebotomy for, 82
  proportions of, 157
  sleeping and diet, 154
  teething in, 171
  violent tempers of, 162
chills, 25, 30, 34, 129, 280
choler, 37
  and vinegar, 148
  bitter humors, 70
choleric humor, 140, 208, 253
choleric (person), and drinking,
    142
Christians, 27
chyle, 67
cider, 27
cinnamon, 31, 247
Cinq liures de la maniere de nour-
    rir and gouuerner les enfans
    des leur naissance, 12
circumcision, xv, 177
City of God, 232
cleanliness, patient kept in absolute,
    56
Clermont, Antoine de, xiii
  Cabrol's letter to, 6
clitoris, 14
clothes, xii
  tight, 155
clots, 40
  dissolved by savory, 76
  in internal organs, 44
cloves, 93
clysters, 97, 122, 130, 251
  and coitus, 160

injection of remedies via, 108
  proper administration of, 109
cock sparrows, and lust, 188
cock sparrow's illness, 183
coitus, 188
  and animals vs. women, 141
  and clysters, 160
  and medication, 92
  and oysters, 111
  and twins, 143
  avoid during dog days, 92
  frequent, 138
  proper amount of, 263
  with a menstruating woman, 161
cold, 170, 180
  change to from hot, 128
  exposure to, 39
  perceived, 128
cold remedies, 32
cold sweats, 26
colds, 26, 30, 249
  causes of other disorders, 41
  disorder called, 39
  in eyes, nose, throat, and ears,
    163
  moon causes, 280
  remedies for prevention of, 149
  running their course, 144
colic, 64, 71, 102, 119, 170-71,
    179, 273
  cure for, 193
  windy, 252
colon, 179
  and clysters, 109
coloring, pale and vile, 68
colors, 233
*Commentarii in sex libros Pedacii
  Dioscoridis adjectis quam
  plurimus plantarum et animalium imaginibus,* 31
common expressions concerning
  illnesses, xv
common sayings, xv
*Compendium scientiae naturalis ex
  Aristotele,* 213
complexion, xii, 232
  cold, 219
  determines fever treatment, 59
  of the quick tempered, 52
  sanguine, 217
  wine affects every, 253
compress, 122
conception,
  from sperm in a bath, 162
  hindered by sadness, 151
  under waxing and waning moon,
    134

*Conciliator differentiarum philoso-
  phorum et praecipue medicorum,* 209
Condrieu, 68
conduct, proper, when taking
  medication, xv
congestion, 249
consommé, 29
constellations, 195
constipation, 108
constitutions,
  moist, 221
  weak, 154
consumption, 42
contagious illness, 138
  and lepers, 136
contraries,
  engender their opposites, 34
  nature of, 32
  proper proportion of, 58
convulsions, 183
coolness (see also cold), 69
copulation (*see* coitus)
Coqueret (school in Paris), 22
coriander water, 31
corpse,
  growth of hair in, 130
  preserved by lightning, 150
cosmetic, health the best, 148
cotton, used in mattresses, 56
coughing, 146
  and ear canal, 157
  and old people, 143
court physician,
  responsibilities of, xvi
covers (excessive), 53
cramps, 206
  gout with, 171
  in stomach and bowels, 64
  intestinal, 78
  stomach, 121
cranial seams, 280
crassule maieur, 225
crocodile, 219
Croesus, 245
crows, 188
  speech of, 237
cures, inept, 191
curtsies, and hunchbacks, 155
custodia, written on prescriptions,
  100
custom, power of, 66
cynanche (synanche), 180
D'Anville, Monseigneur the Maréchal (*see* Damville and
  Montmorency), xii
dame du milieu, 14
Dam(p)ville, Henri I, Comte de, 13

dancing, and the belly, 144
Darius, 5
Dauphiné, 178, 198
David, King, 280
De alimentorum facultatibus, 74, 110-11
De animalibus, 212
De architectura, 219
De causis plantarum, 202
De cognoscendis curandisque animi morbis, 83
De la conduite du fait de chirurgie, 12
De locis affectis, 43
De medicina, 87, 123
De methodo medendi libri XIV, 60, 66, 87
De opeficio dei, 238
De piscibus marinis, 242
De re medica, 99
De regimine sanitatis ad Laurentium Medicem, 225
De sanitate tuenda, 66
De sophisticis elenchis, 205
De temperamentis, 198
De triplici vita, 225
De vanitate scientiarum, 125
De vegetabilis, 212
De venenis eorumque remediis, 209
deaf,
    from birth, 233
deaf-mutes,
    language of child raised among, 231
deafness, 238
death, xii, 195
    and regret, 105
    during the night, 136
decircumcised, 170
decircumcision, 177
Decisiones physionomicae, 209
decoction, 64
deer, 188
deflowered, 170
deflowering (devirgination), 176
dehydration, 217
Deipnosophistai, 213
delivery, 171
    facilitation of, 189
Demonstrations, 99
depression, 108
desantorat, 176
Descartes, René, 212
desensitivation, 97
desieuner, 186
desourat, 176
dessarrier, 175
devil, 185

devirgination, 176
dew,
    and catarrhs, 154
    and rheumatism, 136
dewlaps, 14
diagnosis, 118
diamonds, 190
diaphragm, 177
diarrhea, schoolboy's, 108
Dictionarium historicum ac poeticum, 11
diet, 1, 251, 263
    and rhubarb, 153
    appropriate for the feverous, 51
    proper, xv, 146
    wine in the, xii
digestion, xii, 66, 135, 187
    aided by wine, 252
digestive system, healthy, xv
dining, 185
Dioscorides, 31, 197, 198, 224
disciplines, mathematical, in search of causes, 211
Discours de la méthode, 212
discourse, scientific of the Renaissance, xv
diseases, xii
Diseases, 37
Dispensatory, 108
Distiques, 219
Diverses leçons [Silva de varia lecion], 243
divorce, caused by stinkbug, 130
dizziness, 273
dock, 247
Dodoëns, Rembert, 248
dog days, and purgation, 89
dog's tongue, medicinal value of, 134
dogs, 127, 201
    cold nose of, 152
dolphin, 196
Dorat (d'Aurat), Jean, 22
dormice, 219
doves, 111
dreaming, man vs. animals, 146
dreams, source of, 146
dressings, and lye, 159
drinking, 170, 185
    after soup, 154
    before a journey, 161
    before eating, 148
    frequency of, 146
    water vs. wine, 144
dropsy, 26, 171
    cure for, 193
drugs, 78, 91, 131, 251, 275
    and natural heat, 205

efficacy of odors of, 149
health-restoring, 207
Hippocrates's prescribing of
   strong, 84
not to be used by the healty, 87
penetrative, 64
purgative, 208
purging humors with, 50
vapor of, 95
varying effects of in different
   bodies, 97
drunkards, ailments of, 26
drunkenness, in women vs. old
   people, 150
Du Guillet, Pernette, 197
Du Serain, 72
dysentere, 178
dysentery, 70
   popular expressions for, 170, 178
earaches, 119
ears, 238
   air accesses brain through, 282
   in women, 129
earth nuts, 111
earth sickness, 170, 183
eating,
   in moderation, 263
   living without, 172, 211
   terms for, 170
   when not hungry, 150
   while talking, 142
eau de bouchet, 31
ebullition, 36
ecannez, 184
Ecclesiasticus, 252, 273
eclipses, 227
Ecloges, 203
edemas, 221
eggs, 130
   and the heart, 154
   fresh, 29
   where to crack, 163
egg yolks, as remedy, 109
Egyptians, 232, 246
elderly,
   fussiness of, 144
   have little natural heat, 216
   phlebotomy for, 82
   small appetite of, 219
   tight bowels in, 109
elements (the four), 195
Elias, 228
embonpoint, 148
emerald, and marriage, 131
emissions, nocturnal in animals,
   147
empireume (empyreume), 34
empirics, gross error of, 88

enema, with milk, 154
entrails, heat accumulation in, 73
Epidemics, 37
epidermis, 33
epilepsie, 183
epilepsy, 182, 273
   in Tuscany, 137
   susceptibility to, 143
eprensas, 178
Erasistratus, 77
erection, and flatulence, 111
Erreurs populaires, 127, 255
   1579 edition of, 72
   scandal of, xiv
   vs. Joubert's Latin works, 212
error books, discourse characterizing, xvi
errors,
   based on unsound arguments, 70
   of common folk, 169
escannats, 184
esophagus, 93
espremason, 178
Essais, 125
Estienne, Charles, 11
Europe, 26, 225
   Christian, 27
evacuation, xii, 121
Eve, 233
evil,
   inclination in man, 233
   king's, 137
excoriation, 178
excrement, 46, 207, 220
   and colds, 39
   careful examination of, 274
   disorders caused by retained, 221
   human vs. animal, 145
   molting a form of, 218
   nasal and other, 163
   types of characterizing various
      people, 144
   voided through the skin, 48
   weakens poisons, 208
exercise, 135
   necessity of, 263
exertion, strenuous, 40
exhalation, 33
exhalations, 48
Exogonium jalapa, 99
experience,
   vs. authority, 198, 211
Expositio problematum Aristotelis,
   209
extirpation, 184
extracts, 29
eyes,
   bigger than stomach, 144

green, 153
of sick person, 160
sore, 119
faba inversa, 225
fabulous stories, xii
face, color in, 150
fainting, 94, 170, 185
fall, remedy for victims of, 132
falling sickness, 26, 170, 183
cure for, 193
Fallopio, 14
fasting, 223, 228
and thinking, 161
fever caused by, 217
function of, 221
fat people, longevity of, 161
fat,
from fish, 127
fear, and beans, 152
feather mattresses, 71
featherbed, not recommended, 56
fecundity, 171, 182, 188
types of women and, 144
feeling, loss of, 178
feet,
cold applied to, 107
hot, 129
odor sign of good health, 143
talkativeness and hot, 152
warm, 155
females, smaller than males, 147
fennel, 76, 99
fetus,
eight-month, 140
five-month, 143
harm done to in third or fourth
month, 84
seven-month, 133
fever, xv, 29, 84, 171, 270
and lepers, 136
and worms, 145
burning, 42, 70
colicky, 42
continuous, 36, 58
cure for any type of, 192
cure for quartan, 192
diverse types, 32
during dog days, 89
essence of, 38
fits of, 121
general rules for treating, 59
hectic, 217
in May, 129
inducing of sweating during, 60
intermittent, 34, 37
limited, 32, 58
multiple sources of, 41
persistent, 28

quartan, 135, 178
relation to excrement, 39
susceptibility to, 143
tertian, 70, 90
tertian and constipation, 141
feverous, appropriate diet for, 51
Fevol, Monsieur de, 16
Ficino, Marsilio, 224
figs, 70, 133
as poison, 129
fingernails,
growth of in corpse, 130
in seven-month fetus, 133
of seventh-month children, 156
fingers, cold and pain in, 128
fish, 130
and desire for coitus, 188
best portion of, 143
eating engenders semen, 188
fecundity of, 188
healthy as a, 130
preservation of troublesome, 156
putrefaction of, 145
salted, 127
flatulence, and lust, 110
Fleurs du liure des vertus des
herbes, 210
floor (of patient's room), strewn
with flowers, 55
Florilegium Monacense, 106
flowers (menses), 132
during pregnancy, 85
fluctuation, stomach, 108
fluxion, 31
food, 215, 222
danger of highly refined, 149
eaten in France, 113
on an empty stomach, 111
preparation of, xii
proper chewing of, 133
proper use of during illness, xii
food poisoning, 34
force, vital, 215
forehead,
and headaches, 141
large veins in, 129
foreskin, 177
fowl, 193
digestive potency of, 190
France, 175, 196, 246
François I, 198
frantic, 182
French (language), 178, 246
Frenchmen, 137
frenzy, 28
fright, in children when sleeping,
144
frost, 133

fruit, 248
  and dreams, 151
  astringent after meals, 108
  laxative effect of, 253
  overripe, 99
  ripening of, 129
fuligineux, 25
Fullers thistle (see teasel), 61
Galen, 29, 43, 60, 66, 87, 89, 110-
    12, 120, 198, 205-08, 216-17
  against excessive use of
    phlebotomy, 86
  and excessive bloodletting, 91
  Ars medicinalis, 96
  De alimentorum facultatibus, 74
  on bloodletting, 82, 83
  on oysters and truffles, 112
  on phlebotomy and drugs, 88
gallstones, 158, 273
Gargantua, 180
garlic, 112, 137, 225
  and engendering male children,
    132
garters, and women, 147
Gascons, 136
Gascony, 178, 183
gaster, 197
Genas (maiden-name of Laurent
    Joubert's wife), 116
Genesis, 232
genitalia, female, 13
German (language), 237, 246
Germans, 137
Germany, 213, 246
gestation, and coitus (women vs.
    animals), 141
ghiandozza, 170, 184
Giraud, Monsieur, 200
Girard (two brothers), 16
gizzard, 189
gluttony, 154
gnothi seauton, 272
goat meat, 189
goat milk, 188
goats, 232
  with clouded vision, 79
goatskin, 56
gobbet, 95
God, 229, 252, 255, 273
  and Adam, 233
  jealousy of, 103
goiters, in Savoy, 137
gourds, 112
gout, 27, 30, 71, 119, 137, 154,
    170, 180, 273
  and castration, 129
  and old people, 143
  and the rich, 136

  in Bordeaux, 137
  in capons and roosters, 129
  with cramps cured, 192
gouttes, 180
grape juice, and vision, 130
grapes, 70
  better fresh or dried, 150
Greece (ancient), 213
Greek (language), 233
Greeks (ancient), 30, 49, 204
groin, 184
guiacum, 250
Guise, family, 13
gullet, 181, 184
gynecological terms, xiv, 9
habit, power of, 65
Hadrian (Emperor), 125
hair,
  frequent cutting and shaving of,
    156
  growth of in corpse, 130
  proper time for cutting, 163
  turning white, 138
  used in mattresses, 56
hallucinations, 120, 178
ham, 110
happiness, makes one fat, 144
hares, 193
  blood of, 75
  leprous, 130
Hart, James, 97
head,
  of body likened to prince, 256
  warm, 155
headache, 28, 108, 119, 121, 132,
    133, 156
  and the forehead, 141
  cured by nosebleed, 79
health,
  and the venereal act, 133
  of the prince, 255
hearing,
  and speech, 232
  better at night, 149
  loss of, 183
  nerves providing for, 238
  sense of, 233
  sharpening, 147
heart, 181, 196
  cooling, 73
  growth of, 156
  large, 143
  size of determines complexion,
    144
  suffers effects of fever, 54
heat, 280
  and primal humor, 214
  causes weakness, 30

dilates vessels, 46
effects of on body, 88
exhalation of, 33, 48
foundation of life, 214
natural, 26, 34, 48, 95, 207, 222, 252
troublesome symptoms caused by, 73
vital, 216
heavy-headedness, remedy for, 157
Hebrew (language), 232, 233, 243
hectic state, result of extreme heat, 42
hell, 195
hellebore, 207
hemicranie, 182
hemlock, 96, 207
and wine, 150
hemorrhages, susceptibility to, 143
hemorrhoids, blood exuding from, 79
Henri II, 113
Henri III, 23, 200
sterility of, 4, 68
Henry IV, 4
hens, 142
leprous, 130
without milt, 131
herbati, 209
herbs,
and loose bowels, 150
saxifragial, 190
hernias,
caused by screaming, 139
in Montpellier, 137
repair of causes sterility, 163
Herod, 183
Herodotus, 232, 245
hieroglyphics, 246
high sickness, 170, 183
hip, gout of, 180
hippocras, 31, 61, 112, 247, 249
and quinsy, 130
Hippocrates, 37, 59, 82, 91, 109, 119, 207, 282
Aphorisms, 60, 65, 81, 216, 223
oath of, 11
on bloodletting, 88
on coitus and twins, 143
on diagnosis, 122
on eating and drinking, 66
on fasting, 221
on hellebore, 95
on lethal fasting, 212
on phlebotomy, 84
on purgation, 89
Hippocratis de medicorum astrologia libellus, 209

hippopotamus, 79
Historia plantarum, 202
History of Animals [Historia animalium], 198, 236
Holy Scriptures, translation of into French, 12
Homer, cited by Galen, 74
honey, 248
vs. wine, 133
when to consume, 145
Horace, 195
horehound, 193
horse-parsley, 248
horses, 187, 232
hot, change to from cold, 128
hot complexions, 26
humidity, excessive body, 234
humors, 34, 121, 180-81, 272, 280
abundant, 241
and dreaming, 146
and poison, 97
and purgation, 88
bad, 30, 228
bitter, 70
body needs four different, 37
choleric, 90
coarse, 226, 250
cooling and purifying of, 63
doctrine of the four, 37
expelling bad, 95
freely flowing, 30
how affected by exertion, 45
in the blood, 44
in the stomach, 222
melancholic, 79
move inward in darkness, 101
pernicious, 90
pituitous, 223
superfluous, 217
thick, heavy, 30
thinning of, 249
hunchbacks,
and wet nurses, 155
longevity of, 161
hunger, 216
during famines, 158
quelling of, 145
sign of cleared stomach, 98
hyacinth, 131
hydromel, 31, 93
vs. wine, 133
hydropsy, 43, 68
hymen, 14
hyppocras (*see* hippocras)
hyssop, 76
iatroalipta, 263
ice, 129
ichthyology, 242

idiosyncrasy, 206
ill, care for, xv
illecebra, 225
illnesses,
  and impatience, 155
  caused by youth and wealth, 158
  man's vs. animals' susceptibility
    to, 151
  names of ending in *ique*, 155
  nature of, 121
  popular terms for, 170
  proper use of food during, xii
  susceptibility to, 141
  weight loss during, 162
imbalming, 41
Imbert, Jean, xiii, 168
*In Borbonias consuetudines com-
  mentarius*, 211
*In Dioscoridem corrolariorum
  libri 5*, 213
In sextum decalogi praeceptum, 211
incubus, 138
Indian root, 250
indigestion, 34, 248
  and loose bowels, 107
infection, 34
  transmission of, 128
inflammation, 178
inhalants, 251
Inquisition, 12
insane, in Béarn, 137
insomnia, 121
  and madness, 128
instinct, 215, 232
  man's vs. animals', 142
intemperence, of man, 30
intestines, 187, 208
  effect of chilling, 107
  small, 220, 222, 228
intuition (woman's), 52
iron, 189, 193
ischias, 180
ischiatique, 180
ischion, 180
Italians, 137, 178, 184
Italy, 56
  fowl not bled in, 74
jaundice, 171
  cure for, 192
jay, speech of, 237
jelly, 154
Jesus Christ, 228
  and wine at Holy Supper, 252
Jews, 177
joints,
  gout disorder of, 180
  heat accumulation in, 73
Joubert, François, xiii, 115

Joubert, Isaac, xiv, 172, 200, 211
  translator of the Paradoxes, 4
Joubert, Laurent, 211, 246
  and his *TL*, 168
  father of, 65
  paternal aunt of, 68
Joyeuse, Anne de, 281
judgment, vs. memory, 149
juices, of plants, grains, fruits, 224
julep, 64
julep, Alexanders, 248
kidney beans, 111
kidney stones, 46, 63, 71, 158,
  190, 252, 273
  and tight clothing, 155
  dissolved with goat blood, 74
  pears cause, 144
kidneys, 178
  as food, 75
  cooling of externally, 107
kids (goats), as food, 128
king's evil *(les escrouëlles)*, 162
  in Spain, 137
*Klinikë, or The Diet of the Dis-
  eased*, 97
knees, people with pointed, 161
knots, 221
La Bastie, Monsieur de, 16
La Baume, Monsieur de, 16
La Bruyère, Jean de, 202
La Coste, Monsieur de, 16
*La Dissection des parties du corps
  humain*, 11
La Roche, Monsieur de, 16
La Santé du prince, 68
Labé, Louise, 197
labia, 13
laborers, 217
Lactantius Firmianus, 238
L'Agriculture et maison rustique,
  11
lamb, 111, 232
  as food, 128
landies, 14
L'Angelier, xii
language,
  akin to music, 233
  and practice, 242
  deformations of, 244
  invented by mute individuals, 246
  loss of, 242
  native, 235
  nature of, xiv
  of Adam, 231
Languedoc, 65, 174, 178, 182-85,
  198, 213
lapidaires (lapidaries), 83
lard, 42, 74

larfondement (fat in the excrement),
  42
larfondu (one suffering from *larfon-*
  dement), 42
lark, speech of, 237
larmuses, 198
larynx, 180
Latin (language), 233, 237
laughter, counters aging, 142
laugroles, 198
laxatives, 91, 94, 97
laziness, 217
Le Notaire, 211
learning, and instruction, 234
leaves, mixed with water, 71
lechery, and constricted waist, 141
left-handedness, and bastards, 148
leisure time, 267
lemon juice, 190
lemon peel, 93
Lent, and married people, 92
Leo X, Pope, 213
lepers,
  and immunity, 146
  blood of, 78
  feeling and blood in, 155
  immunity of, 136
  near Limoges, 137
leprosy,
  and cannibalism, 145
  and lust, 136
  in hens and hares, 130
lethargy, 191
  caused by phlegmatic humor, 234
lettuce, 55
  soup, 99
lice,
  and chestnuts, 152
  and lepers, 136
Liébault, Jean, 11
light, danger of bright, 128
lightning, and preservation of
  corpse, 150
limb, body affected by mutilated,
  146
liminal poems, xv
Limousine, 137
linen,
  changing of, xv, 48
  warming, 130
linnet, speech of, 237
lips, swollen or split, 163
liquids,
  drinking of cool, 61
  proper drinking temperature of,
  68
liver, 159
  ailments, 136

as food, 75
calmed by wine, 252
cooling of externally, 107
diseased, 148
excessive heat in, 87
hot, 128
large, 143
love resides in, 75
matter for semen from, 111
receives chyle, 67
lizards, 198, 218
longevity, of man and animals, 145
loubet, 184
Louise de Lorraine, 200
  sterility of, 68
loup, 184
loupes, 221
love, 195
  excessive, 103
lozenges, 251
luck, bad, 130, 156
lunatic, 170, 182
lungs,
  ailments, 136
  as food, 75
  cool the heart, 54
  cooling, 73
  hot, 154
  inflammation of, 77
  shocked by cold air, 39
lust, and leprosy, 136
lye, 41
  and dressing cleaning, 159
lying, 185
Lyon, 15, 197
Lyte, Henry, 248
Macer, Lucinie (Lucius Clodius,
  Æmelius), 210
madness, and insomnia, 128
magistrates, and bloodletting, 88
magnet, facilitates childbirth, 189
magpie, speech of, 237
Maison rustique, 11
mal au coeur, 30
males, larger than females, 147
malmsey, 31
man,
  ability to represent of, 233
  as microcosm, 147
  social and political animal, 255
  susceptible to illness, 145
  variety of species, 202
mange, 132
  and the poor, 136
  on child's scalp, 144
  susceptibility to, 143
manna, 91, 96
March violet water, 55

Marguerite de France, 200, 234
Marguerite de Navarre, 8
Marguerite de Valois (Marguerite
    de France), 9
Marot, Clement, 4
marriages, in May, 127
Martial, 219
masclon, 179
Master Mouche *(Maistre mousche),*
    103
Materia medica, 31
Matinées de l'Ile d'Adam, 113
matrix, 177
Mattioli, Pietro Andreo, 31
mattresses,
    feather, 71
    materials used in, 56
mau de las passeras, 170
mau-loubet, 170, 184
meals, xii
    frequency of, 135
    types of and trades, 142
meat, 130, 143, 157, 188
    boiled, 99
    bullion, 100
    goat, 189
    minced, 154
    of lambs and kids, 74
    salted, 127
    strained, 29
    tenderness of, 128
    wholesome preparation of, 158
mechoachan (jalap), 99
mede, 31
medical arts, 169
medication,
    conduct and diet during, 93
    proper diet when taking, 64
    sleeping after, 95
medicinal pound *(liure medicinale),*
    subdivisions of, 247
medicine, 251
    administered after fasting, 154
    and war, 157
    art of true, 207
    contrary to nature, 62
    intervals for administering, 97
    nature of the art of, 206
    prophylactic, 270
    secrets of art of, 252
melancholic humor, 163, 253
melancholic (person), and eating,
    142
melancholy, 37, 182
    and the company of women, 138
    and vinegar, 148
melicrat, 31
melons, 70, 254

and wine, 133
as poison, 129
memory, 171
    adversely affected, 190
    cause of loss of, 138
    children's vs. old people's, 149
    Mithridates's, 235
    vs. judgment, 149
menses, 182
    during pregnancy, 85
    popular expressions for, 170, 173
    provoking of, 63
    stopping flow of, 189
    unborn child nourished by, 78
menstruation, xv
Mesua (Iahia ibn-Masawayh), 99
Meteorologica, 40
metheglin *(bouchet),* 31
Method (Galen's), 206
Mexía, Pero, 243, 246
Micard, Claude, xii
Micard edition, xii, xiv, 64, 127
    inventory of, xiii
microcosm, man is, 259
midwives,
    depositions of, 13
    handling of children by, 139
    practices of, 189
migraine, 170, 182, 273
milk, 248
    curds, 137
    drying up mother's, 171, 192
    easily digested, 157
    goat, 188
    of black goat, 161
    remedy for mother's, 141
    she-ass, 64
    soured by bread crumb, 145
Millanges, Simon, 3, 255
mint, and war, 145
miracles, 228
miscarriage, 171, 175
    means of avoiding, 189
mithridate, 41
Mithridates, King, 235
moisture,
    and heat, 214
    body heat founded in, 48
    loss of substantific, 215
    natural body, 220
    natural, 222
molting, form of excrement, 218
Momin, Jean, 115
monarchy, 256
Moncontour, battle of, 6
Monin, Jean Edouard du, 21
monkeys, 168, 188
mons Veneris, 13

Montaigne, Michel de, 125
months,
    without an *r*, 92
Montmorency, Anne de, 13
Montmorency, François de, 113,
    247
Montmorency, Henri de, 247
    his beverage, xvi
Montoison, Baron de (see Cler-
    mont, Antoine de), 6
Montpellier, 168, 185, 200
    University of, 11
    University of Medicine of, 222,
    246
Mon[t]perroux la Verune, Monsieur
    de, 16
moon, 182, 195, 280
    and menstrual cycle, 174
morfondement, 32
Moses, 228
mouse, Alpine, 219
Moutet, Monsieur du, 16
mouth, 238
movement,
    during sleep, 144
    loss of, 178
Muhammad, 27
Muhammadans, 252
mules, sterility of, 141
mummy, 41
    abuses of, 158
    as remedy, 132
muscatel (vin musquat), 136
muscles, supporting the clitoris, 14
Muses, 187
mushrooms, as poison, 129
music, language akin to, 233
musk, 93
mustard, 112
    whole, 41
mute,
    from birth, 238
mutes, 246
mutton, and aging, 160
myrobolans, 158
napel, 96
narcotic, 208
nature,
    great providence of, 70
    man's vs. animals', 201
nausea, 64, 78, 108, 222
Navarre, Queen of (Marguerite de
    France), 8
neck, 184
needle, 191
neo-Platonism, 235
nephretic, 170, 178
nephritis, 119

nephros, 178
nerves,
    and continuity between body
    parts, 107
    branching from spinal cord, 238
Neufville, Nicolas de, xiii
    Cabrol's letter to, 4
Nicocles, 106
*Niewe herball or historie of
    plantes*, 248
nightfall,
    causes hair to whiten, 282
    dangers of, xvi
    harmful to those who have shaved
    heads, 282
    nature of, 280
    no evil quality in, 281
    worse in the city than in the
    country, 282
nightingales, 237
nodes, carneous, 14
noli me tangere, 170, 181, 184
nose,
    blowing of as sign of health, 159
    of sick person, 160
    post-nasal flow in, 248
    violent blowing of and health,
    143
nosebleed, 47, 170, 181
nourishment, how long one can live
    without, xiv
*Nouvelles recreations et joyeux
    devis*, 114
numbness, 26
nurses, wet, 109
nymphs, 14
oat chaff (mattress), 72
obstructions, 34
    and tight clothing, 157
    in veins and arteries, 63
    stomach, liver, and spleen, 68
odors,
    after strong exertion, 48
    in hot climates, 224
    of flowers as remedy, 151
    sniffing of as remedy, 143
oil,
    and loose bowels, 107
    olive, 108
    vs. butter, 161
    when to consume, 145
oligophore, 29
olive oil, 108
omelets, 111
*On Scarification (from Celsus's De
    medicina)*, 87
*On Temperament [De temperamen-
    tis]*, 198

On the Conservation of Health [De sanitate tuenda], 66
On the Faculty of Nourishment [De alimentorum facultatibus], 74, 110-11
On the Method (De methodo medendi), 60
On the Nature of Man, 37, 59
On the Triple Life [De triplici vita], 225
On the Virtue of Simple Remedies [Ars medicinalis], 96
onions, 137, 225
opiates, 251
orange peel, 93
order, in every-day activities, 255
organs, internal, 273
orifice, internal, 14
os Bertrand (os Barré, os pubis), 13
os du penil, 13
os sans nom, 13
ostriches, 142, 190
ox blood, 74
oxycrat, 29, 94
oysters, aphrodisiac nature of, xv, 110
Padua, 209
pain,
  caused by colds, 39
  expulsion, 35
  perceived, 128
painters (and poets), 196
palette, 83
palpitations, 68
panada, and loose bowels, 142
panade, 142
Papon, Jean, 211, 226
Paradoxes [Paradoxorum decas prima atque altera], 4, 7, 38, 62-63, 96, 172, 200, 211
  first and second decade of Joubert's, xiv
  first decade of, 7
paralysis, 26
Pardillan, Monsieur de, 16
parelle (parille: sharp-pointed dock), 247
Paris, 15, 169, 189, 200
  University of, 14
paroxysm, from fever, 57
parrot, 236, 241
  speech of, 237
parsley, 41, 74
  and vision, 130
parsnip juice, 41
partridges, 143, 154, 193, 237
  and lice, 139

pathological conditions, common, xv
patient,
  and physician relationship, 159
  excessive care causes death of, 102
  sustaining a weak, 29
  treating, 187
  wishes of, 61
patient's room, walls of, 55
Paul, Saint, 252
Paul of Aegina, 177
peaches, as poison, 129
peacock, 134
pear water, 27
pearls, 190
pears, 94, 144
  cooked, 99
peas, 111, 157
peasants, their affection for wine, 27
Peletier du Mans, Jacques, 197
pelican, 196
pendiculation, 35
penis, man without, 158
pepper, corrective of oysters, 112
perier, 189
Périers, Bonaventure des, 114
Perreau, Pierre, 201, 210
Perron, Jacques Davy du, 23
perroquet (aloe), 225
perspiration (*see* sweating)
Pharmacopaea, 108
philopore, 253
philosophers,
  ancient, 196
  claim wine a necessity, 253
  defining life, 214
philosophy, true definition of, 234
phlebotomy (*see* bloodletting), blamed for death, 80
phlegm, 25, 37, 46, 111, 225, 227
  cause of pain, 102
  caused by improper diet, 63
  cold foods produce, 110
  dissolved by wine, 253
phlegmatic (person), 140, 217
  and sleeping, 142
phoenix, 196
phrenetic, 178
Phrygian (language), 232
phthisis, in Portugal, 137
physicians, 113, 133, 187, 253
  abilities and failings of, xv
  acting freely, 103
  ancient, 45, 89, 196
  and mules, 131
  and patient relationship, 159

average, 35
blamed for prescribing bloodlet-
    ting, 80
combatting illness, 277
duties of toward prince, 255, 269
errors of, 106
fresh-water, 153
from Montpellier, 168
gentle and humane, 28
good and bad, 159
Greek and Roman, 82
heal body and mind, 144
honor of put into question, 29
Joubert's contemporaries, 96
lack of respect for, 62
layman disrespect of, 118
medieval, 82
ministers of nature, 79
mocked, 155
more than one per patient, 125
necessity of trusting, 147
of the prince, 255
ordering bloodletting, 88
prescribe according to case, 54
procedures of blamed, 104, 121
subject to God's will, 106-07
uninformed, 80
Pibrac, Guy du Faur de, 8
picrocholes, 217
Pietro d'Abano (*see* Abano, Pietro
    d'), 209
pigeons, 111, 148
pignolat (teasel), 61
pigs, 201
    as food, 128
    blood of, 75
pilchards (salted), 110
pills, 251
pine-apple (pine-kernell), 61
piss (burning: gonorrhea), 132
pissasphalte, 41
pissing, before resting, 45
pitch, 41, 193
pituitousness (pituity), 208, 221-22,
    282
    foods causing, 110
plague, 178, 205
    and garlic, 132
    and lepers, 136
    and soup, 134
    ideal weather to counter, 143
    immunity from, 130
    proper diet in times of, 145
    transmitted by money and bread,
        162
plague-sore, 170, 184
planets, 195, 227
plantain, 192

Plato, 26, 75, 234
Pléiade, 22
pleurisy, 28, 77
Pliny, 78, 79, 209, 219, 223
    and lethal fasting, 212
plums, 70
Plutarch, 56
poets (and painters), 196
poison, xv, 129
    administering, 172, 201
    and choleric, 140
    as nutriment, 96
    various types of, 204
Polish (language), 237
Polish people, 162
Politiques (Huguenot political
    group), 13
Poliziano, Angelo, 225
Pollio, Vitruvius, 219
pomegranate, 182
*Popular Errors [Les Erreurs
    populaires]*, 7, 115, 169, 255
    praising condition of women, 182
    scandal of, 8
    second book of, 176
pores (skin), 33, 39, 48, 225, 250,
    280
    constriction of, 57
    dilate with heat, 30, 43
    open in summer, 73
    poisons entering through, 204
    role of, 49
potion, 95, 122
poussif (pursy), 39
powders, 122, 251
pox (syphilis), 180
    caught from privy seat, 130
    decline of, 137
Praedium rusticum, 11
pregnancy, 189
preparatories (spermatic vessels),
    111
prescriptions, and common folk,
    119
preserves, 61
prince,
    daily activity regimen, 264
    enchiridion for, xvi
    obligations of, 255
    sound regimen of, 259
Problems, 236
prognosis, xii
Prognostic, 37
propoma, 247
Psalms, 280
Psammetichus, 232
pterigomes, 13
pubes, smelly, 143

pubic hair, 13
pullets, 74
pulse, 274
  weakening of, 94
purée, 29
purgation, xii, xv, 88, 89, 121
  darkness aids, 101
  monthly, 174, 182
  role of nature in, 98
purging, 220
purple (ointment), 108
purslane soup, 99
pursy, 273
  resulting from colds, 39
pus, 178
Quaestiones de febribus, 209
quail, 207
quartan fever, 32, 37
Quatre livres des secrets de
    medecine et de la philosophie
    chimique, 11
queasiness, 64
quince,
  marmalade, 99
  tightens and loosens bowels, 140
quinsy, 77, 170, 180
  and hippocras, 130
rabbit, 193
  brains, 190
Rabelais, François, 177, 180, 197, 228
rabies, 149
Rate, Estienne de, xiii, 168
rats, mountain (Alpine mice), 219
ravens, 188
Receptarium antidotarii, 99
recovery, desire for, 158
Recueil d'arrets notables des cours
    souveraines de France, 211
recutit, 177
reffiron (arrierefosse), 14
Reformation, troubled times of, xv
regimen, self-made, 66
regimen artis, written on prescrip-
    tions, 100
regret, types of, 105
relapses,
  sign of growth, 130
  when more dangerous, 141
religion, Christian, 211
remedies (see also drugs), 118, 263
  contesting ancient, 213
  metaphorical and extravagant, xii,
    169, 171, 188
  purgative, 206
  superstitious, vain, and
    ceremonious, 171, 191
  vain, xii
remission, 121

renal, 179
Renier, Monsieur, 16
rennet, as remedy, 132
restlessness, 121
restrictive virtue of stomach, 108
revulsion, 108
rhein, 174
rheum, 180, 273, 280
Rhodais (Rodez), 174
rhubarb, 91, 95-96,
  and diets, 153
ribs, as food, 75
rice, 157
Rodez (Rhodais), 174
Romans (ancient), 49, 225
Rome, 213
Rondelet, Guillaume, 198, 213,
    242, 253
room (of the patient), 55
rooms (bedrooms), cooling with
    water, 71
roosters, and gout, 129
rose, 174
  ointment, 108
  syrup, 91
  vinegar, 55, 93
  water, 55, 248
rosemary, 76
roses, 55
Rouergue, 174
royal family, members of France's,
    276
rubdowns (and baths), 49
sadness, 34
  hinders conception, 151
saffron, 41
sage, 192
Sagnes, Monsieur de, 16
sailing, and vomiting, 151
Saint John the Baptist, 183
Saint John's illness, 170, 183
salamander, xv, 171, 196, 198, 224
salt, 148, 193
  and fever, 150
  as remedy, 109
  as remedy for vomiting at sea,
    192
  during pregnancy, 156
  in blood sausage, 76
  provokes lust, 110
  water, 41
saltpeter, nature of, 160
sanguine (people, humors), 217
sausages,
  blood, 74
  rapid deterioration of, xv
savages, 204
savory, 41, 76

savory, 41, 76
scabs, 223
scalp, mange on child's, 144
sciatica, 170, 180
sciences, mathematical and true,
    211
scirrhi, 221
scurvy, 135
sea hare, 209
*Second Part of the Popular Errors
    [La Seconde Partie des erreurs
    populaires]*,
    organization of, 64
    secretly printed, xv
seintegne, 178
seleniaques, 182
semen, 40, 171, 188
    food converted into, 111
    oysters and, 110
sempervive, 225
sengreen, 225
senna, 91, 96
senses, loss of, 183
septiques, 204
serpents, 218
serpoulet (thyme), 76
seventh male child, healing powers
    of, 162
sexual drive, in men and women,
    132
shakes, 26
shameful parts, throwing water on,
    137
sharp-pointed dock, 247
she-ass, milk from, 64
sheep, 232
    and tamarisk tree, 131
shit, 153
    value of woodcock's 143
sick (people),
    rapid recovery of, 128
    sleep beneficial for, 129
sight, poisons and sense of, 204
Silva de varia lecion, 243
silver, 193
Simoni, Simon, 38
sin, original, 233
skin, 33
    fair, 161
    of the prince, 274
    pale in girls, 160
sleep, 128
    after milk, soup, 153
    aided by wine, 67
    as part of prescription, 96
    best hours for, 157
    importance of, xii
    importance of mattress, 72

improper times for, 143
motion during, 144
nourishes, 144
outdoors, 73
remedy for nausea, 155
slows digestion, 62
sleeping,
    after medication, 95
    proper position when congested,
    159
sleeping in, 170, 187
smell, poisons and sense of, 204
smoke, cause of leprosy and mis-
    carriage, 162
sneezing, 157
    and the sun, 129
snow, 129
sorrel soup, 99
soul, 232
    conceptions of rational, 233
    Plato's divisions of, 75
soup, 29, 93, 99, 132
    and longevity, 153
    and plague, 134
Spain, 182, 213
Spaniards, 137
sparrows, and lust, 188
spasm, 183, 185
speculum, 14
speech,
    definition of, 235
    differences in, 240
    loss of, 177
    origin of, 232
    vs. voice, 237
    written letter vicar of, 239
spermatic vessels, 111
spider, 192
spinsters, 154
spirits (humors), 50
    and poison, 97
    raised by wine, 252
spitting, 159
    frequent and good health, 143
spleen, as food, 75
squinance, 181
starlings, 207
    speech of, 237
stars, 280
steel, as remedy, 131
sterility, 113
    and different species, 141
    and sexual partners, 132
    of Louise de Lorraine, 68
stinkbug, and divorce, 130
*Stirpium differentiae ex Dioscorida
    secundum locos communes*, 31
Stobaeus, 106

stomach, 30, 159, 179, 190, 193,
    220, 222, 248, 254
  calmed by wine, 252
  cold, 128
  disorders, 273
  eyes bigger than, 144
  governed by sixth couple, 107
  having no ears, 150
  hot, 130
  noises in, 64, 135
  queasy, 206
  rinsing of, 97
  undigested foods in, 63
  upper sphincter of, 94
  upset, 78, 94, 108
  weak, 160
stomachal, 250
stones,
  in the body, 171, 189
  passing of, 179
stool, 178
  retention, 146
  runny, 155
straw, 191
  insulating properties of, 129
  mattress, 72
strigati, 209
stuttering, 240
sudorific agents, 250
sugar, 61, 100, 247
  and worms in children, 139
sulfur, 41
sun, 195
  and rheumatism, 129
Sunday, people born on, 130
sunstroke, 34
superfetation, 143
surgeon, 187, 275
surgery, 187
swallows, blindness and stool of,
    150
sweat, 48, 253
  nature of, 46
sweating, 33, 132
  agents provoking, 250
  inducing of during fever, 60
  provoking of, 63
  substances provoking, 41
sweats (cold), 94
sweetmeats, 61
swimming, and appetite, 142
swooning, 183, 185
synanche (cynanche), 180
syncope, 183
syncopiser, 185
syphilis, 180
syrup,
  preparative agents, 64

  water mixed with, 29
tabula rasa, 234
talking, while eating, 142
tamarinds, 96
tamarisk tree, 131
Tarragon, archbishop of, 12
tartar, 61
taste, poisons and sense of, 204
teasel, 61
teeth,
  children's, 134
  high-pitched sound and pain in,
    142
  people with spaces between, 161
  sensitivity of, 141
teething, 171, 192
Teiseer, 83
telephion, 225
temperature, clothes and breath
    controlling, 151
Temple de Cupido, 4
tennis, best exercise, 264
tentigo, 14
Terence, 62, 124
terra melia, potency of, 159
terra sigillata, 159
tertian fever, 32, 38
testicles, 14, 111, 197
  man without, 158
Textor, Benoît, 31
The Brothers, 124
theologians, 12, 269
theology, 211
Theophrastus, 202
thirst, xii, 120
  nature of, 69
  quelling of, 145
Thomas Aquinas, 212
Thresor des pauvres, 11
throat, 93
  swelling of, 177
throttle, 170, 184
thrush, speech of, 237
thyme, 76
Tiers Livre, 228
Timaeus, 75
Timon, 213
Timothy, 252
tisane, 93
tissues, and poison, 97
tongue, 233
  black, 133
  defect in, 238
toothache, superstitions concerning,
    160
Tournes, Jean de, 196
*Treatise on Laughter [Traité du
    ris],* 211, 245

treatment, 170
tripe, 137
Trois livres de la santé et fecondité
   et maladies des femmes, 11
truffles, 112
   aphrodisiac nature of, xv
truth, human mind in search of,
   211
tumor, 180, 184
Turk, strong as a, 27
Turks, 177, 204
twins,
   and coitus, 143
   infertility in, 156
   vs. other children, 147
Tyard, Pontus de, 197
udder, 232
ulcer, in the bladder, 46
unction, 122
Universalis aquaetilium, 242
urine, 253
   children's as remedy, 138
   deposits in, 47
   holding, 134
   nature of, 46
   retention and odor, 146
   voiding before resting, 45
uterus,
   mouth of, 78
   of pregnant woman, 110
   suffocation of, 68
Vallambert, Simon de, 12
vapors, 25, 33, 46, 48, 224, 251
   and erection, 111
   drug, 98
   in brain, 280
   in the blood, 44
   of drugs, 95
   wine fills the head with, 26
Vaure, Monsieur du, 16
veal, 111
veins, 74, 204
   bursting of, 79
   in forehead, 129
   mesaraic, 102
   stiffened by cold, 40
vena cava, 111
venereal act,
   and health, 133
   as remedy for gallstones and back
      pain, 158
   in hot or cold bath, 162
Venice, 111, 225
venom, 138
   and aconite, 149
   potency of, 161
   remedies protecting from, 149
ventilation, of patient's room, 55

Vergil, 203
verjuice, and pissing vinegar, 155
vessels, spermatic, in women, 14
Vilanova, Arnau de, 12
Villars family (Joubert's aunt), 68
Villeroy, Seigneur de (*see* Neufville, Nicolas de), 4, 17, 116
vin de commeres, 142
vin de Lion, 140
vin de porceau, 140
vin de singe, 140
vine shoots, 55
vinegar, 148, 154, 190
   and choler vs. melancholy, 148
   and verjuice, 155
   cleaning floors with, 55
   makes water penetrate, 29
   mixed with water, 71
   sniffing, 94
   strong, 79
vineyards, 27
violets, 55
viper, xv, 171, 196
virginity, determinable in man, 162
virgins, and illnesses of the womb,
   160
virility, organic products accompanying, 48
vision,
   and grape juice, 160
   and parsley and grape juice, 130
   cure for clouded, 80
   in old people, 148
   loss of, 183
   sharpening, 147
   troubled by drink, 154
vitiligos, 221
Vivarez, 28
voice,
   vs. language, 235
   walnuts ruin, 144
vomiting, 64, 121
   after drunkenness, 137
   and diluted wine, 147
   and sailing, 151
   at sea, 171
   cure for at sea, 192
   how to avoid, 93
   people prone to, 248
Vontais, Monsieur de, 16
vulva, insatiability of, 146
waist,
   constricted, 141
   man's vs. woman's, 147
walnut brandy, 41
walnut oil, 156
walnuts, 144
warts, 171

cure for, 193
washing, recommended frequency
    of, 134
water, 247
    activity and drinking of, 144
    and eyes, liver, stomach, womb,
        135
    at bedtime, 143
    before retiring, 68
    cold, 133
    cooling rooms with, 71
    from springs, 150
    holy, 134
    importance of, 144
    makes one thin, 144
    soothing sound of, 55
    taken after strenuous exertion, 43
    well, 148, 162
    well vs. spring, 152
water camlet, 56
water lily leaves, 55
water-horse (beaver), 171, 197
wearisomeness, 108
weather,
    change felt by plants and animals,
        146
    change in felt, 137
weight,
    caused by sleeping in, 187
    not increased by greasy food, 161
weight loss,
    during illness, 162
well, water from, 148
wet nurses, 112
wheat, 225
wheat chaff (mattress), 72
whipping the buttocks as treatment,
    108
willow branches, 55
windiness (flatulence), 110
    and erection, 111
    cause of pain, 102
winds (the four), 195
wine, 111-12, 129, 249
    aids digestion, 25, 66
    aids sleep, 67
    and good blood, 152
    and hemlock, 150
    and life span, 135
    and loose bowels, 136
    and melancholy, 158
    and natural heat, 28
    appetite and drinking of, 144
    before retiring, 65
    benefits of, 25
    beverage used in place of, 247
    cooling with ice or snow, 71
    cools the body, 43

correcting, 252
damages the mind, 26
dangers of new, 145
dark red, 254
dilute during medication, 99
diluted, 93, 252
effects of quickly felt, 142
engenders blood, 25
evils of, 26
how to dilute, 146
in the diet, xii
internal and external use, 131
makes blood, 144
nourishing food, 25
nutritional and therapeutic value
    of, xv
passing in urine, 135
remedy for old age, 26
salad and fruits alter taste of, 148
sweet or old wives', 142
swine, lion, and monkey, 140
therapeutic value of, 44
undiluted, 41, 43, 146
vomiting and diluted, 147
when to consume, 145
white diuretic, 148
with evening meal, 65
young and sour, 160
wings, supporting ovaries, 14
Wit's Commonwealth, 106
wolves, 127, 141, 148, 184
womb,
    conjuring, 171, 194
    cure for suffocation of, 193
    growth of males vs. females in,
        141
    suffocation of, xv, 170, 171, 177,
        179
    susceptibility to suffocation of,
        143
    virgins and illnesses of, 160
women,
    ability to recover from illness,
        137
    and copulation, 92
    and garters, 147
    and stomachaches and headaches,
        143
    attendants, nefarious role of, xv
    bearded, 148
    clysters for pregnant, 110
    compared to men, 138
    complexion of, 52
    do harm through improper care,
        51
    excessive by nature, 52
    excessive in their affections, 51
    fear cold water, 151

healing powers of, 162
ignorance of in patient care, 102
inconstant nature of, 182
more choleric than men, 150
more talkative than men, 138
nature of, 51
pale enjoy coitus, 144
parts of characterized, 149
pregnant, 82
quickness of mind in, 52
sexual capacity of, 133
skinny, 154
true nature of, 182
types of enjoying coitus, 144
victimized by womb, 93

with small ears, 129
without wombs, 158
woodcock, 143
wool,
  and lice, 128
  used in mattresses, 56
workers, 217
worms, 34
  and fever, 145
  stop milk curdling, 145
  susceptibility to, 143
yeast water, 41
Zangmaistre, Jean-Paul, 108
zodiac, 195
Zopyres, 5

TABLE OF THE PRINCIPAL SUBJECTS
CONTAINED IN THE MICARD EDITION

You will note that preceding all page numbers there is
a 1 or a 2 so you will not be mistaken about the volume

[The following table from the Micard edition is provided to afford a
view of what may have been of interest to the printer's contemporaries;
the page numbers refer to the Micard edition but the subjects may be
found by consulting the index to *Popular Errors* in the case of entries
followed by a *1*, and in the case of entries followed by a *2*, the index
to the present volume.]

A

Abortion, causes of, 1:109
Abortion, and other such terms,
2:155
Abortion, hindered, 2:168
Abortion, what can cause, 1:134
Abstinence, two to three years
without eating or drinking, 1:99
Abuses, and hoaxes of bad
physicians, 1:23
Adam, his speech was not spon-
taneous or natural, 2:214
Aesculapius, 1:3
Africa (and America), countries too
hot for the use of wine, 2:3
Age, old, 1:13
Age, requires diverse treatments,
1:242
Age, not a limitation as is the con-
dition of the body, 1:86 & 87
Age of puberty in males and
females, 1:60 & 63
Aging, cause of, 1:87
Agnelette, 1:160
Air, or sky calls for different treat-
ments, 1:241
Alexander, brother of Olympias,
1:187
Alfonso d'Este, Duke of Ferraro,
1:39
Algemont, first king of the Lom-
bards, 1:97
Aloe, lignum, powdered, 1:201
Amas, mola uteri, mole, "brother
of the Lombards," 1:163 & 164
Ambassador of the dominion of
Venice, 1:51

Ambroise Paré, principal royal surgeon, 1:101
America (and Africa), countries too
hot for the use of wine, 2:3
Ancientness of medicine, 1:3; and
woman, polluted, 1:73
Animals (male), pregnant female
will not allow coupling by,
1:108
Animals, different from trees, 1:91
Animals, produce less excrement
than man, 1:192
Animals, of the same species have
the same complexion, 1:111
Animals, have a fixed time for
coupling, 1:108
Animals, diversity in quadrupeds,
reptiles, aquatic, birds, 1:110
Animals (female), refuse coupling
with male when pregnant,
1:108
Antipater, had his wife put to
death, 1:185
Apollo, founder of the art of
medicine, 1:3
Apothecaries, evil and arrogant,
1:58
Appetites, of pregnant women,
1:136 & 137
Arriere-faix (biggin, secundine),
1:102 & 160
Artabanus, king of the Epirotes,
1:187
Arts, human, 1:1
Asia, moderate climate of, 2:3
Athenians, effeminate, 1:182

Attendants, and servants, of the
    sick, 1:58
Augustus, chambermaid of had five
    children, 1:101
Avarice, of the physician, 1:18
Awake, what it is to be, 1:78
    B
Barley porridge, and broths, given
    at midnight, 2:43
Baths, as a means of becoming
    pregnant, 1:89
Bear, 2:178
Beard, and body hair, 1:201
Beauville, an illustrious household
    in the region of Agen, 1:95
Beauville, history of Mademoiselle
    de [see Mon(t)luc], 1:95 & 96
Beaver, also called a castor, 2:178
Bed, and covers necessary for a
    patient, 2:5
Bedtime, liquids drunk at are
    harmful, 2:48
Benefit, of the stomach, 2:94 & 95
Bernoise, mother of five children in
    a single burden, 1:103
Biggin (secundine, arriere-faix),
    preserves from harm, 1:161 &
    62
Birdsong, learned to a certain
    extent, 2:217
Birthmarks, red, cause of in
    children, 1:69
Blaise de Mon(t)luc, Maréchal de
    France, 1:95
Blood, clotting of, 2:21
Blood, of animals, 2:56
Blood, of man, 2:59
Blood, menstrual, 2:61
Bloodletting, of pregnant women,
    2:67
Bloodletting, of children and the
    elderly, 2:65 & 66
Bloodletting, good and necessary
    practice, 2:60, 61 & 62
Bloodletting, how and when to be
    done, 2:70, 71 & 72
Body hair, and beard, 1:201
Body, temper of determines con-
    duct of the mind, 1:66
Bondwoman, of a man from Siena,
    had seven children at once,
    1:103
Breast-feeding (nursing), prescribed
    duration, 1:241-246
Breasts, drying up of due to heating
    the milk, 1:225, 226 & 227
Breasts, communication between
    womb and, 1:218

Broths, and barley porridge given
    at midnight, 2:43
Broths, laxative, taken before
    meals, 2:81 & 82
Buckling, or infibulation, 1:215
Butter, and honey, given to Jewish
    children, 1:192
    C
Calendar, observed by elderly, 1:84
Camillus, Roman captain, 1:135
Castor (beaver), 2:178
Catalans, 2:147
Catalogue of Various Common
    Sayings and Popular Errors,
    2:139
Celsus, from the time of Augustus,
    2:68
Cervix (neck of the uterus), 2:213
Chambermaid of Augustus, had
    five children, 1:101
Change of voice, 1:201
Chestnuts, cause both men and
    women to become aroused,
    2:97
Child, nourishment of while in the
    womb, 1:142 & 143
Child, with too much intelligence
    will not live long, 1:140
Child, must be nursed any time it
    wishes, 1:234-235
Child, its diaper must be changed
    as soon as soiled, 1:212-233
Children, legitimate and bastard,
    1:76
Children, must abstain from wine,
    2:2
Children, of Laurent Joubert and
    Catherine de Genas, 1:166 &
    167
Children, of François Joubert and
    Loyse Guichard, 1:167
Clotting, of blood, 2:21
Clyster, softening, 2:94
Coitus, filth, indecency of
    menstruating women engaging
    in, 1:73
Cold, applied to the feet causes the
    bowels to move, 2:92
Cold, morfondement, and its
    remedies, 2:15, 16 & 17
Cold, external, how it causes fe-
    vers, 2:11
Colic, windy, 2:158 & 159
Common folk, highly ignorant, un-
    just, and iniquitous judges, 1:41
Communication, between the
    breasts and the womb, 1:218

Complexion, bodies must be maintained in their, 1:221
Complexion, different types of, 1:91
Complexion, and body temper, 1:15
Complexions, the nine, 1:110
Conception, the most propitious moment for, 1:80
Conception, and generation of the child, 1:60
Conditions, professional, of physician, 1:7 & 18
Conditions, required for semen, 1:74
Conduct, of the mind follows the temper of the body, 1:66
Conjuration, of a fallen uterus, 1:174
Cooling, of the bed-ridden patient's room, 2:53
Copulation, rare or frequent, 1:74 & 75
Copulation, carnal, forbidden times for, 2:76
Cornelius Scipio (Asianus), 1:185
Coupling, animals have a fixed time for, 1:108
Courtesans, worn and aged before their time, 1:87
Crepasi of Agen, collegial church of Saint, 1:95
Crupper, 1:147 & 148
Crying, and weeping in children is harmful, 1:239
Cuckold, 1:148
Curruca [hedge-sparrow], *verdalie,* 1:148
D
Daughters, and sons, how they are engendered, 1:80-81
Deaf, from birth also mute, 2:218
Death, never comes without regret, 2:90 & 91
Deflowering, 2:156
Delivery, best methods for, 1:149 & 150
Delivery, easy, 2:168
Delivery, easier for women, 1:149
Delivery, date, depends on child's and mother's complexion, 1:113
Democritus, lengthened his life, 1:11
Depositions, by midwives (one from Paris, one from Béarn), 1:202

Diet, proper, is a good remedy and good medicine, 1:44
Difference, between children's speech and singing of birds, 2:218
Difference, between speech and voice, 2:217
Diseases, internal and external, 1:21
Dog days, 2:76
Dormouse, 2:200
Drinks, mild, 2:7
Dropsy, 2:20 & 173
Drugs, medicine, not to be spurned, 1:52
Drugs, medicine, only for unhealthy people, 1:55
Drugs, medicine, how to be properly taken, 2:77
Duration, of our life, 1:13
Dysentery, 2:158
E
Elderly, wine is most fitting for, 2:2
Elderly, calendar observed by, 1:84
Elizabeth, conceived Saint John miraculously, 1:86 & 99
Escannar (strangle), 2:163
Este, Alfonso d', Duke of Ferraro, 1:39
Estourneau, noble family in the Perigord region, 1:151
Europe, the smallest part of the world, 2:3
Excrement, 2:26
Excrement, child's, cause harm physically and mentally, 1:237
Eyes, sunken, cause of, 1:88
Eyes, change quickly with diverse conditions, 1:88
Ezechias, had his life prolonged, 1:9
F
Fabulous stories, 2:175
Faculty, nutritive, 1:13
Fainting, swooning, and spasms, 2:164
Falling sickness, 2:162
Fasting, cases of miraculous, 1:99
Fasting, of Jesus Christ, Elias, and Moses, 2:209
Favorinus, Athenian philosopher, 1:176
Female, is a mutilated and imperfect male, 1:71
Ferrante da Sanseverino, prince of Salerno, 1:63

Fever, a fierce heat, cold is its precursor, 2:9
Fever, and quartan fever, 2:173
Fever, reason for return of, at same hour on same day, 2:13-15
Fever, continuous, source of, 2:10
Feverous, must drink liquids, 2:41
Fevers, why they are so called, 2: 13 & 33
Fevers, continuous and intermittent, 2:13
Fevers, tertian and continuous, duration of, 1:2-9
Fevers, intermittent, 2:11
Flow, of blood, 2:171
Flowers, and other synonyms, 2:154
Flowers, why they are so called, 1:59
Food, and drink is broken down and digested in the stomach, 1:143
Forgetting, everything including one's name, 2:223
Fortune, what it consists of, 1:12

G

Galen, lived 140 years, 1:10
Garlic, hot quality of, 2:98
Gathering of Common Expressions and Popular Errors, 2:118
Gathering of Common Sayings and Popular Errors, 2:113
Genethliacs, casters of nativities, basis of, 1:120
Genoa, women of, for the most part lascivious and loose, 1:146
Girls, must not be given in marriage too young, 1:67
Girls, more lascivious when devirginated very young, 1:67
Girls, who have children at nine and ten years of age, 1:63
Girls, who marry when much older have difficult deliveries, 1:147
Gonnella, famous buffoon, 1:39
Gout, cramping, 2:172
Gout, source of, 1:176 & 2:159
Gracchi, famous valiant Roman captains, 1:185

H

Hadrian (the Emperor) on the plethora of physicians, 1:42
Happiness, is a gift from God, 1:35
Harpies, what type of animals they are, 1:[page reference blank]
Healing, against popular opinion is two-edged, 1:29
Health, preservation of, 1:15

Hearing, precondition for reading or writing intelligibly, 2:220
Heat, of the night, 2:53
Heat, natural, 2:25
Hedge-sparrow [verdalie], curruca in Latin, 1:148
Herbs, Saint John's, 1:89
Hercules, and Iphicles, born as twins, 1:106
Hermaphrodites, also called Androgynes, or women-people, 1:101
Herodicus, lived a hundred years, 1:10
Hippocrates, and his successors, 1:5
Hippopotamus, 2:26
History, of Mademoiselle de Beauville [see Mon(t)luc], 1:95 & 96
Honey, and butter, given to Jewish children, 1:192
Human, arts, 1:1
Hungry stomach has no ears, 1:236
Hydromel, 2:8
Hymen, dame du milieu, cloister of virginity, 1:205, 210 & 211

I

Idleness, consumes the body, 1:87
Ignorance, leads to suspicion of poisoning and witchcraft, 2:183
Ignorance, of the physician, 1:17
Ignorant, are unjust and unreasonable, 2:104
Illnesses, accompanying pregnancy, not to be scorned, 1:129, 131
Imagination, strong, has great power to leave an impression, 1:50
Imagination, can be an element in curing but not everything, 1:50
Imaginings, of pregnant women, 1:138
Importunate, suspicious, calumniate physician's procedures, 2:107
Indulgence, of physician, 1:21
Infibulation, or buckling, 1:215
Ingratitude, odious to God and to men, 1:25
Institutions, life's, lead to diverse courses of treatment, 1:241
Interval, during which men and women can conceive, 1:86
Isaac, called a child of promise, 1:99
Italians, 2:147

J

Jane du Peirie [Jeanne da Peirié], 1:63 & 67

Jaundice, 2:172

Jean Momin, Doctor of Medicine at Univ. of Montpellier, 2:102

Jeanne da Peirié [Jane du Peirie], 1:63 & 67

Jews, children of, given honey and butter, 1:192

Judging, the competence of physicians by their success, 1:133

Jurisdiction, high-middle-low, physician, surgeon, midwife, 1:153

Jurisprudence, 1:2

K

Knots, in afterbirth indicate number of future children, 1:159

L

Laborers, manual, are less gouty and have more children, 1:76

Language, of a child who never heard speech, 2:212

Larfondement [voiding of grease or fat in one's excrement], 2:18

Latin, people, 2:159

Laxative broths, taken before meals, 2:81 & 82

Lechers, susceptible to gout and other diseases, 1:77

Leprosy, a contagious disease, 1:92

Life, can be shortened and lengthened, 1:8, 9, 10 & 11

Life, whether sustainable for several years without food, 2:191

Life, full of opposition, 1:45

Life, how it can be lengthened, 1:13 & 14

Life, length of our, 1:13

Lignum aloe, powdered, 1:201

Limits, of man's life fixed, 1:8

Limits, life, supernatural, natural, and accidental, 1:12

Linens, sheets, nightshirts of feverous changed often, 2:27, 29

Liquids, drunk at bedtime are harmful, 2:48

Liquids, drinking of necessary for feverous, 2:41

Loss, of milk, 2:172

Lunatic, and being under the influence of the moon, 2:161

M

Machaon, and Podalirius, 1:3

Macrina, wife of the Roman Consul Torquatus, 1:135

Magistrates, base child's legitimacy on death date, 1:119

Magistrature, 1:2

Maldeme(u)re, lady from Seaux had 6 children at once, 1:101

Male, more esteemed, excellent, and perfect than the female, 1:70

Male, hotter than the female, 1:221

Males, and females, how formed and conceived, 1:71

Malice, of the physician, 1:20

Man, why it is that he learns to talk so much later, 2:220

Man, the excellence of, 1:2

Man, able to engender several children, 1:105

Man, the most perfected animal in the world, 1:107

Man, elderly, not totally unable to engender sons, 1:82 & 83

Man, more differences within the species than in the others, has no need of a physician if in good health, 1:55

Margaret, Countess of Holland, 1:98

Marks, visible, source of on children, 1:136 & 137

Masclon [colic in males], 2:174

Matinées de l'Isle d'Adam, 2:99

Mattresses, and thick mats, 2:54

Mau-loubet [chancre], imprecation, 2:163

Mead [*melicrat*], 2:8

Meals, on the day medicine is taken, 2:83 & 84

Meals, (drinking and snacking), 2:164

Medication, patient should stay in room when taking, 2:85 & 86

Medicine, the Art of, prolongs life, 1:10

Medicine, necessity of the Art of, 1:4

Medicine, divided into three branches, 1:5

Medicine, the Art of, obscure and profound science, 1:33

Medicine, the Art of, excellence of above all human arts, 1:1-2

Medicine, is a conjectural art, 2:109

Medicine, the Art of, subject to calumny, 1:16

Medicine, drugs, how to be properly taken, 2:77

Medicine, drugs, only for unhealthy people, 1:55
Medicine, ancientness of, 1:3
Medicine, the Art of, ordained by God to cure the sick, 1:25
Medicine, drugs, are not to be spurned, 1:52
Melicrat [mead], 2:8
Memory, sharp and prompt conceptualization undesirable, 1:140
Memory, 2:170
Men, some have more strength than others in certain organs, 1:84
Men, women, who have lived several years without eating, 2:193
Meslanges (Gathering) of common sayings and popular errors, 2:113
Methods, best for delivery, 1:149 & 150
Midwives, depositions by (Paris, Béarn, Carcassonne), 1: 202 & 203
Midwives, 1:151, 153
Migraine, 2:161
Miguel Verin [Michele Verino], Spaniard, 1:66
Military arts, subject to calumny, 1:16
Milk, is the proper food for the infant, 1:245
Milk, in the breasts of women and virgins, 1:193, 194, 195 & 196
Milk, found in the breasts of some men, 1:197
Milk, from male child mother is colder than from female, 1:222
Milk, losing one's, 2:172
Milk, from the natural mother is always more fitting, 1:224 & 229
Milk, wet-nurses', its properties and qualities, 1:178 & 179
Milk, thick and clotted, called *colostrum* by the Romans, 1:190
Milk, of parturient women, 1:173
Mind, conduct of, follows the temper of the body, 1:66
Miracles, natural and supernatural, 1:99 & 2:211
Mohammed, and his sect, 2:3
Mole, *mola uteri, amas,* "brother of the Lombards," 1:163 & 164
Moment, the most propitious for conception, 1:80
Momin, Jean, Doctor of Medicine at Univ. of Montpellier, 2:102

Mon(t)luc, Blaise de, Maréchal de France, 1:95
Monkey, of the physician in Montpellier, 2:150
Months, of pregnancy, how counted, 1:119
Moon, directs child's conception, nourishment, and birth, 1:120
Morfondement, cold, and its remedies, 2:15, 16 & 17
Mothers, [1]:7, 9, 11, 12, 36, & 363
Mothers, vicious and ill-complexioned must not breast-feed, 1:182
Mothers, of several children in one burden, 1:196, 197 & 198
Mothers, ought to breast-feed their children, 1: 176
Mule, from Montpellier that had a colt, 1:100
Mute, from birth, whether consequently deaf, 2:219
N
Natural heat, 2:25
Necessity, of the Art of Medicine, 1:4
Neck (cervix), of the uterus, 2:213
Neck, measured from the chin to the top of the head, 1:201
Negligence, of the physician, 1:4
Nephritis, 2:158
Nero, killed his mother, 1:185
Nipple, small end of, changing color (in deflowering), 1:200
Noli me tangere [chancre on the face], 2:161
Nosebleed, 2:161
Nourishment, when to be given to women lying-in, 1:170
nursing (breast-feeding), prescribed duration, 1:241-246
O
Oil, of sweet almonds, and rock candy, 1:168-169
Oil, olive, fatty broth, lots of butter, laxative effect of, 2:93
Olympias, mother of Alexander the Great, 1:187
Opinion, of physician, patient's is an aid in healing, 1:49
Orgeol [*orgelet,* sty], type of ailment, 1:133
Os Bertrand [*os pubis,* pubic bone], 1:145 & 146
Overconfident, presumptuous, danger of with the sick, 2:110

Oysters, are cold and worthless in love's games, 2:26 & 97

P

Paillasse, & Balouffe [mattress stuffing], 2:54

Pain, severe, of parturient women, 1:169 & 174

Pain, severe, caused by drugs, 2:87

Pain, not the main concern in treatment, 1:54

Paré, Ambroise, principal royal surgeon, 1:101

Parturient women, do not overfeed, 1:172; can piss milk, 1:173

Passereaux [sparrows], lecherous and wanton, not long-lived, 1:77

Passerilles [sun-dried raisins], in Latin *uva passa,* 1:141

Patients, most cared for die the most often, 2:88 & 89

Peasants, 1:87

Peirie, Jane du [Jeanne da Peirié], 1:63 & 67

People of letters, and of finance, 1:87

Pepper, heating quality of, 2:98

Philosophy, moral, 1:2

Philtres, lovers' potions, 1:156 & 157

Physician, pleasant, unpleasant, 1:50

Physician, object of calumny, 2:103

Physician, created by God for His glorification, 1:24

Physician, negligence of, 1:4

Physician, fortunate to arrive as illness wanes, 1:32 & 2:106

Physician, avarice of, 1:18

Physician, professional conditions of, 1:7 & 18

Physician, assiduous in patient care is great blessing, 1:44

Physician, the good, what type of person he must be, 1:18

Physicians, judging their competence by their success, 1:133

Physicians, called the hands of God, 1:27

Physicians, most famous, 1:49

Physicians, must sometimes be called to deliveries, 1:152 & 153

Physicians, good and bad, 1:7

Physicians, greater in number than any other estate, 1:39

Physicians, honored and supported in Rome, 1:4

Physicians, several on a case not good or profitable, 1:41, 2:112

Pissing, before resting, 2:22 & 23

Plague, [*male bosse*], imprecation, 2:163

Plato, and Lycurgus, enjoin women to nurse their children, 1:187

Pleasure, children give to their wet-nurses, 1:184

Podalirius, and Machaon, 1:3

Poison, whether it can have a delayed effect, 2:181

Poison, can never be considered a food, 2:81

Porcelets, from the city of Arles in Provence, 1:97

Pores, holes in man's skin, 2:40

Potter, envious of another, 1:42

Pox, a contagious disease, 1:93

Pregnancy, cases of miraculous, 1:99

Pregnancy, months of, how counted, 1:119

Pregnant women, appetites of, 1:136 & 137

Prescriptions, physicians', must be followed, 1:52

Preservation of health, two main objectives to observe in, 1:15

Privileges, given to Roman women by the senate, 1:135 & 136

Prudence, principle activity of a temperate man, 1:140

Psammetichus, king of the Egyptians, 2:212

Puberty, age of in males and females, 1:60 & 63

Pubic bone [*Os Bertrand, os pubis*], 1:145 & 146

Purgation, can be fitting in any season, 2:72 & 73

Q

Quince, marmalade, its strength and properties, 1:139

R

Raisins, sun-dried [*passerilles*], in Latin *uva passa,* 1:141

Reading, or writing intelligibly contingent upon hearing, 2:220

Reffiron, or *arriere-fosse* [cervix], 1:213

Regimen, to be observed by the feverous, 2:29

Remedies, metaphoric and extravagant, 2:167

Remedies, superstitious, vain, & ceremonious, 2:171

Remedies, the most recent prefer-
    red to all others, 1:31 & 2:106
Reproach, and false accusations
    expressed by patients, 1:35
Retaillat [decircumcision], 2:157
Return, of fever, reason for, at
    same hour on same day, 2:13-
    15
Rheum, & catarrh, 2:159
Romans, 2:149
Romans, did without physicians for
    600 years, 1:4
Rule, observed by wet-nurses with
    respect to infants, 1:232-234
        S
Saint Crepasi of Agen, collegial
    church of, 1:95
Saints, and physicians, both cure
    but very differently, 2:210
Salamander, 2:178
Salt, given to flocks makes them
    more fecund, 2:96
Sancerre, besieged in the year
    1573, 1:34
Sarah, at 69 years of age conceived
    a child, 1:99
Sausage, custom of giving as
    present, 2:57
Sausage, unstable nature of, 2:57
Sciatica, 2:160
Scipio, Cornelius (Asianus), 1:185
Scrova, magnificent family in Pa-
    dua, 1:97
Scurf, a contagious disease, 1:93
Secundine (biggin, *arriere-faix*),
    1:102 & 160
Semen, from different occasions
    unite in single pregnancy, 1:106
Semen, of the woman joins with
    that of the man, 1:104
Semen, increased and in abun-
    dance, 2:167
Semen, is neither masculine nor
    feminine, 1:71
Seven months, vital term, 1:102
Sex, diverse, diversely maintained,
    1:242
Sexual arousal, chestnuts cause in
    both men and women, 2:97
Sheep, 2:26
Shivering, in the feverous, the
    cause of, 2:12
Sickroom, how it should be main-
    tained, 1:34
Sickroom, patient taking medication
    should remain in, 2:85 & 86
Signs, of an intact maidenhead,
    1:212

Signs, of a woman bearing two
    children at once, 1:127
Signs, of virginity, 1:200
Singing, of birds, learned to a cer-
    tain extent, 2:217
Sky, or air calls for different treat-
    ments, 1:241
Sleeping, not prohibited after taking
    medication, 2:79
Snack, supper, etc., 2:164-165
Sons, and daughters, how they are
    engendered, 1:80-81
Soul, knows no natural language,
    2:215
Soul, possesses nothing of itself in
    terms of knowledge, 2:214
Spaniards, 2:147
Sparrows [*passereaux*], lecherous
    and wanton, not long-lived,
    1:77
Spartans, manly and courageous,
    1:182
Speech, difference between voice
    and, 2:217
Speech, what it is, how developed,
    and why, 2:216
Speech, difference between bird-
    song and children's, 2:218
Speech, learned, taught, 2:212
Squinance [quinsy], Adam's apple,
    2:160
Sterility, & its causes, 1:91
Stomach, for the benefit of, 2:94 &
    95
Stomach, healthy, 2:94 & 95
Stones, in the body, 2:169
Stork, compassionate and charita-
    ble, 1:240
Strength, the source of a man's,
    1:88
Success, often due to luck rather
    than physician's skill, 2:103
Suffocation, of the womb, 2:157 &
    174
Superfetation, accepted by Aristot-
    le, 1:106
Superstition, foolish, of a few im-
    beciles, 1:23
Syrian man, nursed his child over 6
    months with his milk, 1:197
Syrup, for parturient women, 1:192
    & 193
        T
Tandrieres [fissures in nipples],
    remedies for, 1:231 & 232
Teeth, in small children, 2:172
Temper, of the body, determines
    conduct of the mind, 1:66

Terms, of 7, 9, 10 & 11 months as vital, 1:109

Theology, 1:1 & 2

Thomistes, seventh king of the Lacedaemonians, 1:186

Time, predetermined, for sexual intercourse in humans, 1:107 & 108

Treatment, of the patient, 2:66

Treatment, called for by sky or air, 1:241

Trees, different from animals, 1:91

Tunic, or shirt, covering the child's shoulders, 1:160

Tunique agnelette [amnion], 1:102

Turks, drink no wine, 2:3

Twins, born a few days apart, 1:107

U

Udders, of animals become dry if the milk spills into fire, 1:230

Umbilical cord, 1:157

Urine, not a sure indication of pregnancy, 1:121

Urine, must not be retained, 2:22 & 23

Urine, what it can indicate with certainty, 1:121 & 123

Usefulness, of the Art of Medicine, 1:4

Uterus, neck of, 2:213

V

Vapors, and sweat exiting from the body, 2:26

Vedille [navel], of the infant, how to care for, 1:155

Venereal Act, worse by day and more sure by night, 1:79

Venus, engendered by the foam of the sea, 2:96

Venus is cold without bread and wine, 1:74

Verdalie [hedge-sparrow], *curruca* in Latin, 1:148

Verin, Miguel [Michele Verino], Spaniard, 1:66

Vices, and imbalanced complexions, source of in children, 1:188

Viper, 2:177

Virboflaë, county in Cracow, 1:98

Virgin, can have milk in considerable quantities, 1:193 & 194

Virginity, of a maiden is difficult to ascertain, 1:199

Visits, by physicians, 1:46

Voice, change in, 1:201

Voice, difference between speech and, 2:217

Voice, is natural, speech is not, 2:216

Vomiting, of medicine, how to prevent, 2:78

Vomiting, at sea, 2:172

W

Warts, 2:173

Wet-nurses, ought to enjoy love's games rather than burn, 1:226

Wet-nurses, why loved more than their mothers by children, 1:185

Wet-nurses, why impassioned and in love with children, 1:183

Windows, open at night, 2:54

Wine, increases heat and thirst in the feverous, 2:4

Wine, not as necessary as believed, 2:2

Wine, most profitable and most dangerous, 2:1

Wine, with meals, 2:46

Wine, heated, cooled, 2:50, 51 & 52

Wine, forbidden to the sick but allowed by physicians, 2:5

Wine, very penetrating, 2:7

Wine, aids digestion and assimilation of other foods, 2:6

Wine, gives off heat when heady, subtle, and penetrating, 2:98

Wine, how it can be refreshing, 2:20

Woman, well disposed to conceive, 1:75

Woman, hunchbacked, had 5 children in Rouen, 1:104

Woman, type likely to conceive many children, 1:103

Woman, from Nîmes with copious milk, 1:225

Woman, does not conceive during her flowers, 1:68

Woman, can conceive without ever having had her flowers, 1:61-62

Woman, always ready, 1:108

Womb, communication between breasts and, 1:218

Womb, empty, what meat it calls for, 1:172

Womb, in women, 1:101

Womb, in animals, 1:100

Womb, suffocation of, 2:157 & 174

Womb, conjuration of a fallen, 1:174

Women, are influenced by the
    moon, 1:194
Women, pregnant (appetites of),
    1:136 & 137
Women, who have borne
    2,3,4,5,6&7 children at once,
    1:101
Women, ignorant around the sick,
    1:57

Women, who have borne dead
    children more than four years,
    1:100
Women, hot and cold, 1:90
Women, Egyptian, often bear 5
    children at once, 1:101
Women, quick and clever, 2:30-31
World, divided into four parts, 2:2
Writing, or reading intelligibly
    contingent upon hearing, 2:220

END

IN ROUEN

From the printshop of
GEORGE L'OYSELET